Biochemical, Pharmacological, and Clinical Aspects of Nitric Oxide

Biochemical, Pharmacological, and Clinical Aspects of Nitric Oxide

Edited by

Ben Avi Weissman, Nahum Allon, and Shlomo Shapira

Israel Institute for Biological Research
Ness-Ziona, Israel

Plenum Press • New York and London

Library of Congress Cataloging-in-Publication Data

Biochemical, pharmacological, and clinical aspects of nitric oxide /
  edited by Ben Avi Weissman, Nahum Allon, and Shlomo Shapira.
        p.   cm.
    "Proceedings of the 38th OHOLO Conference on Biochemical,
  Pharmacological, and Clinical Aspects of Nitric Oxide, held April
  17-21, 1994 in Eilat, Israel"--T.p. verso.
    Includes bibliographical references and indexes.
    ISBN 0-306-45113-1
    1. Nitric oxide--Physiological effect--Congresses.   I. Weissman,
  Ben Avi. II. Allon, Nahum. III. Shapira, Shlomo, 1943-   .
  IV. OHOLO Conference on Biochemical, Pharmacological, and Clinical
  Aspects of Nitric Oxide (1994 : Eilat, Israel)
    [DNLM: 1. Nitric Oxide--physiology--congresses. 2. Nitric Oxide-
  -pharmacology--congresses.   QV 126 B614 1995650]
  QP535.N1B54 1995
  612'.01524--dc20
  DNLM/DLC
  for Library of Congress   95-37450
                                                                  CIP

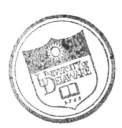
Proceedings of the 38th OHOLO Conference on Biochemical, Pharmacological, and Clinical Aspects of
Nitric Oxide, held April 17–21, 1994, in Eilat, Israel

ISBN 0-306-45113-1

© 1995 Plenum Press, New York
A Division of Plenum Publishing Corporation
233 Spring Street, New York, N. Y. 10013

10 9 8 7 6 5 4 3 2 1

PREFACE

A decade ago, for most scientists investigating various issues in life sciences the word "NO" was used in a negative context. It is astounding to observe how recently researchers are addressing the issue of NO, namely, nitric oxide, in over fifty publications weekly. *Science* journal, while naming nitric oxide: "Molecule of the Year" (December 1992), said it all: "NO news is good news."

For a long period of time NO was considered as a pollutant and every ecology-minded person tried to eliminate it. It was the discovery of NO involvement in the process of host killing by macrophages and several years later the finding that EDRF is none else but NO, that promoted this field. Nitric oxide's major role in the control of blood pressure is merely one factor of an extensive list of effects and functions attributed to it. NO is implicated in long-term potentiation (LPT), a principal process involved in memory consolidation and it is considered as the main biochemical substance responsible for penile erection. It should be noted that additional roles for NO are discovered continuously as many laboratories join the quest for the mystery of this small molecule. The observation that NO is involved in various biological processes is not unique, as other second messengers (i.e., cyclic AMP), participate in a diverse set of functions. Yet, the chemical nature of nitric oxide, that is, a labile and toxic gas, has no analogous counterpart in physiology or biochemistry. Carbon monoxide may emerge as a candidate for a similar title.

It is common knowledge today that enzymes producing NO differ in various tissues and organs. Nitric oxide synthase (NOS) is present in macrophages, endothelial cells, neurons, fibroblasts, and many other cell types. NOS presence in the central nervous system may indicate that in addition to NOs role in LTP it could take part in mood and behavior. Moreover, regulation of NOS in blood vessels offers therapeutic approaches for the treatment of cardiovascular disorders such as high blood pressure, as well as for conditions involving excessive NO production (e.g., septic shock). As mentioned above, impotence may become an easily corrected syndrome due to the development of specific NO donors or NOS stimulating agents.

Certain aspects of biochemistry and pharmacology of NO are discussed in this book. Special attention has been given to issues related to NOS characterization, in terms of co-factor(s) requirements, substrates, and novel specific inhibitors. While several authors describe the importance of NO in the vascular bed, including the corpus cavernosum, others address items related to learning, cardiac and cerebral circulation, memory, and aging. Although many aspects of NO actions are not reported herein, this book may serve as a stepping stone for scientists wishing to enter the are of NO research.

B.A. Weissman
IIBR, Israel

The organizing committee of the 38th OHOLO Conference gratefully acknowledges the generous support of the following organizations:

Amgen Center, Thousand Oaks, California, USA

Israel Academy of Sciences and Humanities, Jerusalem, ISRAEL

Joseph Meyerhof Fund Inc., Baltimore, Maryland, USA

Ministry of Science and the Arts, Jerusalem, ISRAEL

Pharmos Ltd., Rehovot, ISRAEL

Rhone-Poulenc Rorer, Antony Cedex, FRANCE

Sandoz Pharma Ltd., Basel, SWITZERLAND

Smithkline Beecham Pharmaceuticals, Harlow, Essex, UK

Teva Pharmaceutical Industries, Petach Tikva, ISRAEL

The British Council, Tel-Aviv, ISRAEL

Yad Avi Ha-Yishuv, Jerusalem, ISRAEL

CONTENTS

NITRIC OXIDE AND THE RESPIRATORY AND CARDIOVASCULAR SYSTEMS

NITRIC OXIDE AND BRAIN FUNCTIONS

THE NITRIC OXIDE SIGNAL TRANSDUCTION SYSTEM

Ferid Murad

Molecular Geriatrics Corporation
Lake Bluff, Illinois 60044, USA

INTRODUCTION

The nitric oxide-cyclic GMP signal transduction system has emerged in recent years as a very ubiquitous pathway for intracellular and intercellular communication. This review is intended to describe and summarize some of our observations and those of other laboratories that have helped lead us and others to our present understanding of the nitric oxide-cyclic GMP signal transduction system. Readers are also referred to some of our earlier reviews for references and information[1-6].

Although cyclic GMP was considered a potentially important second messenger in hormonally induced effects for many years, there was considerable disappointment with much of the early work in defining a definitive role for this cyclic nucleotide in signal transduction. The significance of cyclic GMP in cellular regulation comes from our work and that of others with nitrovasodilators, endothelial-dependent vasodilators, atrial natriuretic peptides (ANP), and *Escherichia coli* heat-stable enterotoxin (ST).

Nitric oxide is a simple, but unique, gaseous molecule and free radical that can serve many diverse functions including an intracellular second messenger as well as an intercellular messenger (paracrine substance, autacoid, or hormone) to regulate neighboring and perhaps distant cells. The important interrelationships of nitric oxide and cyclic GMP that began in the mid and late 1970s and that have expanded remarkable in recent years, have led to our present understanding of a fundamentally ubiquitous and important signal transduction system. In addition to its function as an intracellular second messenger and local extracellular agent for intercellular communication, I would like to suggest that nitric oxide might also be viewed as a more classical humoral substance. Effects of nitric oxide at some distant target site could occur if there were complexes or carrier states for nitric oxide. For example, if a carrier(s) or complex(es) of nitric oxide was formed that was inactive and that could release nitric oxide at a distant target site (perhaps selectively with specific uptake or transport, then nitric oxide could be viewed also as a classical humoral substance. Many hormones are inactive when bound or complexed with carrier proteins and become active in information transfer after their release or dissociation at their distant target. With the rapid recirculation times in the cardiovasculature, a complex of nitric oxide would only need to

Biochemical, Pharmacological, and Clinical Aspects of Nitric Oxide
Edited by B. A. Weissman *et al.*, Plenum Press, New York, 1995

survive for seconds to serve as a humoral substance downstream from its formation or at a distant target site. However, this hypothesis will be rather difficult to prove definitively. Because of the ubiquity of nitric oxide in more cell types, it will be virtually impossible to prove that nitric oxide generated at one site is the same molecule that functions at a distant site, particularly since radionuclides of NO are not available. The ubiquity and reactivity of nitric oxide with thiols, proteins, sugars, metals, heme proteins, etc., permit us to predict with some degree of certainty that nitric oxide complexes and adducts will, undoubtedly, be present in various extracellular fluids. The question is, do any of these complexes serve a humoral function. We suspect that they will, considering the very low concentrations (nanamolar) of nitric oxide required to activate guanylyl cyclase and elevate cyclic GMP levels in tissues (see below).

Nitric oxide is formed by most, but not all, cells. Its formation and release by central and peripheral neurons permit the molecule to function as a neurotransmitter of "nitrinergic" neurons. Thus, nitric oxide may function as an intracellular second messenger and an intercellular messenger (autacoid, neurotransmitter, or hormone). Such a diverse role for a single molecule has not been described previously. Perhaps the agents that come closest to fulfilling all of these roles are some of the eicosanoids. However, multiple members of this molecular class together share these diverse roles in signal transduction.

The discoveries of the effects of nitric oxide and particularly how they relate to cyclic GMP synthesis will be reviewed below.

EFFECTS OF NITRIC OXIDE ON CYCLIC GMP SYNTHESIS AND SMOOTH MUSCLE RELAXATION.

Like many laboratories working with cyclic GMP in the late 1960s and early 1970s, we were adding various hormones and drugs to different intact cells and tissues and attempting to correlate cyclic GMP accumulation in these tissues with some possible physiological and biochemical functions. Frankly, this descriptive cataloging, although leading to a number of publications by us and others, provided no significant insight into the mechanisms of humoral regulation of cyclic GMP synthesis or possible biochemical or physiological functions of cyclic GMP. We then turned to the characterization of the enzyme that synthesized cyclic GMP from GTP, guanylyl cyclase[7-10]. We had hoped that biochemical characterization of the enzyme would provide us with insights regarding mechanisms of hormonal regulation of guanylyl cyclase and cyclic GMP functions. This approach, needless to say, has certainly paid off with regard to our current understanding of mechanisms of hormone action, role of nitric oxide, and some cyclic GMP functions. We quickly learned that there were soluble and particulate isoforms of guanylyl cyclase in most tissues[7-10]. The kinetic and physiochemical properties of the cytosolic (soluble) guanylyl cyclase were quite different from the membrane associated (particulate) guanylyl cyclase. With regard to the substrate GTP, the crude soluble isoform gave typical and linear Michaelis-Menton kinetics, whereas the crude particulate isoform showed curvilinear plots or cooperativity. We though initially that the apparent cooperativity in these crude preparations could be attributable to contaminating ATPases and phosphatases that modified the GTP concentrations in incubations. Therefore, we added various inhibitors to our crude guanylyl cyclase incubations such as fluoride, pyrophosphate, and azide. We accidentally found that azide activated some, but not all, preparations of guanylyl cyclase[11,12]. In addition to azide, nitrite and hydroxylamine also activated our preparations[11,12]. This was an exciting turn of events for us because it was the first group of agents that would activate the enzyme in both intact cell and cell-free preparations. We reasoned that if we understood this activation mechanism, perhaps we would some day be clever enough to reconstitute a hormone effect on GMP synthesis in cell-free systems[1-4,6,13].

The effects of azide in some, but not all, preparations permitted us to develop assay systems and various classical biochemical mixing experiments to help us understand the mechanisms of activation. The lag time for azide activation and the absence of azide effects in all preparations convinced us that another intermediate was being generated in our experiments that was responsible for guanylyl cyclase activation, and we were committed to identifying this active intermediate. We also found that the azide effect was dependent on the presence of some heme-containing proteins such as catalase, peroxidase, or cytochromes in our preparation that probably convert azide to the active intermediate[14,15]. In addition, other heme proteins such as hemoglobin and myoglobin blocked the azide activation of guanylyl cyclase[16]. The requirements for some heme proteins to set the azide activation and the inhibitory effects of hemoglobin and myoglobin could explain the apparent tissue selectivity for the effects of azide (i.e.., some tissue extracts lacked the required proteins for azide conversion to the active molecule while other tissue extracts contained large amounts of inhibitors of the azide effect).

Fortunately, at the same time our laboratory was working with tracheal smooth muscle and gastrointestinal smooth muscle preparations. We suspected that cyclic GMP might contract smooth muscle and we set out to test the hypothesis. After finding the stimulatory effects of azide, nitrite, and hydroxylamine on guanylyl cyclase, we added these agents to various intact tissues including brain and our smooth muscle preparations. These agents elevated cyclic GMP and caused smooth muscle relaxation rather than contraction[17,18]. We logically tried other smooth muscle relaxants such as nitroprusside and nitroglycerin and found that they too activated guanylyl cyclase and elevated cyclic GMP[17-19]. We coined the term "nitrovasodilators" for this broad class of guanylyl cyclase activators and found that their effects were mediated by the formation of nitric oxide[19,20]. Thus, it appeared that azide, hydroxylamine, nitrite and other nitrovasodilators such as nitroglycerin and nitroprusside could be converted enzymatically or nonenzymatically, based on the prodrug used, to the reactive intermediate. We also learned that nitric oxide formation could explain the effects of this broad class of nitrovasodilators. Furthermore, the redox state of tissues and extracts could have a profound effect on the formation of nitric oxide from some prodrugs and/or the inactivation of nitric oxide by its oxidation to nitrogen dioxide, which was inactive. The effects of oxidizing and reducing agents and nitric oxide scavengers, such as methylene blue, potassium ferricyanide, and hemoglobin, subsequently became important research tools in characterizing the formation and effects of endothelial-derived relaxing factor (see below).

To our knowledge, guanylyl cyclase has been the first and only enzyme whose activity is increased with a free radical activation mechanism. Nitric oxide can activate homogeneous preparations of guanylyl cyclase in the absence of other macromolecules[21,22]. Furthermore, the activation was reversible, as would be expected if this regulatory mechanism were physiologically relevant. Although the precise mechanisms of nitric oxide activation are not totally understood, it is apparent from the work in Bohme's and Ignarro's laboratories[23,24] that heme functions as a required prosthetic group. Although several hypotheses have been offered to explain the mechanism of activation, large quantities of purified enzyme (milligrams) are required for detailed ESR/EPR studies with simultaneous monitoring of catalytic activity. Until recently, such studies have not been possible and this was one of the reasons we initiated our cloning and expression studies with the enzyme. To date, such studies have not been conducted by us or other laboratories. It may be that other mechanisms also participate in the activation process since thiol groups in the enzyme also appear to be critical for activation[25].

Although the soluble isoform of guanylyl cyclase is clearly activated in a reversible manner with nitric oxide under physiological conditions at low concentrations (K_a is about 1-10 nm), other isoforms of guanylyl cyclase are also activated by azide, nitroprusside, or nitric oxide. Our earliest studies in this regard were with particulate guanylyl cyclase from rat intestinal mucosa, a tissue in which the enzyme is predominantly or exclusively particulate. With washed, high-speed particulate fractions from rat intestinal mucosa, nitrovasodilators activated guanylyl cyclase. Most tissues, however, contain greater quantities of soluble isoenzyme. However, many crude particulate guanylyl cyclase preparations from these tissues are often contaminated with entrapped soluble enzyme. Unfortunately, detergents, which are required for the solubilization and purification of the particulate enzyme, inhibit the activation. Therefore, we prepared tryptic fragments of particulate guanylyl cyclase from rat liver membranes and also found that these preparations were activated with nitric oxide[26]. Recently, we also purified the cytoskeletal isoform of guanylyl cyclase from bovine rod outer segments and also found that this isoform could be activated with nitroprusside[27]. Thus, several isoforms of guanylyl cyclase can be activated with nitric oxide and perhaps these isoforms also contain heme prosthetic groups. Obviously, a number of additional studies are required.

When guanylyl cyclase is activated by nitrovasodilators, the properties of the enzyme change dramatically. The V_{max} may be increased as much as 100- to 200-fold under some conditions. Although the native, basal enzyme prefers Mn^{2+} as its cation cofactor, the activated enzyme can utilize Mn^{2+} or Mg^{2+} equally well, which makes more sense considering the K_a values and cellular concentrations of these cations[28]. The K_m for GTP is markedly decreased and the enzyme generally becomes more labile to storage. The enzyme can also synthesize cyclic AMP from ATP[29]. Although the activated enzyme prefers to make cyclic GMP from GTP, the formation of cyclic AMP from ATP can be appreciable (as much as 5 to 15% of the rate of cyclic GMP formation under some conditions). This alternate pathway for cyclic AMP synthesis has undoubtedly led to misinterpretations of some experiments and data where adenylyl cyclase regulation was expected.

In many cell types, including vascular smooth muscle, the increases in cyclic GMP lead to cyclic GMP-dependent protein kinase activation and altered phosphorylation of many endogenous proteins, including the dephosphorylation of myosin light chain and relaxation[1,6,30,31] (see Fig. 1). The decreased phosphorylation of myosin light chain probably occurs with cyclic GMP inhibition of phospholipase C activity, which appears to be cyclic GMP-dependent protein kinase mediated[32]. Decreased phospholipase C activity and decreased inositol tris-phosphate formation lead to decreased cytosolic calcium, which is required for myosin light chain kinase activity.

Although most of the cyclic GMP mediated effects to date are probably mediated through increased cyclic GMP-dependent protein kinase activity, other effects of cyclic GMP on phototransduction and phosphodiesterase regulation appear to be independent of the kinase.

EFFECTS OF ENDOTHELIAL-DERIVED RELAXING FACTOR (EDRF) ON CYCLIC GMP FORMATION.

The studies by Furchgott's laboratory described relaxation of vascular preparations with a variety of agents when the endothelium was intact but not after the endothelium was damaged or removed[33]. These endothelium-dependent vasodilators produced an endothelial-derived relaxant factor (EDRF) required for the relaxant effects. The lability of this factor and the similarities of these effects to those of nitrovasodilators and *E. coli* heat-stable enterotoxin suggested to us that these effects may also be mediated through cyclic GMP formation. This was indeed the case. We found that a variety of endothelium-dependent vasodilators increased cyclic GMP accumulation in the smooth muscle compartment of vascular preparations[31]. The effects of endothelium-dependent vasodilators on cyclic GMP accumulations were also dependent on the integrity and/or presence of the endothelium in preparations. Furthermore, the effects of EDRF were virtually identical to those of nitrovasodilators with regard to cyclic GMP-dependent protein kinase activation and altered protein phosphorylation including the dephosphorylation of myosin light chain and relaxation[34,35] (see Fig. 1). Due to the similar biochemical and pharmacological effects of EDRF and nitrovasodilators, we viewed EDRF as the "endogenous nitrovasodilator"[1]. Subsequently, Ignarro and Furchgott suggested that EDRF was nitric oxide[36,37]. From the reactivity of nitric oxide and the low concentrations of nitric oxide required for guanylyl cyclase activation, we have always suspected that EDRF is a nitric oxide complex(es) or adduct(s) that can liberate nitric oxide. Although this view has subsequently been shared by some other laboratories, the chemical identity of EDRF cannot be proven with current technologies because of the lability of EDRF and the apparent low concentrations in tissues. Nevertheless, most investigators today would agree that EDRF is either nitric oxide or a nitric oxide-like complex and that nitric oxide certainly mediates the effects of EDRF via guanylyl cyclase activation and cyclic GMP formation. It has also been shown that EDRF/NO can also cause other vascular and nonvascular effects such as platelet adhesion, platelet aggregation, and decreased vascular smooth muscle proliferation.

NITRIC OXIDE FORMATION

Working with brain preparations and neuroblastoma cell cultures, DeGuchi's laboratory found that an endogenous substance could activate guanylyl cyclase preparations[38]. This endogenous material was identified as L-arginine. The activation of guanylyl cyclase by L-arginine was similar in many respects to the activation observed with various nitrovasodilators since the effects were not additive and were inhibited by similar compounds.

Subsequent studies from the laboratories of Hibbs found that murine macrophages could form nitrite and nitrate and the apparent precursor of the synthesis was arginine[39]. Furthermore, arginine analogs such as L-methyl arginine blocked the pathway. Similar observations were noted by Marletta's laboratory. Subsequently, Moncada's laboratory extended these observations to endothelial preparations[40]. They found, similar to the studies of Hibbs, that one of the guanidino nitrogens of L-arginine could be oxidized and converted to nitric oxide. The other product of the reaction was citrulline. We, and others, found that numerous cell types, in addition to macrophages and endothelial cells, could also carry out the same reactions[5,13,41]. To date, there are few cell types that do not possess this enzyme pathway (see Fig. 2).

The enzymes that catalyze this reaction are nitric oxide synthases (NOS); they have also been called EDRF synthase or guanylyl cyclase-activating factor synthase (GAF synthase). These studies rapidly led to the characterization, purification, and cloning of the family of enzymes from many tissues and cell types by many laboratories. Today three gene products from cloning studies have been described (Table I). From purification and characterization studies, additional isoforms and gene products seem

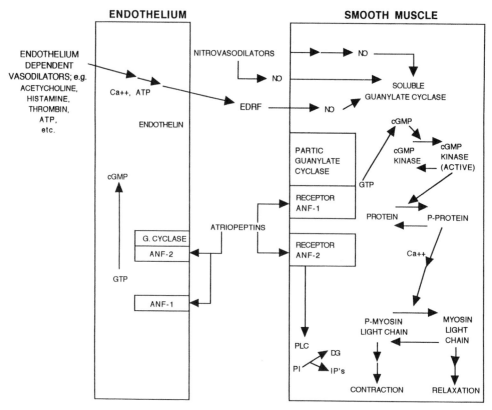

Figure 1. The effects of some vasodilators on cyclic GMP formation and vascular relaxation. (Modified form Ref. 1)

likely. Furthermore, there are various post-translational modifications of the enzyme(s), including myristylation and phosphorylation[42,43]. Post-translational modifications with myristylation and/or phosphorylation can alter enzyme activity and/or subcellular localization in the membranous or cytosolic compartments. These are currently very active areas of investigation. It seems likely that while six isoforms have been described to date, with at least three different gene products, more isoforms will undoubtedly be described in the future. Generally, within a given species, the isoforms are 50 to 70% homologous from cloning studies and deduced amino acid sequencing. However, a specific isoform can be highly homologous between species. For example, the human and rat brain enzymes (Type 1A) are more than 90% identical in sequence. Some isoforms are soluble or particulate and some can be induced with endotoxin and/or cytokines. Some isoforms are also calcium- and calmodulin-dependent[44-48]. All isoforms to date require NADPH, tetrahydrobiopterin, FMN, and FAD as cofactors. Some isoforms appear to be monomeric, whereas others appear to be active as homodimers.

Polyclonal and/or monoclonal antibodies developed to the various isoforms in our laboratory and other laboratories have been useful in immunohistochemical localization of the various isoforms in different cell types and tissues[42,49,50]. For example, neuronal Type 1A isoform can be found in discrete central and peripheral neurons where nitric oxide may function as a neurotransmitter of these "nitrinergic neurons". NOS-containing neurons include the nonadrenergic-noncholinergic (NANC) neurons in airway smooth muscle, gastrointestinal tract, and corpus cavernosum. Type 1A isoform is also found in pancreatic islets and endometrium[50]. The Type III endothelial isoform has only been reported in endothelial cells and kidney epithelial cells to date, and is the enzyme responsible for EDRF/NO production in vascular preparations[46-48,51-53]. Both Type Ia and III isoforms are calcium- and calmodulin-dependent. Type II isoform is inducible with endotoxin and/or various cytokines and is present in a variety of cell types, including macrophages, smooth muscle, fibroblasts, and liver after appropriate induction. The inducible Type II isoform is calcium-calmodulin independent. The independency of

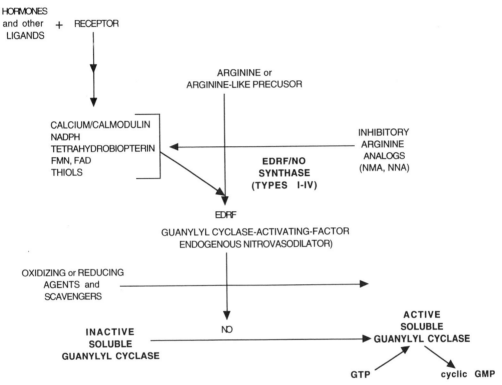

Figure 2. The nitric-oxide/cyclic GMP signal transduction pathway.
The nitric oxide formed from the oxidation of the guanidino nitrogen of arginine can act as an intracellular or intercellular messenger to regulate cyclic GMP synthesis. Some effects of nitric oxide may be mediated independently of cyclic GMP synthesis.

the inducible Type II NOS to calcium and calmodulin is probably incorrect in that recent studies have demonstrated that calmodulin is tightly bound to purified preparations of enzyme. Perhaps the inducible enzyme is already in the active state with tightly associated calmodulin. Although Type I and III isoforms are thought to be constitutive or housekeeping enzymes, we have found that their expression can also be regulated in some cell culture models.

The different physiochemical properties, cofactor requirements, and regulation of the various isoforms of NOS have provided some hope that selective pharmacological regulation of specific isoforms may lead to useful, new therapeutic agents. For example, selective inhibition of the inducible isoforms is expected to be therapeutically useful in managing hypotension in endotoxin-induced shock with sepsis or some inflammatory diseae. Selective inhibitors of the Type I neuronal synthase could alter the progression of some neurodegenerative disease while selective inhibition of the endothelial Type III isoform could be useful in managing migraine. Thus, the work with nitric oxide synthases is expected to expand dramatically.

Table I. Isoforms of NO synthase. All isoenzymes use L-arginine as a substrate and all are inhibited by N^G-methyl-L-arginine and N^G-nitro-L-arginine. The Type Ia, II, and III have been cloned by several laboratories, show about 50 to 60% homology and, obviously represent separate gene products. Some isoforms may also represent post-translational modifications. It is also recognized that this classification if probably incomplete as additional isoforms are expected from future purification, cloning and post-translational modification experiments.

Type	Cosubstrates Co-Factors	Regulated by	Mr	Present in
Ia (soluble)	NADPH BH$_4$ FAD/FMN*	Ca^{2+} calmodulin	155 kDa	brain, cerebellum, N1E-115 neuroblastoma cells
Ib (soluble)	NADPH	Ca^{2+}/calmodulin	135 kDa	endothelial cells
Ic (soluble)	NADPH BH$_4$ FAD	Ca^{2+}/calmodulin	150 kDa	neutrophils
II (soluble)	NADPH BH$_4$ FAD/FMN	unknown (induced by endotoxin/cytokines)	125 kDa	macrophages and other cells
III (particulate)	NADPH BH$_4$ FAD/FMN	Ca^{2+}/calmodulin	135 kDa	endothelial cells
IV (particulate)	NADPH	unknown (induced by endotoxin/cytokines)	?	macrophages and other cells

A literature search has revealed an exponential number of publications annually since our first publications on the effects of nitric oxide in 1977. An understanding of the complex chemistry of nitric oxide formation, oxidation states and reactivity with thiols, Fe/S centers and superoxide anion could offer many new avenues for rational drug development with a diverse spectrum of diseases.

SUMMARY

The understanding of guanylyl cyclase regulation by nitrovasodilators has provided a great deal of information explaining the mechanisms of action of these cardiovascular drugs that have been in clinical use for the past century. The biochemical characterization of guanylyl cyclases and their regulation by NO have also permitted us, and others, to understand the mechanism of action of endothelium-dependent vasodilators and, subsequently, the roles for the nitric oxide-cyclic GMP signal transduction system in numerous cells and tissues. Some of those studies have also permitted us to understand the mechanisms of action of other agents such as the atriopeptins and enterotoxins which are presumably not nitric oxide dependent. The potential importance of this signal transduction cascade is probably not fully appreciated since numerous additional studies obviously need to be performed. Also, as in many areas of science, serendipitous experiments and observations have added critical data to our present understanding in this field.

Acknowledgments

I thank the numerous trainees and collaborators who, over the years, have been critical to this laboratory's productivity, and many different funding agencies who provided the support for this work during the past two decades.

REFERENCES

1. F. Murad. Cyclic guanosine monophosphate as a mediator of vasodilation, J. Clin. Invest. 78:1-5 (1986).
2. F. Murad. Modulation of the guanylate cyclase-cGMP system by vasodilators and the role of free radicals as second messengers, in: Vascular Endothelium, J.D. Catravas, C.M. Gillis, and U.S. Ryan, eds., Plenum Publishers, (1989).
3. F. Murad. Mechanisms for hormonal regulation of the different isoforms of guanylate cyclase, in: Molecular Mechanisms of Hormone Action. Y. Gehring, E. Helmreich, and G. Schultz, eds., Springer-Verlag, Heidelberg, (1989).
4. F. Murad, D. Leitman, S. Waldman, C.H. Chang, J. Hirata, K. Kohse, Effects of nitrovasodilators,, endothelium-dependent vasodilators and atrial peptides on cGMP, Proc. Cold Spring Harbor Symposium on Quantitative Biology, Signal Transduction 53:1005-1009 (1988).
5. F. Murad, K. Ishii, L. Gorsky, U. Forstermann, J.F. Kerwin, and M. Heller, Endothelium-derived relaxing factor is a ubiquitous intracellular second messenger and extracellular paracrine substance for cyclic GMP synthesis, in: Nitric Oxide from L-Arginine: A Bioregulatory System. S. Moncada and E.A. Higgs, eds., Chapter 32, pp 301-315, London (1990).
6. S.A. Waldman and F. Murad, Cyclic GMP synthesis and function, Pharm. Rev. 39:163-196 (1987).
7. H. Kimura and F. Murad, Evidence for two different forms of guanylate cyclase in rat heart, J. Biol. Chem, 249:6910-6919 (1974).
8. H. Kimura and F. Murad, Two forms of guanylate cyclase in mammalian tissues and possible mechanisms for their regulation, Metab. Clin. Exp., 24:439-445, (1975).
9. H. Kimura and F. Murad, Localization of particulate guanylate cyclase in plasma membranes and microsomes of rat liver, J. Biol. Chem., 250:4810-4817, (1975).
10. H. Kimura and F. Murad, Increased particulate and decreased soluble guanylate cyclase activity in regenerating liver, fetal liver, and hepatoma, Proc. Natl. Acad. Sci., USA, 72:1965-1969, (1975).
11. H. Kimura, C.K. Mittal, and F. Murad, Activation of guanylate cyclase from rat liver and other tissues with sodium azide, J. Biol. Chem. 250:8016-8022 (1975).
12. H. Kimura, C.K. Mittal, and F. Murad, Increases in cyclic GMP levels in brain and liver with sodium azide, an activator of guanylate cyclase, Nature 257:700-702 (1975).
13. F. Murad, K. Ishii, U. Forstermann, L. Gorsky, J. Kerwin, J. Pollock, and M. Heller, EDRF is an intracellular second messenger and autacoid to regulate cyclic GMP synthesis in many cells, Adv. Cyclic Nucl. Res. 24:441-448 (1990).
14. C.K. Mittal, H. Kimura, and F. Murad, Requirement for a macromolecular factor for sodium azide activation of guanylate cyclase. J. Cyclic Nucleotide Res., 1:261-269, (1975).
15. C.K. Mittal, H. Kimura, and F. Murad, Purification and properties of a protein required for sodium azide activation of guanylate cyclase, J. Biol. Chem., 252:4348-4390, (1977).
16. C.K. Mittal, W.P. Arnold, and F. Murad, Characterization of protein inhibitors of guanylate cyclase activation from rat heart and bovine lung, J. Biol. Chem., 253:1266-1271, (1978).
17. S. Katsuki, W.P. Arnold, C.K. Mittal, and F. Murad, Stimulation of formation and accumulation of cyclic GMP by smooth muscle relaxing agents, Proc. Jpn. Cyclic Nucleotide Conf., pp. 44-50, (1977).
18. S. Katsuki, W.P. Arnold, and F. Murad, Effect of sodium nitroprusside, nitroglycerin and sodium azide on levels of cyclic nucleotides and mechanical activity of various tissues, J. Cyclic Nucl. Res. 3:239-247 (1977).

19. S. Katsuki, W. Arnold, C.K. Mittal, and F. Murad, Stimulation of guanylate cyclase by sodium nitroprusside, nitroglycerin and nitric oxide in various tissue preparations and comparison to the effects of sodium azide and hydroxylamine, J. Cyclic Nucl. Res. 3:23-35 (1977).

20. W.P. Arnold, C.K. Mittal, S. Katsuki, and F. Murad, Nitric oxide activates guanylate cyclase and increases guanosine 3'5'-monophosphate levels in various tissue preparations, Proc. Natl. Acad. Sci. USA 74:3203-3207 (1977).

21. J.M.. Braughler, C.K. Mittal, and F. Murad, Purification of soluble guanylate cyclase from rat liver, Proc. Natl. Acad. Sci., USA, 76:219-222, (1979).

22. J.M.. Braughler, C.K. Mittal, and F. Murad, Effects of thiols, sugars and proteins on nitric oxide activation of guanylate cyclase, J. Biol. Chem. 254:12450-12454 (1979).
    F. Murad, C.K. Mittal, W.P. Arnold, S. Katsuki, and H. Kimura, Guanylate cyclase: Activation by azide, nitro compounds, nitric oxide, and hydroxyl radical and inhibition by hemoglobin and yoglobin, Adv. Cyclic Nucl. Res. 9:145-158 (1978).

23. R. Gerzer, E. Bohme, F. Hoffman, and G. Schultz, Soluble guanylate cyclase purified from bovine lung contains heme and copper, FEBS. Lett., 132:71-74, (1981).

24. L.J. Ignarro, J. Adams, P. Horwitz, and K.S. Wood, Activation of soluble cyclase by NO-hemeproteins involves NO-heme exchange: Comparison of heme containing and heme deficient enzymes, J. Bio. Chem., 261:4997-5002, (1986).

25. H.J. Brandwein, J.A. Lewicki, and F. Murad, Reversible inactivation of guanylate cyclase by mixed disulfide formation, J. Biol. Chem., 256:2958-2962, (1981).

26. S.A. Waldman, J.A. Lewicki, H.J. Brandwein, and F. Murad, Partial purification and characterization of particulate guanylate cyclase from rat liver after solubilization with trypsin, J. Cyclic Nuc. Res. 8:359-370 (1982).

27. Y. Horio and F. Murad, Solubilization of guanylate cyclase from bovine rod outer segments and effects of Ca++ and nitro compounds, J. Biol. Chem., 266:3411-3415, (1991).

28. H. Kimura, C.K. Mittal, and F. Murad, Appearance of magnesium guanylate cyclase activity in rat liver with sodium-azide activation, J. Biol. Chem., 251:7769-7773, (1976).

29. C.K. Mittal, J.M. Braughler, K. Ichihara, and F. Murad, Synthesis of adenosine 3',5'-monophosphate by guanylate cyclase, a new pathway for its formation, Biochim. Biophys. Acta, 585:333-342, (1979).

30. R.M. Rapoport, M.B. Draznin, and F. Murad, Endothelium-dependent vasodilator and nitrovasodilator-induced relaxation may be mediated through cyclic GMP formation and cyclic GMP-dependent protein phosphorylation, Trans. Assoc. Am. Physicians, 96:19-30, (1983).

31. R.M. Rapoport and F. Murad, Agonist-induced endothelial-dependent relaxation in rat thoracic aorta may be mediated through cyclic GMP, Circ. Res. 52:352-357 (1983).

32. M. Hirata, K. Kohse, C.H. Chang, T. Ikebe, and F. Murad, Mechanism of cyclic GMP inhibition of inositol phosphate formation in rat aorta segments and cultured bovine aortic smooth muscle cells, J. Biol. Chem. 265:1268-1273 (1990).

33. R.F. Furchgott and J.V. Zawadski, The obligatory role of endothelial cells in the relaxation of arterial smooth muscle to acetylcholine, Nature 288:373-376 (1980).

34. R.M. Rapoport and F. Murad, Endothelium-dependent and nitrovasodilator-induced relaxation of vascular smooth muscle: Role for cyclic GMP, J. Cyclic Nucl. and Protein Phosphor. Res. 9:281-296 (1983).

35. R.M. Rapoport, M.D. Draznin, and F. Murad, Endothelium-dependent vasodilator-and-nitrovasodilator-induced relaxation may be mediated through cyclic GMP formation and cyclic GMP-dependent protein phosphorylation, Trans. Assoc. Amer. Phys. 96:19-30 (1983).

36. L.J. Ignarro, G.M. Buga, K.S. Wood, R.E. Byrns, and G. Chaudhuri, Endothelium-derived relaxing factor produced and released from artery and vein is nitric oxide, Proc. Natl. Acad. Sci. 84:9265-9269 (1987).

37. R.F. Furchgott. Studies on relaxation of rabbit aorta by sodium nitrite: The basis for the proposal that acid-activatable inhibitory factor from bovine retractor penis is organic nitrite and EDRF is nitric oxide, in: "Vasodilation: Vascular Smooth Muscle, Peptides, Autonomic Nerves and Endothelium". P.M. Vanhoutte, ed., Raven Press, New York (1988).

38. T. DeGuchi and M.H. Yoshioko, L-Arginine identified as an endogenous activator for soluble guanylate cyclase from neuroblastoma cells, J. Biol. Chem. 257:10147-10151 (1982).

39. J.R. Hibbs, R.R. Taintor, and Z. Varrin, Macrophage cytotoxicity: Role for A-arginine deiminase and amino nitrogen oxidation to nitrite, Science 235:473-476 (1987).

40. R. Palmer, D. Ashton, and S. Moncada, Vascular endothelial cells synthesize nitric oxide from L-arginine, Nature 333:664-665 (1988).

41. K. Ishii, L. Gorsky, U. Forstermann, and F. Murad, Endothelium-derived relaxing factor (EDRF): The endogenous activator of soluble guanylate cyclase in various types of cells, J. Applied Cardiology 4:505-512 (1989).

42. J.S. Pollock, V. Klinghofer, U. Forstermann, and F. Murad, Endothelial nitric oxide synthase is myristoylated, FEBS Lett. 309:402-404 (1992).

43. M. Nakane, J.A. Mitchell, U. Forstermann, and F. Murad, Phosphorylation by calcium calmodulin-dependent protein kinase II and protein kinase C modulates the activity of nitric oxide synthase, Biochem. Biophys. Res. Commun. 180:1396-1402 (1991).

44. D.S. Bredt and S.H. Snyder, Isolation of nitric oxide synthetase, a calmodulin-requiring enzyme, Proc. Natl. Acad. Sci. USA 85:682-685 (1990).

45. U. Forstermann, L. Gorsky, J. Pollock, K. Ishii, H.H.H.W. Schmidt, M. Heller, and F. Murad, Hormone induced biosynthesis of endothelium-derived relaxing factor-nitric oxide-like material in N1E115 neuroblastoma cells required calcium and calmodulin, Mol. Pharmacol., 38:7-13, (1990).

46. U. Forstermann, L. Gorsky, J.S. Pollock, H.H.H.W. Schmidt, K. Ishii, M. Heller, and F. Murad, Subcellular localization and regulation of the enzymes responsible for EDRF synthesis in endothelial cells and N1E 115 neuroblastoma cells, Eur. J. Pharmacol. 183:1625-1626 (1990).

47. U. Forstermann, J. Pollock, H.H.H.W. Schmidt, M. Heller, and F. Murad, Calmodulin-dependent endothelium-derived relaxing factor/nitric oxide synthase activity is present in the particulate and cytosolic fractions of bovine aortic endothelial cells, Proc. Natl. Acad. Sci. 88:1788-1792 (1991).

48. U. Forstermann, H.H.H.W. Schmidt, J.S. Pollock, H. Sheng, J.A. Mitchell, T.D. Warner, M. Nakane, and F. Murad, Isoforms of EDRF/NO synthase: Characterization and purification from different cell types, Biochem. Pharmacol. 41:1849-1857 (1991).

49. S.H. Snyder and D.S. Bredt, Nitric oxide as a neuronal messenger, Trends Pharmacol. Sci. 12:125-130 (1991).

50. H. Schmidt, G. Gagne, M. Nakane, J. Pollock, M. Miller, and F. Murad, Mapping of neural NO synthase in the rat suggests frequent colocalization with NADPH diaphorase but not soluble guanylyl cyclase and novel paraneural functions for nitrinergic signal transduction, J. Histo. Cytochem. 40:1439-1456 (1992).

51. U. Forstermann, H.H.H.W. Schmidt, J.S. Pollock, M. Heller, and F. Murad, Enzymes synthesizing guanylyl cyclase activating factor (GAF) in endothelial cells, neuroblastoma cells and rat brain, J. Cardiovasc. Pharmacol., 17, Suppl. 3:557-564, (1991).

52. J.S. Pollock, U. Forstermann, J.A. Mitchell, T.D. Warner, H.H.H.W. Schmidt, M. Nakane, and F. Murad, Purification and characterization of particulate EDRF synthase from cultured and native bovine aortic endothelial cells, Proc. Natl. Acad. Sci. USA, 88:10480-10484, (1991).

53. R. Tracey, J. Pollock, F. Murad, M. Nakane, and U. Forstermann, Identification of an endothelial-like nitric oxide synthase in LLC-PK1 kidney epithelial cells, Amer. J. Physiol., 226:C22-C28, (1994).

MECHANISMS OF MAMMALIAN NITRIC OXIDE BIOSYNTHESIS

Paul L. Feldman[1], Dennis J. Stuehr[2], Owen W. Griffith[3], and Jon M. Fukuto[4]

[1]Glaxo Inc. Research Institute, Research Triangle Park, NC 27709
[2]The Cleveland Clinic, Cleveland, OH 44195, Case Western Reserve
University School of Medicine, Cleveland, OH 44106
[3]Department of Biochemistry, Medical School of Wisconsin, Milwaukee,
WI 53226
[4]Department of Pharmacology, UCLA School of Medicine, Los Angeles,
CA 90024, USA.

INTRODUCTION

In mammals nitric oxide (NO) synthesis is catalyzed by the enzyme(s) nitric oxide synthase (NOS).[1] NOS oxidizes one of the two equivalent terminal guanidino nitrogens of the protogenic amino acid L-arginine (Arg) to yield NO and the co-product L-citrulline (Cit).[2] NOS constitutes a family of enzymes of which two distinct types, inducible NOS (iNOS) and constitutive NOS (cNOS), have been cloned and characterized. Both iNOS and cNOS are dimeric enzymes containing two identical subunits with molecular weights in the range of 130-150 kD. They have similar specific activities of about 0.8-1.3 μmole/min-mg of protein at 37°C with a turnover rate of about 2.5-3.2 molecules/sec for each subunit. Both forms of NOS are dependent upon the cofactors tetrahydrobiopterin (BH$_4$), flavin adenine dinucleotide (FAD), flavin mononucleotide (FMN), and heme for enzymatic activity. Each subunit contains one molecule of each of the flavins, heme, and BH$_4$. Although all four of these cofactors are widely utilized by various enzymes in nature to catalyze various oxidative and reductive reactions, NOS is the only known mammalian enzyme to contain all four groups. Given the importance of understanding the physiology and biochemistry of NO-mediated processes and translating that understanding to therapeutic benefit, we have studied NOS enzymology with the goal to determine the mechanism of NO biosynthesis.

Prior to our work three mechanisms for NOS-mediated biosynthesis of NO had been published.[2] One proposal invoked an enzyme catalyzed hydrolytic deimination of Arg to generate Cit and ammonia with subsequent oxidation of the ammonia to give NO.[2a] In the two other postulated mechanisms, depicted in scheme 1, L-N^G-hydroxyarginine (NOHArg) is implicated as the first oxidation product of Arg. As shown in path a further oxidation of NOHArg followed by homolytic bond cleavage yields NO and the N^E-carbodiimide of ornithine, which upon hydration yields Cit.[2b] An alternative pathway

Biochemical, Pharmacological, and Clinical Aspects of Nitric Oxide
Edited by B. A. Weissman *et al.*, Plenum Press, New York, 1995

13

proposed to NO from NOHArg, path b, is via the hydrolysis of NOHArg to yield hydroxylamine and Cit followed by oxidation of hydroxylamine to NO.[2c] All three of the proposed mechanisms require that the oxygen of the urea be derived from water. In 1990, it was demonstrated using $^{18}O_2$ labeling experiments that the oxygen of the urea group is derived from dioxygen rather than water, and thus an alternative mechanism for NO synthesis must be operating.[3]

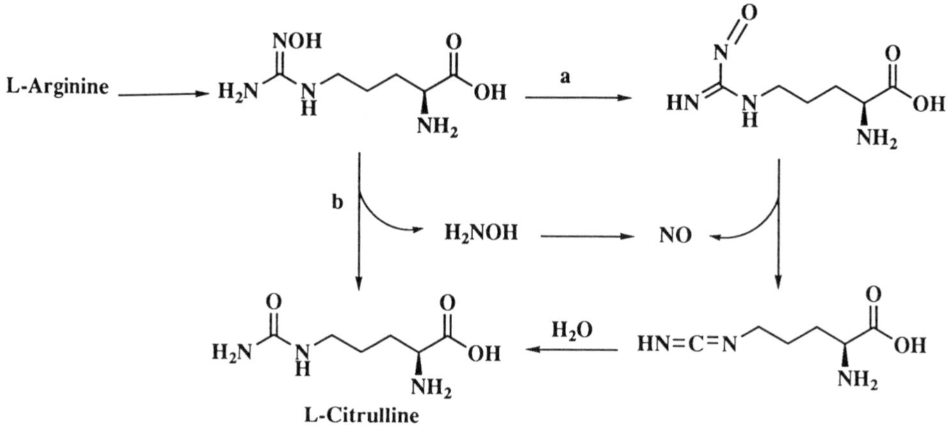

Scheme 1. Two of the early proposals of the mechanism of NOS mediated NO biosynthesis from L-arginine included the hypothesis that L-N^G-hydroxyarginine is an intermediate.

Although portions of all of these mechanisms published were proven to be incorrect, it seemed reasonable that the proposed initial two electron oxidation product of Arg, NOHArg, could be an intermediate in NO biosynthesis. In order to elucidate whether NOS oxidizes Arg to NOHArg and subsequently to NO and Cit, we synthesized NOHArg, and its ^{15}N labeled analogs, shown in Figure 1, using L-ornithine as the enantiopure educt.[4]

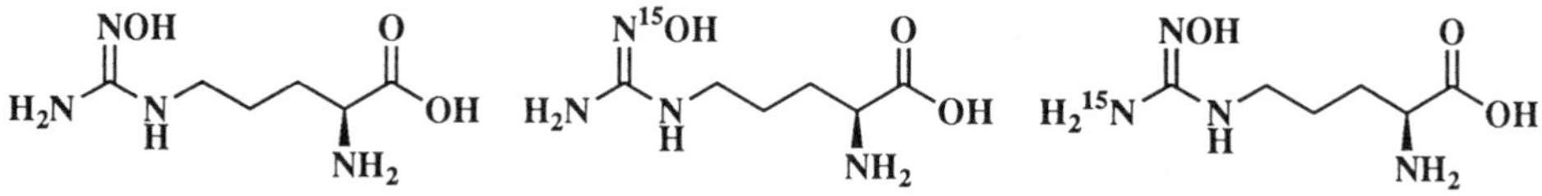

Figure 1. Synthesized L-N^G-hydroxyarginine and its ^{15}N-labeled congeners were used to determine the intermediacy of L-N^G-hydroxyarginine in mNOS mediated NO biosynthesis from L-arginine.

We first compared NOHArg with Arg as a substrate for murine macrophage NOS (mNOS).[5] NOHArg has an apparent K_m of 6.6 µM versus 2.3 µM for Arg and a apparent V_{max} of 99 nmol/min-mg versus 54 nmol/min-mg for Arg. NO synthesis using NOHArg as a substrate was completely inhibited in the presence of the flavoprotein inhibitor diphenylene iodonium (10 µM) and inhibited by the known arginine-based NOS inhibitors L-N^G-aminoarginine (IC_{50}= 8µM) and L-N^G-methylarginine (IC_{50}= 13µM). Furthermore, D-NOHArg was not a substrate for NOS at concentrations as high as 1 mM.

Although these initial experiments demonstrated that NOHArg is an enantiospecific substrate for NOS, further experiments were required to support its intermediacy in the Arg to NO biosynthetic pathway. It had previously been shown that the oxygen of the urea function of Cit is derived dioxygen, not water, when Arg is the substrate for NOS. For

14

NOHArg to be an intermediate in the biosynthesis of NO, it too must be processed such that the urea oxygen of Cit is derived from dioxygen. When NOHArg is used as the substrate for NOS in the presence of 95% [^{18}O] water and [^{16}O] oxygen, the Cit urea oxygen contains less than 5% ^{18}O. Thus, as with Arg, the oxygen of the urea function of the co-product Cit is derived from dioxygen and not water. See scheme 2.

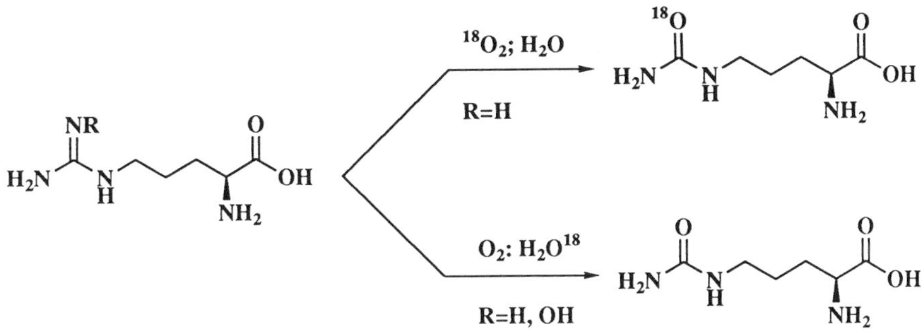

Scheme 2. In mNOS mediated NO biosynthesis the urea oxygen of the co-product L-citrulline is derived from water, not water, when either L-arginine or L-N^G-hydroxyarginine is used as the substrate.

In the biosynthesis of NO from Arg NOS oxidizes one of the two equivalent terminal guanidino nitrogens to NO. Since the two N^G-nitrogens of NOHArg are chemically distinct, we used differentially ^{15}N-labeled NOHArgs to determine which nitrogen NOS oxidized. If NOHArg is an intermediate in NO biosynthesis from Arg, then only the hydroxylated nitrogen would be oxidized. Indeed, analysis of the nitrogen oxide products produced using the labeled NOHArgs as substrates for NOS demonstrated that NOS exclusively utilized the hydroxylated nitrogen of NOHArg for NO synthesis. Furthermore, HPLC analysis showed that Cit, and not L-N^G-hydroxycitrulline, was generated as the co-product. See scheme 3.

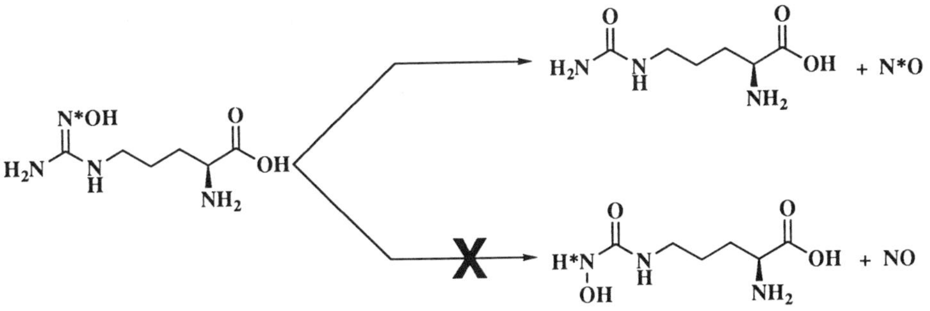

Scheme 3. mNOS oxidizes the hydroxylated terminal guanidino nitrogen, not the reduced guanidino nitrogen, of L-N^G-hydroxyarginine to generate NO and L-citrulline.

Experiments were also conducted to determine which cofactors (NADPH, dithiothreitol, BH$_4$, FAD) were essential for NO synthesis using Arg or NOHArg as the substrate. All of the cofactors were required for either substrate, however, the synthesis of 1mol of NO from Arg was coupled to the oxidation of 1.5mol of NADPH; whereas with NOHArg as the substrate only 0.5mol of NADPH was oxidized per mole of NO formed. Therefore, although NOS requires all of the cofactors to mediate NO synthesis from Arg or NOHArg, NOHArg utilizes less NADPH for NO synthesis than Arg which is consistent with it being derived from Arg.

Further evidence that NOHArg is an intermediate in the biosynthesis of NO was obtained by incubating NOS with excess NOHArg in the presence of [^{14}C]Arg. NOS

15

generated a metabolite of $[^{14}C]$Arg that co-chromatographed with authentic NOHArg in three different solvent systems. The metabolite, like authentic NOHArg, generated $[^{14}C]$Cit upon alkaline hydrolysis.

The combination of all the data collected establishes NOHArg as an intermediate in mNOS mediated biosynthesis of NO from Arg. Furthermore, we have shown that the initial hydroxylation of Arg to generate NOHArg is coupled to the oxidation of 1mol of NADPH and subsequent oxidation of NOHArg to NO and Cit is coupled to 0.5mol of NADPH. Following this work we could now write the reaction scheme depicted in scheme 4 for mNOS mediated NO biosynthesis.

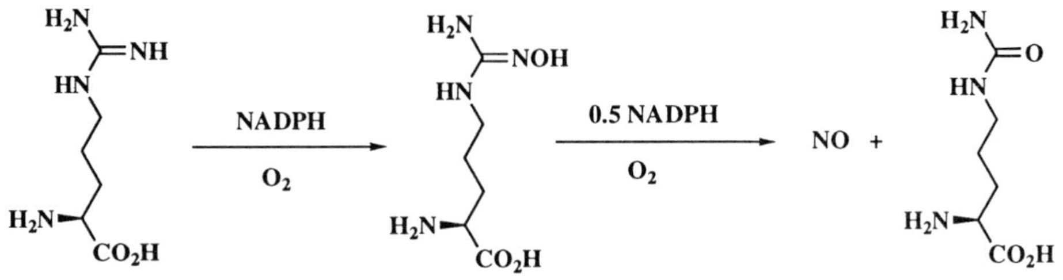

Scheme 4. Biosynthetic scheme for mNOS mediated NO synthesis from L-arginine.

Following our work with NOHArg, molecular cloning of several NOS isoforms revealed important insights into how the primary structure of NOS might relate to its function.[6] Each NOS subunit appears to be comprised of a reductase and oxygenase domain, each representing roughly one-half of the protein. The reductase domain contains binding sites for NADPH, FAD, and FMN. The oxygenase domain does not contain any clear consensus sequences, but is presumed to contain binding sites for heme, H_4biopterin, and Arg. Between these two domains is a binding sequence for the allosteric protein calmodulin. The amino acid sequence of the reductase domain is similar to sequences present in the mammalian protein cytochrome P450 reductase.[6] The similarity of the NOS reductase domain to cytochrome P450 reductase suggests that the function of the flavins is to store and transfer electrons from NADPH to a catalytic site in the oxygenase domain.

Subsequent to the cloning of NOS several groups disclosed that NOS is a heme containing protein.[7] As in the cytochrome P450s, the NOS heme in its resting state contains a five coordinate ferric iron and is bound to the protein through coordination of the heme iron to a thiolate anion from a cysteine. The iron's sixth open coordination site is available to bind dioxygen when in its reduced to its ferrous form. By analogy to the cytochrome P450 enzymes, this site is likely to bind and activate dioxygen, which then reacts with Arg to produce NO and Cit.

Based on our mechanistic work with NOHArg and these recent disclosures we and others have proposed a two-step mechanism for the oxidation of Arg to produce NO and Cit which is shown in scheme 5.[1b, 8] One intriguing aspect of the proposed mechanism is that the heme generates distinct oxidants to form and metabolize the intermediate, NOHArg. Thus, the heme first generates an electrophilic species $[FeO]^{3+}$ which hydroxylates a nucleophilic nitrogen of Arg to form NOHArg, and then generates a nucleophilic oxygenating species $[FeOO]^+$ that attacks the electron deficient carbon of the guanidino group of NOHArg to ultimately form NO and Cit. A nucleophilic peroxy-heme has been proposed as an oxidant in other enzymes such as aromatase.[9]

Two lines of evidence indirectly support the use of a nucleophilic oxidant in the second step of NO synthesis. We have found that the guanidino carbon of NOHArg is susceptible to attack by hydroxide ion (yielding Cit) and ammonia (yielding Arg).[5] Second, we have carried out chemical model studies to show that N-hydroxyguanidines are transformed to their urea analogs in good yields by peracids.[10] Oxidation of N-(N-hydroxyamidino)piperidine (NHAP) by m-chloroperbenzoic acid in benzene under

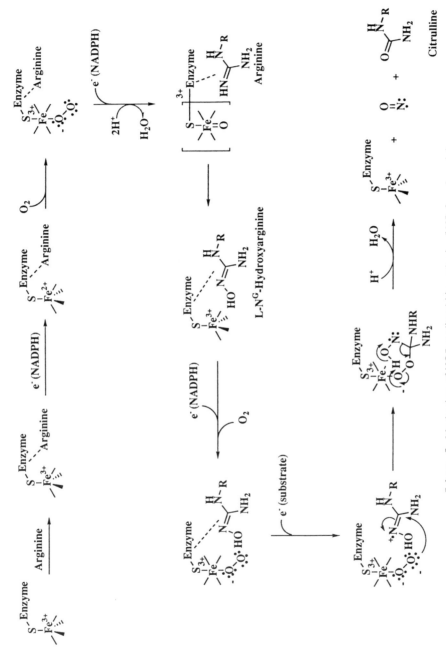

Scheme 5. Mechanism of NOS mediated biosynthesis of NO from L-arginine.

17

anaerobic conditions gave significant amounts of piperidinecarboxamide (PCA) and relatively minor amounts of 1-piperdinecarbonitrile (PCN). Analysis of the gases evolved from the reaction mixture by gas chromatography-thermal conductivity (for N_2O detection) and by chemiluminescence (for NO detection) indicated that N_2O was the major gaseous product. Only trace amounts of NO were detected (<0.1%). N_2O generation is an indication of HNO production since HNO is a metastable species that rapidly decomposes to give N_2O. Since all of the oxidants used in this study are two electron oxidizers, the formation of HNO as the major nitrogen oxide product was expected. The formation of HNO from a N-hydroxyguanidine is a two electron oxidation process. Several mechanisms accounting for the formation of PCA and HNO can be formulated. All of the mechanisms require initial nucleophilic attack by the oxidant on the N-hydroxyguanidine functional group which is commensurate with our proposed mechanism for the formation of NO and Cit from NOHArg. See scheme 6.

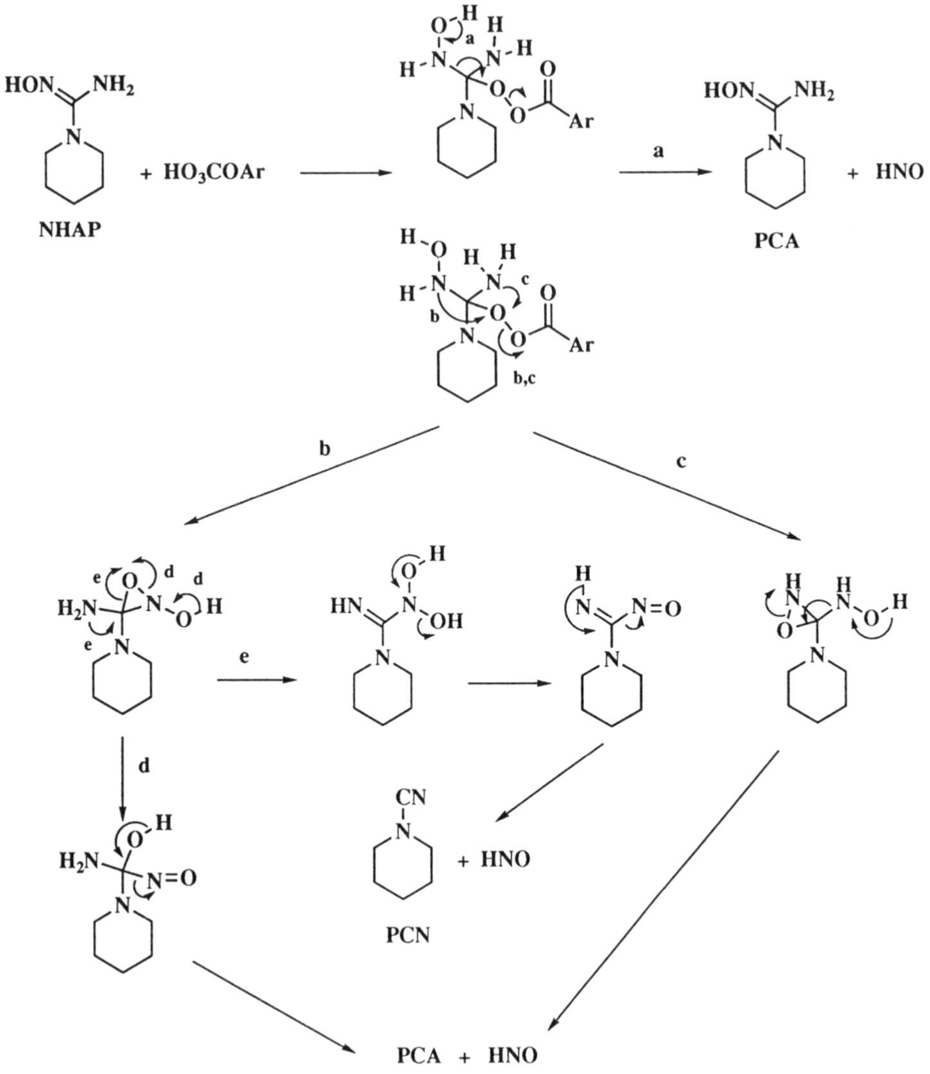

Scheme 6. Possible mechanisms for PCA, PCN, and HNO generation from peracid oxidation of NHAP. A chemical model for NOS oxidation of L-N^G-hydroxyarginine to NO and L-citrulline.

Another important, yet still speculative, aspect of our proposed mechanism is the hypothesis that the heme obtains an electron from the intermediate NOHArg to generate the oxidant in the second step.[1a] This proposal is based on the surprising finding that NOS obtains only one electron from NADPH to carry out the oxidation of NOHArg. This one electron transfer from substrate would enable the heme to generate a nucleophilic oxygenating species while obtaining only one electron from NADPH. This mechanism also provides a means to understand how NOS carries out a three electron oxidation of NOHArg to generate NO, an odd electron product. There are several possible junctures for electron donation back to the enzyme by substrate, and the exact point where NOS obtains an electron from an intermediate is unknown.

In summary, we have shown that NOHArg is a likely intermediate in the NOS mediated biosynthesis of NO from Arg. Coupled with the recent data on the structure of NOS, its similarity with cytochrome P450 reductase, and the discovery that NOS is a heme containing protein we have proposed a two step mechanism for NO biosynthesis. Furthermore, based on our proposal we have carried out chemical model studies that are consistent with the idea that a nucleophilic peroxo-iron species of NOS attacks the N-hydroxyguanidine functional group of NOHArg ultimately converting it to NO and Cit. These mechanistic studies on NOS should serve as a useful framework from which new, interesting, and therapeutically useful NOS inhibitors can be designed.

Acknowledgements. The authors would like to thank the following people for their contributions to the collaborative work described in this manuscript: Nyoun Soo Kwon, Carl F. Nathan, Jeffrey Wiseman, Hui Hong, Michael P. Bova, and Patrick Wong.

REFERENCES

1. For recent reviews of NOS biochemistry see: a. Stuehr, D. J.; Griffith, O. W.; Mammalian nitric oxide synthases, *Adv. Enzymol. Mol. Biol.* **1992**, 346, 287. b. Marletta, M. A.; Nitric oxide synthase structure and mechanism, *J. Biol. Chem.* **1993**, 268, 12231. c. Kerwin, Jr., J. F.; Heller, M.; The arginine-nitric oxide pathway a target for new drugs, *Medicinal Res. Rev.* **1994**, 14, 24. d. Feldman, P. L.; Griffith, O. W.; Stuehr, D. J. The surprising life of nitric oxide, *Chem. and Engin. News* **1993**, December 20, 26.

2. A. Hibbs, Jr., J. B.; Taintor, R. R.; Vavrin, Z.; Macrophage cytotoxicity: Role for L-arginine deiminase and imino nitrogen oxidation to nitrite, *Science* **1987**, 235, 473. b. Marletta, M. A.; Yoon, P. S.; Iyengar, R.; Leaf, C. D.; Wishnik, J. S.; Macrophage oxidation of L-arginine to nitrite and nitrate: Nitric oxide is an intermediate, *Biochemistry* **1988**, 27, 8706. c. DeMaster, E. G.; Raij, L.; Archer, S. L.; Weir, E. K.; Hydroxylamine is a vasorelaxant and a possible intermediate in the oxidative conversion of L-arginine to nitric oxide, *Biochem. Biophys. Res. Commun.* **1989**, 163, 527.

3. Kwon, N. S.; Nathan, C. F.; Gilker, C.; Griffith, O. W.; Matthews, D. E.; Stuehr, D. J.; L-Citrulline production from L-arginine by macrophage nitric synthase: The ureido oxygen derives from dioxygen, *J. Biol. Chem.* **1990**, 265, 13442.

4. Feldman, P. L.; Synthesis of the putative L-arginine metabolite L-N^G-hydroxyarginine, *Tetrahedron Lett.* **1991**, 32, 875.

5. Stuehr, D. J.; Kwon, N. S.; Nathan, C. F.; Griffith, O. W.; Feldman, P. L.; Wiseman, J.; N$^\omega$-Hydroxy-L-arginine is an intermediate in the biosynthesis of nitric oxide from L-arginine, *J. Biol. Chem.* **1991**, 266, 6259.

6. The first report describing the cloning of a cNOS and its homology with cytochrome P450 reductase is: Bredt, D. S.; Huang, P. M.; Glatt, C. E.; Lowenstein, C.; Reed, R. R.; Snyder, S. H.; Cloned and expressed nitric oxide synthase structurally resembles cytochrome P-450 reductase, *Nature* **1991**, 351, 714.

7. a. Stuehr, D. J.; Ikeda-Saito, M.; Spectral characterization of brain and macrophage nitric oxide synthases: Cytochrome P-450-like hemeproteins that contain a flavin semiquinone radical, *J. Biol. Chem.* **1992**, 267, 20547. b. White, K. A.; Marletta, M. A.; Nitric oxide synthase is a

cytochrome P-450 type hemoprotein, *Biochemistry* **1992**, 31, 6627. c. McMillan, K.; Bredt, D. S.; Hirsch, D. J.; Snyder, S. H.; Clark, J. E.; Masters, B. S. S. Cloned, expressed rat cerebellar nitric oxide synthase contains stoichiometric amounts of heme, which binds carbon monoxide, *Proc. Natl. Acad. Sci. U. S. A.* **1992**, 89, 11141.

8. Feldman; P. L.; Griffith; O. W.; Hong, H.; Stuehr, D. J.; Irreversible inactivation of macrophage and brain nitric oxide synthase by L-N^G-methylarginine requires NADPH-dependent hydroxylation, *J. Med. Chem.* **1993**, 36, 491.

9. Vaz, A. D. M.; Roberts, E. S.; Coon, M. J.; Olefin formation in the oxidative deformylation of aldehydes by cytochrome P-450. Mechanistic implicatios for catalysis by oxygen-derived peroxide, *J. Am. Chem. Soc.* **1991**, 113, 5886.

10. Fukuto, J. M.; Stuehr, D. J.; Feldman, P. L.; Bova, M. P.; Wong, P.; Peracid oxidation of an N-hydroxyguanidine compound: A chemical model for the oxidation of N$^\omega$-hydroxy-L-arginine by nitric oxide synthase, *J. Med. Chem.* **1993**, 36, 2666.

NITRIC OXIDE SYNTHASE INHIBITORS: MECHANISM OF ACTION AND IN VIVO STUDIES

Owen W. Griffith

Department of Biochemistry
Medical College of Wisconsin
Milwaukee, WI 53226 USA

INTRODUCTION

Nitric oxide synthase (NOS) catalyzes the NADPH- and O_2-dependent oxidation of L-arginine to citrulline and nitric oxide (NO) (1,2). At least three distinct isoforms of NOS occur in mammals including a brain isoform (bNOS) that produces NO having a poorly defined role in neurotransmission (3,4), an isoform in vascular endothelial cells (eNOS) that produces NO having a vasodilatory role in normal blood pressure homeostasis (5,7), and an inducible isoform (iNOS) that is expressed in many tissues in response to lipopolysaccharide (LPS) and various cytokines (e.g. tumor necrosis factor (TNF), interleukin-1 (IL-1), interleukin-2 (IL-2) (8). Although iNOS has a physiological role in the control of intracellular pathogens including viruses (9) and may play a role in the cytostatic/cytotoxic reaction of macrophages to tumor cells (10,11), overproduction of NO by iNOS expressed in vascular smooth muscle (VSM) and endothelial cells has been shown to be a major hypotensive mediator in septic and cytokine-induced shock (7,12-15). Recent evidence also suggests iNOS-derived NO accounts in part for the tissue damage seen in inflammatory disorders including arthritis (16-18). Elucidation of these potentially pathological roles of iNOS and speculation that bNOS has a role in the post-ischemic damage of stroke (4) has stimulated efforts to selectively inhibit the NOS isoforms.

Both bNOS and eNOS are constitutive enzymes and are physiologically regulated by Ca^{++}/calmodulin (1,2,7). Although iNOS contains tightly bound calmodulin, it is fully active at endogenous levels of Ca^{++}; iNOS is therefore mainly, perhaps exclusively, regulated at the transcriptional and translational levels (19). In terms of selective pharmacological control, bNOS and eNOS, but not iNOS, are inhibited *in vitro* by Ca^{++} chelators and by calmodulin antagonists (1). The diversity of Ca^{++}/calmodulin-dependent enzymes present in tissues severely limits the utility of such approaches. Although iNOS can in principle be controlled by prevention of expression (7), the efficacy of this approach in shock is limited (see later). It is thus notable that to date it has not been possible to pharmacologically regulate NO production by manipulating physiological control mechanisms.

Biochemical, Pharmacological, and Clinical Aspects of Nitric Oxide
Edited by B. A. Weissman *et al.*, Plenum Press, New York, 1995

All three NOS isoforms have been cloned from animal and human cell lines, and the amino acid sequences deduced (20). Although homology among the three isoforms is only modest (50-60% identity), the C-terminal sequences of all three are homologous to cytochrome P_{450} reductase. The similarity is of mechanistic significance because all isoforms also share with cytochrome P_{450} reductase a requirement for FAD and FMN (1,2). In fact, this and other observations suggest that the C-terminal region of NOS acts in a cytochrome P_{450} reductase-like manner to bind NADPH and shuttle NADPH-derived electrons via the flavins to the heme cofactor-binding N-terminal portion of the protein. Although the N-terminal portion of NOS isoforms shows little homology with known cytochromes P_{450}, that domain binds arginine (21) and mediates the cytochrome P_{450}-like monooxygenations necessary to form N^{ω}-hydroxy-L-arginine (NOH-ARG) and convert that tightly-bound intermediate to citrulline and NO (Scheme 1)(1,22). Appreciation of the functional similarity between NOS and a cytochrome P_{450} reductase - cytochrome P_{450} hybrid allows important insights into the mechanism by which several NOS inhibitors block catalytic activity.

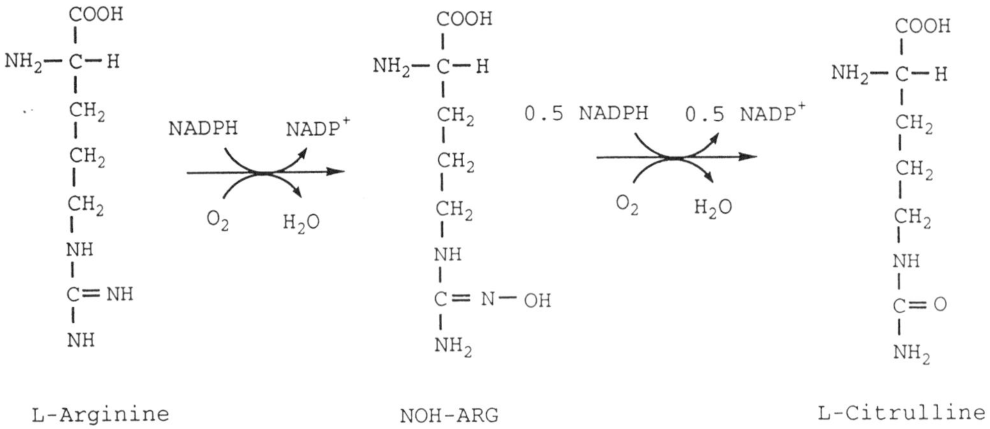

Scheme 1 (structures):

L-Arginine: COOH — CH(NH$_2$) — CH$_2$ — CH$_2$ — CH$_2$ — NH — C(=NH) — NH

NADPH, O$_2$ → NADP$^+$, H$_2$O

NOH-ARG: COOH — CH(NH$_2$) — CH$_2$ — CH$_2$ — CH$_2$ — NH — C(=N—OH) — NH$_2$

0.5 NADPH, O$_2$ → 0.5 NADP$^+$, H$_2$O

L-Citrulline: COOH — CH(NH$_2$) — CH$_2$ — CH$_2$ — CH$_2$ — NH — C(=O) — NH$_2$

Scheme 1.

Despite modest sequence homology, the three NOS isoforms each catalyze the reaction sequence shown in Scheme 1 using exactly the same cofactors; the detailed chemistry of the complex 5 electron oxidation of arginine is apparently highly conserved. Notwithstanding this similarity of chemistry, the diverse biological functions of the individual NOS isoforms strongly supports efforts to develop isoform-selective NOS inhibitors. To date, progress in the design and synthesis of potent, general NOS inhibitors has been much better than progress in obtaining isoform-selective (or, ideally, isoform-specific) inhibition. The present report considers several general approaches to limiting or preventing the adverse effects of NO overproduction; NOS inhibitors and arginine depletion strategies are discussed in detail. The physiological activity of specific NOS inhibitors and their pharmacological use are also discussed.

GENERAL APPROACHES TO THE CONTROL OF NO OVERPRODUCTION

Table 1

I.	Prevention of Nitric Oxide Synthase Induction A. Anti-cytokine or Anti-endotoxin Antibodies/Receptor Antagonists B. Blockade of Tetrahydrobiopterin Synthesis
II.	Inhibition of NO Formation by Nitric Oxide Synthase A. Enzyme Inhibitors - Arginine Antagonists B. Arginine Depletion
III.	Prevention of NO Action A. NO Scavengers B. Guanylyl Cyclase Inhibitors

Prevention of iNOS Induction

Table 1 lists six distinct therapeutic interventions that may prevent or minimize the hypotension associated with the overproduction of NO by vascular cells (15). Since the NO accounting for clinical shock is iNOS-derived, the first two approaches listed are directed at preventing active iNOS expression. As indicated, expression can be decreased by blocking the cytokine cascade responsible for iNOS induction. Antibodies to TNF and endotoxin as well as IL-1 receptor antagonist show some efficacy in limiting iNOS activity (15,23). With respect to the septic shock, they may have an advantage over the other approaches in that not only NO overproduction but other cytokine-dependent aspects of sepsis might be prevented. Unfortunately, recently reported clinical trials suggest cytokine interception is of limited utility in septic patients (23,24). With respect to NO-mediated hypotension, it is likely that the problems are three-fold.

First, prevention of iNOS expression requires an anticipation that is not always clinically possible. That is, cytokine interception has no effect on iNOS already expressed, and given the $t_{1/2}$ of iNOS activity *in vivo*, prevention of further expression will not usefully affect NO synthesis for 48 to 72 hrs, a long delay for a severely hypotensive patient. Slowness of response would, of course, be of less concern in treating inflammatory disorders attributable to NO overproduction (e.g. arthritis).

A second problem with using cytokine interception strategies in shock is their apparently poor efficacy even with extended treatment. Poor efficacy may be due in part to the difficulty of fully blocking the action of specific cytokines or LPS. That is, in an amplifying cascade a little cytokine signal "leaking" past the blockade may allow iNOS induction to levels causing production of highly vasoactive amounts of NO. In this regard, it should be noted that vasorelaxation requires only nM concentrations of NO whereas full induction of iNOS in VSM and endothelial cells can lead to μM NO; even 90% inhibition of iNOS expression may not fully prevent iNOS-mediated hypotension. This issue also would be of less concern in chronic inflammatory disorders where it is the cytotoxic consequences of NO overproduction rather than vasoactive effects that are important. Cytotoxic effects, seen only at high levels of NO, may diminish in fairly direct proportion to the extent that NO production is diminished.

Poor efficacy of cytokine-directed antibodies and receptor antagonists in shock may also be due to the variety of signals able to induce NOS expression. In VSM or endothelial cells, LPS, TNF, IL-1, IL-2 and IFN-γ have all been shown to stimulate iNOS induction (19,25,26). Blocking only one or two of these factors may reduce iNOS expression, but is unlikely to fully prevent induction. As noted a little iNOS expression is sufficient to cause severe vasodilatation.

Whereas expression of the iNOS apoenzyme is controlled by cytokines, expression of active iNOS is additionally dependent on availability of the required cofactors FAD, FMN, tetrahyrdobiopterin (THB) and heme. In vascular smooth muscle cells, THB can be limiting and, as pointed out by S.S. Gross *et al.* (27), inhibition of THB synthesis has the effect of limiting iNOS activity. Inhibitors and strategies appropriate to this goal are known and under development. Because inhibition of THB synthesis may have only modest effect on existing iNOS, overproduction of NO will not be immediately altered, a limitation shared with cytokine interception strategies. However, unlike interception strategies, inhibitors of THB synthesis act directly on the enzymes involved, and there is no amplification problem. It is also notable that inhibition of THB synthesis affects only iNOS activity and not the full spectrum of cytokine-induced events. This limitation may be a disadvantage in treating septic shock, but may be important if the goal is prevention of the hypotension associated with therapeutic use of cytokines (e.g. TNF or IL-2) without abrogating their beneficial effects.

Inhibition of iNOS Activity

Table I lists two approaches to the inhibition of iNOS once it has been expressed in the vasculature - direct inhibition using arginine antagonists and substrate deprivation. Both approaches are capable of providing rapid reversal of NO-mediated hypotension; their efficacy has been established in animal models of both cytokine-induced and septic shock. The mechanism of action of both established and novel NOS inhibitors is a major focus of our work and is discussed in detail in the next section; substrate depletion is discussed here.

Of the three NOS substrates (NADPH, O_2 and L-arginine), only arginine can be made rate-limiting without causing major nonspecific derangement of cellular metabolism. Arginine depletion strategies have a further advantage of potentially being iNOS selective. That is, the physiological role of both eNOS and bNOS requires the formation of only small amounts of NO and therefore should require only small amounts of arginine. In contrast, cells expressing iNOS typically produce high levels of NO and consume substantial arginine. We anticipated that in shock NO production by VSM and endothelial cells would deplete cellular stores of arginine thereby making continued NO synthesis dependent on the ability of such cells to produce or take up additional arginine. Cells can obtain arginine by degradation of protein, by recycling the citrulline produced by NOS to arginine via argininosuccinate, and by uptake of exogenous arginine. Since extensive protein degradation in the absence of resynthesis is incompatible with cell survival, only the latter two sources of arginine are likely to play an important role in iNOS-mediated overproduction of NO.

At present, the relative importance of citrulline recycling and arginine uptake in the continued overproduction of NO is unknown. Recent studies show that argininosuccinate synthase, the rate-limiting enzyme for citrulline recycling, is co-induced with iNOS in cultured VSM cells (28) and macrophages (29). That finding suggests that recycling is important in at least those cells.

That recycling alone can not sustain overproduction of vasoreactive NO *in vivo* is illustrated by the results shown in Figure 1. In this study, the effect of arginase on the blood pressure of control and endotoxemic pithed rats was examined. As shown, arginase administration, which decreased plasma arginine > 90%, had no effect on the blood pressure of control rats but increased the blood pressure of the hypotensive, endotoxemic rats by 20% (30). The study indicates that basal formation of NO by eNOS can be sustained without recourse to the uptake of plasma arginine (control rat studies), but in endotoxemic shock overproduction of NO by iNOS is limited (but not prevented) when uptake of arginine is reduced by arginase-mediated depletion of extracellular stores. It is important to note that arginase hydrolyzes arginine to urea and ornithine, products which can not be converted to arginine by VSM or endothelial cells. We anticipate that conversion of arginine to citrulline (e.g. by administration of arginine deiminase) would be less effective due to the aforementioned citrulline recycling pathway. Arginase-mediated depletion of plasma arginine also restores vascular responsivity to α-adrenergic pressor agents, a result consistent with diminished NO synthesis (30).

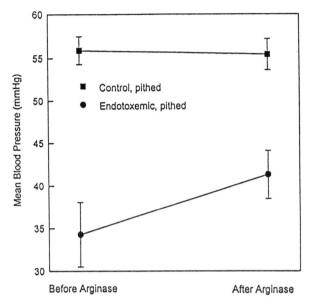

Figure 1. Effect of arginase on the blood pressure of control and endotoxemic pithed rats. Rats were instrumented to measure blood pressure and were pithed to eliminate central control of blood pressure. Arginase (300 I.U./min for 20 min) was given intravenously. Endotoxemic rats received LPS (15 mg/kg, intraperitoneally) (S.S. Gross, K. Aisaka, K.H. Park, R. Levi and O.W. Griffith, unpublished).

Prevention of NO Action

The third major approach to shock encompasses strategies directed at preventing the vasoactive effect of NO (Table 1). The two most promising possibilities are destruction of NO after it is formed using NO scavengers and inhibition of soluble guanylyl cyclase, the enzyme normally activated by vasoactive NO. For the latter approach, better inhibitors are needed. Although some of the vasopressor response to methylene blue may be attributable to its inhibition of guanylyl cyclase (31,32), the dye is neither a specific inhibitor (32) nor physiologically benign (e.g. in the presence of NO, superoxide generation by methylene blue (31) leads to peroxynitrite, a potentially toxic metabolite). More specific inhibitors are likely, however, to be effective drugs. NO scavengers (e.g. hemoglobin or spin traps) have shown some promise *in vitro* in reversing endotoxin-mediated hyporeactivity to pressors (33); further development is anticipated. To the extent that pathological vasorelaxation is due to iNOS induction in VSM cells and autocrine activation of guanylyl cyclase occurring in the same cell, extracellular NO scavengers might be expected to have limited efficacy. In fact, the diffusability of NO is sufficiently large that extracellular NO sinks appear to deplete intracellular NO (33).

MECHANISM OF ESTABLISHED AND NOVEL NOS INHIBITORS

N^ω-Alkyl-L-Arginines and N^δ-Iminoalkyl-L-Ornithines

In 1987, Hibbs *et al.* reported that N^ω-methyl-L-arginine (L-NMA) blocked the arginine-dependent anti-tumor activity of macrophages (10). Following that initial report, L-NMA has been widely used as a NOS inhibitor *in vitro* and *in vivo*. Although not isoform specific, NMA shows better activity against iNOS and lesser activity toward bNOS and eNOS than either N^ω-nitro-L-arginine (L-NNA) or N^ω-nitro-L-arginine methyl ester (L-NAME), the other readily available, widely used NOS inhibitors (1,34,35). Because it has little toxicity in normal animals, NMA is currently in clinical trial for both cytokine-induced and septic shock.

The mechanism by which L-NMA inhibits NOS is complex. Initial inhibition is strictly reversible and competitive with L-arginine; the Ki values for L-NMA are significantly smaller than the Km for L-arginine, consistent with the ability of L-NMA to achieve good inhibition in the presence of moderate, but not large, concentrations of L-arginine. Longer incubation of NOS with L-NMA results in NADPH-dependent irreversible inactivation of the enzyme (36,37). Recent investigation of the mechanism of such irreversible inhibition established that L-NMA, like L-arginine, is processed by the enzyme to form a monohydroxylated derivative, N^ω-hydroxy-N^ω-methyl-L-arginine (NOH-NMA). As shown in Figure 2, further processing of that derivative by a pathway analogous to that followed by NOH-ARG is expected to yield citrulline and nitrosomethane radical cation (CH_3NO^+) (36). The latter derivative has not been characterized in solution, but it is anticipated that NO would be a strong leaving group allowing CH_3NO^+ to methylate enzymatic nucleophiles or to react spontaneously with water, forming NO and methylated enzyme or methanol, respectively. Subsequent to our report, Olken and Marletta (38) confirmed the formation of NOH-NMA from L-NMA and suggested alternative metabolisms for both L-NMA and NOH-NMA leading to citrulline, NO, and formaldehyde. Formaldehyde formation would be dependent on the formation of carbon-free radical intermediates, species which might inhibit the enzyme irreversibly by destruction of the heme cofactor or active site residues. Further studies are necessary to establish which of these pathways actually account for inactivation of the enzyme; at present it appears that all of the proposed pathways of L-NMA metabolism are operative to some extent.

In addition to L-NMA, we have shown that a variety of N^ω-monoalkyl substituted L-arginine derivatives are NOS inhibitors (39). Similarly, arginine analogs in which the hydroxylated guanidino nitrogen is replaced by CH_3- or higher alkyl groups (N^δ-iminoethyl-L-ornithine (L-NIO, (40) and its homologies) are structurally analogous and also inhibit. Detailed structure-function studies carried out with K. Narayanan establish that the active site region occupied by the reactive guanidino nitrogen is able to accommodate substituents as large as n-propyl and, to a lesser extent, n-butyl. Interestingly, the NOS isoforms are not identical in their structural constraints on inhibitor binding, suggesting that isoform selective inhibition may be possible.

L-Thiocitrulline

Whereas most previously described NOS inhibitors are arginine analogs, we recently reported that L-thiocitrulline (N^δ-thioureido-L-norvaline) is a potent inhibitor of both iNOS and bNOS (41). Additional studies establish that inhibition by L-thiocitrulline is competitive with L-arginine and, unlike L-NMA and L-NIO, fully reversible even following prolonged incubation. Spectral studies carried out in collaboration with K. McMillan and B.S.S. Masters, show that addition of L-thiocitrulline to a solution of bNOS results in a type II difference spectrum consistent with conversion of heme iron from a pentacoordinate high spin state to a hexacoordinate low spin state. This result is interpreted as showing that L-thiocitrulline represents a novel class of NOS inhibitors which bind both to the arginine/citrulline binding site and to the heme cofactor (42, 43). In view of the well established affinity of heme iron for sulfur, we believe L-thiocitrulline is bound in a configuration which juxtaposes sulfur and heme iron (i.e. sulfur occupies the site normally occupied by the guanidino nitrogen subject to hydroxylation and eventual metabolism to NO). L-thiocitrulline is a potent pressor agent in both normotensive control rats and hypotensive, septic rats.

S-Methyl-L-Thiocitrulline

S-Methyl-L-thiocitrulline is an extremely potent inhibitor of both bNOS and iNOS (41,44). This compound, which is structurally reminiscent of L-NMA, is also a competitive inhibitor with respect to L-arginine. Its Ki values with bNOS and iNOS are substantially lower that those for L-NMA, however, and it is, to our knowledge, the most potent NOS inhibiting arginine antagonist reported to date (44). Higher S-alkyl homologs of S-methyl-L-thiocitrulline are also potent inhibitors of NOS. Binding specificity with respect to S-alkyl groups closely parallels that seen with N-alkyl groups in L-NMA homologs, a finding suggesting that the sulfur of S-methyl-L-thiocitrulline occupies the active site position normally filled by the hydroxylated guanidino nitrogen of L-arginine and L-NMA (K. Narayanan and O.W. Griffith, unpublished). Like L-thiocitrulline, S-methyl-L-thiocitrulline is a potent pressor agent (44).

PHARMACOLOGY OF NOS INHIBITORS

Effects in Normotensive Animals

R.F. Furchgott and J.V. Zawadski reported in 1980 that norepinephrine-contracted arterial rings and strips from several species relaxed in response to acetylcholine only if the endothelial cell layer was not removed (45). The presumptive endothelium-derived relaxing factor (EDRF) was identified as NO in 1986 (1). Three years later, K. Aisaka et al. reported that L-NMA (10 mg/kg i.v.) shortened the duration and decreased the magnitude of the vasodilatory response to acetylcholine in guinea pigs made hypertensive with norepinephrine (46). In normotensive guinea pigs, L-NMA shortened the duration of the response to acetylcholine but did not alter the magnitude (Figure 3). Interestingly, administration of L-arginine (30 mg/kg bolus + 10 mg/kg infusion) increased the duration of the response to acetylcholine but did not alter resting blood pressure (Figure 3) (46).

In contrast to the result with L-arginine, K. Aisaka et al. (5) and D.D. Rees et al. (6) had previously shown that bolus injection of L-NMA markedly elevated blood pressure in guinea pigs and rabbits, respectively. As shown in Figure 4, diastolic pressure in guinea pigs was sensitive to L-NMA in doses as low as 1 mg/kg (4 µmol/kg); the maximum pressor response at a 10-fold higher dose was 25 mm Hg, an increase of nearly 50% (5). Rabbits are apparently less sensitive to L-NMA, a dose of 100 mg/kg being required to elevate mean blood pressure about 20 mm Hg (29%) (6). Subsequent studies have consistently shown L-NMA has a pressor effect in all species examined including man.

The observation that NOS inhibitors have a pressor effect in otherwise untreated normotensive animals indicated that vasoactive NO is formed in vivo at a physiologically significant basal rate and that its formation is an important aspect of normal blood pressure homeostasis (5). Additional studies with isolated vessels or vascular beds establish the eNOS-derived NO plays a role in the control of organ perfusion (7). It is likely that shear stress on the endothelial cells of resistance vessels plays an important role in controlling eNOS activity and thereby vessel diameter and blood pressure (47).

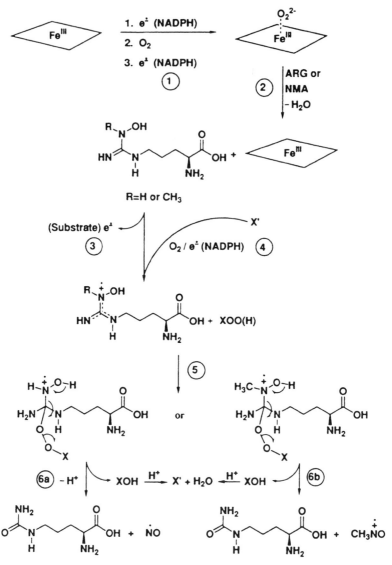

Figure 2. The oxidation of ARG or NMA to NO or the radical cation of nitrosomethane is accounted for by the steps shown. Step 1 is a formal representation of the activation of dioxygen utilizing the model of cytochrome P_{450} activation of dioxygen. The combination of steps 1 and 2 lead to the now-established intermediates NOH-ARG or NOH-NMA. Steps 3 and 4, representing one-electron donations by hydroxylated substrate and NADPH, respectively, produce the oxidizing species XOO(H), probably an oxy-heme species similar to that produced in step 1. Step 5 shows the nucleophilic attack of XOO(H) on the radical cation of NOH-ARG or NOH-NMA; steps 6a and 6b show the further reaction to final products. Note the electron transfers shown in steps 6a and 6b constitute a two-electron oxidation of the hydroxylated nitrogen; the overall scheme thus accounts for a five-electron oxidation. Although NOH-ARG and NOH-NMA are depicted as donating an electron in step 3, it is possible that oxidation occurs later in the scheme. (From (36) with permission).

28

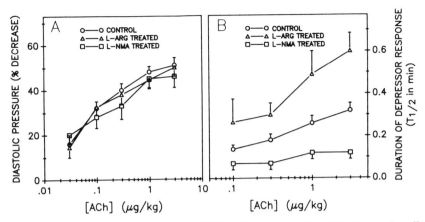

Figure 3. L-NMA abbreviates and L-arginine (L-ARG) prolongs the duration of the hypotensive effect of acetylcholine (ACh) in the anesthetized guinea pig. Depressor responses to ACh administered by bolus i.v. injection were recorded in the absence or presence of L-ARG and L-NMA. L-ARG was infused i.v. at a rate of 10 mg/kg/min immediately after a bolus i.v. injection of 30 mg/kg. NMA was administered as a 10 mg/kg bolus i.v. injection. Depressor responses to ACh (Panel A) are expressed as the maximum percent fall in diastolic blood pressure; duration of ACh depressor responses (Panel B) is expressed as the time to half-recovery ($T_{1/2}$) in minutes from the maximum fall in diastolic pressure. Points are means ($\pm$ S.E.) obtained from 17 control, 8 L-ARG- and 5 L-NMA-treated animals with diastolic blood pressures of 46 $\pm$ 3, 44 $\pm$ 3 mm Hg, respectively. (From (46) with permission).

Effects in Hypotensive Animals

The report by R.G. Kilbourn and P. Belloni in 1989 (25,48) that iNOS was expressed in cultured vascular endothelial cells exposed to LPS and various cytokines immediately suggested that cytokine-induced (49) and sepsis-induced circulatory shock might be due to similar induction of iNOS *in vivo* followed by overproduction of vasoactive NO. This hypothesis was quickly confirmed in studies in which the slowly developing hypotension of anesthetized dogs administered TNF was immediately reversed ($t_{1/2} < 2$ min) by giving L-NMA (4.4 mg/kg). A typical experiment is shown in Figure 5 (12). Note that the pressor response to L-NMA (L-MeArg in the Figure) was reversed by subsequent administration of L-arginine (100 mg/kg) consistent with L-NMA acting as a competitive NOS inhibitor. Pooled results from four dogs showed that systemic arterial pressure (mean $\pm$ S.D.) was 127 $\pm$ 13 before TNF, 66 $\pm$ 21 after TNF and immediately before L-NMA administration, 120 $\pm$ 13 within minutes after giving L-NMA, and 71 $\pm$ 25 after giving excess L-arginine. All of the changes in blood pressure were statistically significant (p = 0.01-0.02) (12). Subsequent studies showed that NOS inhibitors restore blood pressure in dogs made hypotensive with IL-1 (13), IL-2 (15,48,49), and endotoxin (14). Similarly, the hypotension seen in patients receiving IL-2 therapy for renal cell carcinoma responds to L-NMA given in the absence of other pressor drugs (R.G. Kilbourn *et al.*, *Crit. Care Med.*, in press).

Animals or patients made hypotensive by administration of iNOS-inducing cytokines or by bacterial infection (sepsis) are difficult to treat because they are characteristically poorly responsive to α_1-adrenergic pressors (e.g. dopamine, norepinephrine). Studies by I. Fleming *et al.* established that responsivity to such pressors is markedly improved by administration of L-NMA (51) and the view has emerged that the hyporesponsivity to

29

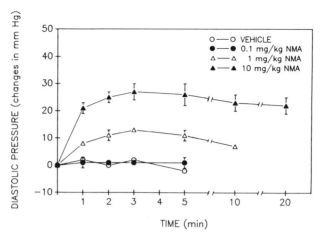

Figure 4. Pressor effect of L-NMA in the anesthetized guinea pig. L-NMA was dissolved in saline (vehicle) and administered i.v. by bolus injection at the doses indicated. Points are mean changes in diastolic arterial pressure (± S.E.: n = 5 animals). Control systolic and diastolic blood pressures were 75 ± 3 and 51 ± 3 mm Hg, respectively. (From (5) with permission).

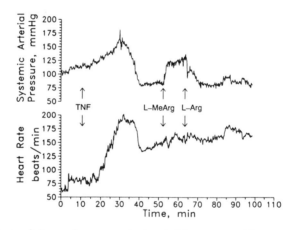

Figure 5. Time course of changes in mean systemic arterial pressure and heart rate in a pentobarbital-anesthetized dog following i.v. administration (arrows) of TNF, (10 µg/kg), L-MeArg (4.4 mg/kg), and L-arginine (100 mg/kg). (From (12) with permission).

pressors seen in cytokine-induced and septic shock is due to overproduction of NO (15,52). It is likely that exposure of VSM cells to high levels of NO increases cGMP levels and thereby decreases Ca^{++} levels to a point where strong contraction is not possible; a useful pressor response remains impossible until Ca^{++} levels are normalized following NOS inhibition.

Toxicology of NOS Inhibitors

Although virtually all studies reported to date show that NOS inhibitors can reverse the hypotension and hyporesponsivity to α_1-adrenergic pressors seen in cytokine-induced and septic shock, several concerns have been raised regarding the clinical use of inhibitors (23). In considering those concerns, it is important to evaluate the results on the basis of the NOS inhibitor used, the dose used, the protocol followed, and the relevance of the specific animal model to NO-mediated shock in patients.

As noted earlier, none of the commonly used arginine antagonists are highly specific for the iNOS isoform; adverse effects attributable to eNOS and bNOS inhibition must therefore be considered. That said, specificity data on commercially available inhibitors strongly encourages use of L-NMA over L-NNA or L-NAME since the former is a relatively stronger iNOS inhibitor and weaker bNOS and eNOS inhibitor (34). In addition, L-NNA and L-NAME are lipophilic relative to L-NMA and may, on that basis, be more likely to cross the blood brain barrier and cause central effects. In rats, cerebellar bNOS activity was decreased 95% by administration of L-NNA (50 mg/kg b.i.d.) for four days and activity remained low for five days after the drug was discontinued (53).

Similar studies with L-NMA have apparently not been reported, but the toxicology of L-NMA was studied in mice, rats and dogs prior to initiation of clinical trials. Little toxicity was seen. The LD_{10} for a single i.v. dose of L-NMA acetate in mice is 1750 mg/kg; no LD_{50} could be determined. Sub-chronic administration of L-NMA to rats by i.v. infusion for 14 days caused no toxicity at doses up to 900 mg/kg per day. A similar absence of acute toxicity was seen in dogs; occasional gastrointestinal ulcers were seen when administration was continued for 14 days (R.G. Kilbourn, O.W. Griffith *et al.*, manuscript in preparation). Although these findings raise some concerns regarding the very long term systemic administration of L-NMA for inflammatory disorders, it is anticipated that treatment of shock will require only short term (1-6 days) use of L-NMA. Such use is apparently not associated with toxicity at vasoactive doses.

It should be emphasized that similar screening has not to our knowledge been reported for other arginine antagonists. Nevertheless at least one potent NOS inhibitor, N^{ω}-amino-L-arginine (34,35,54), was found to be well tolerated by mice and rats but to cause seizures in dogs at vasoactive doses (13,55). Such toxicity is apparently not related to NOS inhibition *per se* since equipotent doses of L-NMA do not cause seizures, and seizures were not prevented by excess L-arginine. The findings do, however, suggest caution in evaluating reports based on studies with aminoarginine concluding that NOS inhibition decreases survival in shock (23,55).

NOS inhibitors including L-NMA differ from conventional pressor drugs in that their action is limited to blocking the synthesis of an endogenous depressor, NO. Once iNOS is fully inhibited, no further pressor action is possible. It follows that doses of NOS inhibitors in excess of those needed to block NOS (e.g. to block iNOS in shock) are inappropriate and likely to increase toxicity without improving efficacy. Although pharmacokinetic data for L-NMA and other NOS inhibitors are limited or unavailable, several considerations should guide the development of dose regimens and the evaluation of published reports. First, the Ki for L-NMA (37,38) is ~ 6 μM for iNOS and the Ki for other useful inhibitors is lower (41). The Km for arginine, with which they compete, is typically several-fold higher. The required dose of L-NMA (or other inhibitor) is thus dependent on the intracellular concentration of arginine, which is generally unknown. Nevertheless, it is clear that L-NMA and arginine are taken up by the same mechanisms with similar affinity (56,57) and that the plasma L-NMA/L-arginine ratio should approximate the tissue ratio. For rapid inhibition of iNOS in VSM and endothelial cells, it is appropriate to administer L-NMA doses that achieve initial plasma concentrations 5- to 10-fold higher than plasma arginine levels. The latter are typically 50-200 μM in experimental animals and patients, subject to nutritional fluctuations. Assuming a 10% blood volume, L-NMA doses of 20 mg/kg (~80 μmol/kg) are likely to achieve the necessary plasma levels. Consistent with this estimate, we find in normotensive anesthetized rats that the pressor response to 20 mg/kg L-NMA is essentially maximal; no further increase is seen with doses of 30 or 40 mg/kg. (L. Spack and O.W. Griffith, unpublished). R.G. Kilbourn *et al.* has made similar observations in dogs (50) and patients (personal communication). Duration of effect shows considerable interspecies variation; the pressor response to a single bolus infusion of L-NMA (20 mg/kg) typically lasts ~ 30 min in rats, ~ 20 min in dogs, and ~ 60 min in man. In cases where longer term blockade of NOS is desired, low dose infusion is preferable to high dose bolus injection. Although studies have been reported in which L-NMA was given at doses as high as 300 mg/kg (58,59), data establishing the need for such doses was not reported; resulting conclusions regarding the toxicity of L-NMA when used in shock should be viewed with caution (59).

Whereas there is good data establishing the relatively low toxicity of L-NMA in normotensive control animals, it does not necessarily follow that L-NMA is similarly non-toxic in hypotensive animals overproducing NO. There are, in fact, several reports indicating that L-NMA increases morbidity or mortality in septic (endotoxemic) shock. Thus T.R. Billar *et al.* found that hepatic damage increased in endotoxemic mice given NMA; they suggested that NO might react with and detoxify superoxide (60). In subsequent studies, R.G. Kilbourn *et al.* have not seen evidence of increased hepatotoxicity in endotoxemic dogs or in septic or IL-2-treated patients given L-NMA (R.G. Kilbourn, *et al.*, *Crit. Care Med.*, in press).

Although a protective role for iNOS-derived NO in liver remains speculative, there can be no question that organ perfusion is affected by NO arising in the vasculature and perhaps other tissues. Systemic blockade of iNOS and eNOS using currently available inhibitors may adversely affect organ perfusion even if blood pressure is normalized. Our early studies in dogs given TNF or endotoxin, in fact, showed a significant drop in cardiac output (CO) following L-NMA administration (12,14). While some drop in CO is anticipated as a baroreflex to increased blood pressure, it has been argued that L-NMA has a negative inotropic effect, possibly due in part to decreased cardiac perfusion. The clinical importance of these observations is species dependent. Septic shock in dogs is typically characterized by low CO; any decrease in CO is thus likely to cause adverse hemodynamic effects or even death. On the other hand, CO is often elevated in septic patients or in cancer patients administered IL-2. Preliminary studies indicate that administration of L-NMA to such patients tends to normalize both CO and blood pressure (R.G. Kilbourn *et al.*, *Crit. Care Med.*, in press). It should also be noted that inotropic agents (e.g. dobutamine) are able to maintain CO in dogs given L-NMA.

The comments above notwithstanding, maintenance of organ perfusion remains a concern when using NOS inhibitors to combat the hypotension of cytokine-induced and septic shock (15,23). It is established, for example, that endotoxin induces both NO and endothelin-1 synthesis; following NOS inhibition, the unopposed vasoconstrictive action of endothelin on the renal arteries (61) is likely to account for the observed decrease in renal perfusion. Pulmonary hypertension may occur in shock (23,61) and is likely to be made worse by NOS inhibition. Where sepsis is due to a nidus of infection, local induction of iNOS is likely to cause beneficial hyperemia and perhaps extravsation of lymphocytes; NOS inhibitors would abrogate these effects. Finally, even vasoconstriction and increased vascular resistance, the intended effects of NOS inhibitors, may cause increased vascular leak and edema. Preliminary patient studies suggest edema can be minimized by limiting the amount of fluids given prior to NOS inhibition; the high pressor efficacy of L-NMA, in fact, argues against giving large preliminary doses of saline or colloids. L-NMA-treated patients may nevertheless gain weight; careful management using a flow-directed pulmonary artery catheter to avoid fluid overload prior to giving NOS inhibitors is recommended (R.G. Kilbourn, personal communication). Whether these and related adverse effects can be mitigated therapeutically or, if not, will over balance the beneficial effects of NOS inhibitors on blood pressure and α_1-adrenergic agent hyporesponsivity remains to be determined. Clinical trials should certainly be approached with caution and should be designed with full appreciation of pharmacology of NOS inhibitors.

SUMMARY

Studies reported in the past 5 years clearly establish that iNOS-mediated overproduction of NO is a major cause of the hypotension seen in cytokine-induced and septic (endotoxemic) shock. More recent studies indicate that iNOS produces cytotoxic quantities of NO which account for some of the pathology seen in inflammatory disorders such a rheumatoid arthritis. Although not discussed here in detail, S. Snyder *et al.* have proposed that brain ischemia (stroke) allows Ca^{++} influx into bNOS containing neurons which, when supplied with oxygen following reperfusion, produce NO in cytotoxic amounts (4). All of these considerations argue for the development and testing of NOS inhibitors as therapeutic agents. At present, there is no dearth of agents to test. Initial work by J. Hibbs and coworkers identified L-NMA as a useful inhibitor (10), and this agent has progressed to clinical trials in the U.S. and Europe. More potent inhibitors continue to be reported including L-thiocitrulline and S-methyl-L-thiocitrulline (41) discussed herein. Isoform selective inhibition, particularly iNOS selective inhibition, remains problematic although in this area progress is also being made. Selective limitation of iNOS activity may also be possible by arginine depletion. With both established and novel NOS inhibitors, substantial work remains to be done with respect to their pharmacology and therapeutic utility in shock and other disorders of NO overproduction.

REFERENCES

1. D.J. Stuehr and O.W. Griffith, Mammalian nitric oxide synthases, *Adv. Enzymol. Relat. Areas Mol. Biol.* 65:287 (1992).
2. M.A. Marletta, Nitric oxide synthase structure and mechanism, *J. Biol. Chem.* 268:12231 (1993).
3. K.L. Crossin, Nitric oxide (NO): a versatile second messenger in brain, *Trend. Pharmacol. Sci.* 16: (1991).
4. S.H. Snyder and D.S. Bredt, Nitric oxide as a neuronal messenger, *Trend. Pharmacol. Sci.* 12:125 (1991).
5. K. Aisaka, S.S. Gross, O.W. Griffith and R. Levi, N^G-methylarginine, an inhibitor of endothelium-derived nitric oxide synthesis, is a potent pressor agent in the guinea pig: does nitric oxide regulate blood pressure *in vivo*? *Biochem. Biophys. Res. Commun.* 160:881 (1989).
6. D.D. Rees, R.M.J. Palmer and S. Moncada, Role of endothelium-derived nitric oxide in the regulation of blood pressure, *Proc. Natl. Acad. Sci.* 86:3375 (1989).
7. S. Moncada and A. Higgs, The L-arginine nitric oxide pathway, *New. Eng. J. Med.* 329:2002 (1993).
8. C.F. Nathan and J.B. Hibbs, Jr., Role of nitric oxide synthesis in macrophage antimicrobial activity, *Curr. Opinion Immunol.* 3:65 (1991).
9. G. Karupiah, Q.W. Xie, R.M. Buller, C. Nathan, C. Duarte and J.D. MacMicking, Inhibition of viral replication by interferon-γ-induced nitric oxide synthase, 261:1445 (1993).
10 J.B. Hibbs, Jr., Z. Vavrin and R.R. Taintor, L-arginine is required for expression of the activated macrophage effector mechanism causing selective metabolic inhibition in target cells, *J. Immunol.* 138:550 (1987).
11 D.J. Stuehr and C.F. Nathan, Nitric oxide, a macrophage product responsible for cytostasis and respiratory inhibition in tumor target cells, *J. Exp. Med.* 169:1543 (1989).
12. R.G. Kilbourn, S.S. Gross, A. Jubran, J. Adams, O.W. Griffith, R. Levi and R.F. Lodato, N^G-methyl-L-arginine inhibits tumor necrosis factor-induced hypotension: implications for the involvement of nitric oxide, *Proc. Natl. Acad. Sci. U.S.A.* 87:3629 (1990).
13. R.G. Kilbourn, S.S. Gross, R.F. Lodato, J. Adams, R. Levi, L.L. Miller, L.B. Lachman and Griffith, O.W., Inhibition of interleukin-1-α-induced nitric oxide synthase in vascular smooth muscle and full reversal of interleukin-1-α-induced hypotension by N omega-amino-L-arginine, *J. Natl. Cancer Inst.* 84:1008 (1992).

14. R.G. Kilbourn, A. Jubran, S.S. Gross, O.W. Griffith, R. Levi, J. Adams and R.F. Lodato, Reversal of endotoxin-mediated shock by N^G-methyl-L-arginine, an inhibitor of nitric oxide synthesis, *Biochem. Biophys. Res. Commun.* 172:1132 (1990).

15. R.G. Kilbourn and O.W. Griffith, Overproduction of nitric oxide in cytokine-mediated and septic shock, *J. Natl. Cancer Inst.* 84:827 (1992).

16. F.N. McCartney, J.B. Allen, D.E. Mizel, J.E. Albina, Q.W. Xie, C.F. Nathan and S.M. Wahl, Suppression of arthritis by an inhibitor of nitric oxide synthase, *J. Exp. Med.* 178:749 (1993).

17. J.B. Weinberg, D.L. Granger, D.S. Pisetsky, M.F. Seldin, M.A. Misukonis, S.N. Mason, A.M.Pippen, P. Ruiz, E.R. Wood and G.S. Gilkeson, The role of nitric oxide in the pathogenesis of spontaneous murine autoimmune disease: Increased nitric oxide production and nitric oxide synthase expression in MRL-1pr/1pr mice, and reduction of spontaneous glomerulonephritis and arthritis by orally administered N^G-monomethyl-L-arginine, *J. Exp. Med.* 179:651 (1994).

18. M. Stefanovic-Racic, J. Stadler and C.H. Evans, Nitric Oxide and Arthritis, *Arthritis Rheum.* 36:1036 (1993).

19. C. Nathan and Q.W. Xie, Regulation of biosynthesis of nitric oxide, *J. Biol. Chem.* 269:13725 (1994).

20. W.C. Sessa, The nitric oxide synthase family of protein, *J. Vasc. Res.* 31:131 (1994).

21. E.A. Sheta, K. McMillan and B.S. Masters, Evidence for a biodomain structure of constitutive cerebeller nitric oxide synthase, *J. Biol. Chem.* 269:15147 (1994).

22. D.J. Stuehr, N.S. Kwon, C.F. nathan. O.W. Griffith, P.L. Feldman and J. Wiseman, N^ω-hydroxy-L-arginine is an intermediate in the biosynthesis of nitric oxide from L-arginine, *J. Biol. Chem.* 266:6259 (1991).

23. C. Natanson, W.D. Hoffman, A.F. Suffredini, P.Q. Eichacker and R.L. Danner, Selected treatment strategies for septic shock based on proposed mechanisms of pathogenesis, *Ann. Intern. Med.* 120:771 (1994).

24. J.E. Parrillo, Pathogenetic mechanisms of septic shock, *New. Eng. J. Med.* 328:1471 (1993).

25. R.G. Kilbourn and P. Belloni, Endothelial cell production of nitrogen oxides in response to interferon γ in combination with tumor necrosis factor, interleukin-1 or endotoxin, *J. Natl. Cancer Inst.* 82:772 (1990).

26. D. Beasley and M. Eldridge, Interleuken-1 β and tumor necrosis factor-α synergistically induce NO synthase in rat vascular smooth muscle cells, *Amer. J. Physiol.* 266:R1197 (1994).

27. S.S. Gross, R. Levi, A. Madera, K.H. Park, J. Vance and Y. Hattori, Tetrahydrobiopterin synthesis is induced by LPS in vascular smooth muscle and is rate-limiting for nitric oxide production, *Adv. Exp. Med. Biol.* 338:295 (1993).

28. Y. Hattori, E.B. Campbell and S.S. Gross, Argininosuccinate synthetase mRNA and activity are induced by immunostimulants in vascular smooth muscle. Role in the regeneration or arginine for nitric oxide synthesis, *J. Biol. Chem.* 269:9405 (1994).

29. A.K. Nussler, T.R. Billiar, Z.Z. Lui, and S.M. Morris, Jr., Coinduction of nitric oxide synthase and argininosuccinate synthetase in a murine macrophage cell line. Implications for regulation of nitric oxide production, *J. Biol. Chem.* 269:1257 (1994).

30. O.W. Griffith, K.H. Park, R. Levi and S. Gross, The role of plasma arginine in nitric oxide synthesis: studies with arginase-treated guinea pigs and rats, *in:* "The Biology of Nitric Oxide (1) Physiological and Clinical Aspects," S. Moncada, ed., Portland Press, London (1992).

31. D. Paya, G.A. Gray and J.C. Stoclet, Effects of methylene blue on blood pressure and reactivity to norepinephrine in endotoxemic rats, *J. Cardiovas. Pharm.* 21:926 (1993).

32. J.F. Keaney, Jr., J.C. Puyana, S. Francis, J.F. Loscalzo and J.S. Stamler, Methylene blue reverses endotoxin-induced hypotension, *Circ. Res.* 74:1121 (1994).

33. R.G. Kilbourn, G. Joly, B. Cashon, J. DeAngelo and J. Bonaventura, Cell-free hemoglobin reverses the endotoxin-mediated hyporesponsivity of rat aortic rings to α-adrenergic agents, *Biochem. Biophsy. Res. Commun.* 199:155 (1994).

34. S.S. Gross, D.J. Stuehr, K. Aisaka, E.A. Jaffe, R. Levi and O.W. Griffith, Macrophage and endothelial cell nitric oxide synthesis: cell-type selective inhibition by N^G-methylarginine, *Biochem. Biophys. Res. Commun.* 170:96 (1990).

35. L.E. Lambert, J.P. Whitten, B.M. Baron, H.C. Cheng, N.S. Doherty and I.A. McDonald, Nitric oxide synthesis in the CNS, endothelium and macrophages differs in its sensitivity to inhibition by arginine analogues, *Life Sci.* 48:69 (1991).

36. P.L. Feldman, O.W. Griffith, H. Hong and D.J. Stuehr, Irreversible inactivation of macrophage and brain nitric oxide synthase by L-N^G-methylarginine requires NADPH-dependent hydroxylation, *J. Med. Chem.* 36:491 (1993).

37. N.M. Olken, K.M. Rusche, M.K. Richards and M.A. Marletta, Inactivation of macrophage nitric oxide synthase activity by N^G-methyl-L-arginine, *Biochem. Biophys. Res. Commun.* 177:828 (1991).

38. N.M. Olken and M.A. Marletta, N^G-methyl-arginine functions as an alternate substrate and mechanism-based inhibitor of nitric oxide synthase, *Biochem.* 32:9677 (1993).

39. O. Fasehun, S. Gross, E. Pipili, E. Jaffe, O.W. Griffith and R. Levi, N^G-substituted arginine analogs: structure-activity relationship for inhibition of nitric oxide biosynthesis in vascular rings and endothelial cells, *FASEB J.* 4:A309 (1991).

40. T.B. McCall, M. Feelisch, R.M.J. Palmer and S. Moncada, Identification of N-iminoethyl-L-ornithine as an irreversible inhibitor of nitric oxide synthase in phagocytic cells, *Br. J. Pharmacol.* 102:234 (1991).

41. K. Narayanan and O.W. Griffith, Synthesis of L-thiocitrulline, L-homothiocitrulline, and S-methyl-L-thiocitrulline: a new class of potent nitric oxide synthase inhibitors, *J. Med. Chem.* 37:885 (1994).

42. K. Narayanan, C. Frey and O.W. Griffith, Inhibitors of nitric oxide synthase: structural constraints on binding and mechanisms of action, *in*: "Third International Meeting on The Biology of Nitric Oxide," S. Moncada and E.A. Higgs, ed., Elsevier Science Publishers, Amsterdam (In Press).

43. C. Frey, K. Narayanan, K. McMillan, L. Spack, S.S. Gross, B.S. Masters and O.W. Griffith, L-Thiocitrulline: a stereospecific, heme-binding inhibitor of nitric oxide synthases, *J. Biol. Chem.* (1994) in press.

44. K. Narayanan, L. Spack, M. Hayward and O.W. Griffith, S-methyl-L-thiocitrulline: a potent inhibitor of nitric oxide synthase with strong pressor activity *in vivo*, *FASEB J.* 8:A360 (1994).

45. R.F. Furchgott and J.V. Zawadski, The obligatory role of endothelial cells in the relaxation of arterial smooth muscle by acetycholine, *Nature*, 288:373 (1980).

46. K. Aisaka, S.S. Gross, O.W. Griffith and R. Levi, L-arginine availability determines the duration of acetylcholine-induced systemic vasodilation *in vivo*, *Biochem. Biophys. Res. Commun.* 163:710 (1989).

47. G.M. Burg, M.E. Gold, J.M. Fukuto and L.J. Ignarro, Shear stress-induced release of nitric oxide from endothelial cells grown on beads, *Hypotension* 17:187 (1991).

48. R.G. Kilbourn and P. Belloni, Endothelial cells produce nitrogen oxides in response to interferon-γ, tumour necrosis factor and endotoxin, *in*: "Nitric Oxide from L-Arginine: A Bioregulatory System," S. Moncada and E.A. Higgs, ed., Elsevier Science Publishers, Amsterdam (1990).

49. R.G. Kilbourn, Antagonsim of tumour necrosis factor-induced hypotension by N^G-monomethyl-L-arginine, *in*: "Nitric Oxide from L-Arginine: A Bioregulatory System," S. Moncada and E.A. Higgs, ed., Elsevier Science Piblishers, Amsterdam (1990).

50. R.G. Kilbourn, L. Owen-Schaub, S.S. Gross, O.W. Griffith and C. Logothetis, Interleukin-2-mediated hypotension in the awake dog is reversed by inhibitors of nitric oxide formation, *in:* "The Biology of Nitric Oxide," S. Moncada, M.A. Marletta, J.B. Higgs, Jr. and E.A. Higgs, ed., Portland Press, London and Chapel Hill (1992).

51. I. Fleming, G.A. Gray, G. Julou-Schaeffer, J.R. Parratt and J.C. Stoclet, Incubation with endotoxin activates the L-arginine pathway in vascular tissue, *Biochem. Biophys. Res. Commun.* 171:562 (1990).

52. S.M. Hollenberg, R.E. Cunnion and J. Zimmerberg, Nitric oxide synthase inhibition reverses arteriolar hyporesponsiveness to catecholamines in septic rats, *Am. J. Physiol.* 264:H660 (1993).

53. M.A. Dwyer, D.S. Bredt and S.H. Snyder, Nitric oxide synthase: irreversible inhibition by L-N^G-nitroarginine in brain *in vitro* and *in vivo*, *Biochem. Biophys. Res. Commun.* 176:1136 (1991).

54. J.M. Fukuto, K.S. Wood, R.E. Byrns and L.J. Ignarro, N^G-amino-L-arginine: a new potent antagonist of L-arginine-mediated endothelium-dependent relaxation, *Biochem. Biophys. Res. Commun.* 168:458 (1990).

55. J.P. Cobb, C. Natanson, W.D. Hoffman, R.F. Lodato, S. Banks, C.A. Koev, M.A. Solomon, R.J. Elin, J.M. Hosseini and R.L. Danner, N^ω-amino-L-arginine, an inhibitor of nitric oxide synthase, raises vascular resistance but increases mortality rates in awake canines challenged with endotoxin, *J. Exp. Med.* 176:1175 (1992).

56. O.W. Griffith, R.D. Allison, R. Rouhani, M. Handlogten and M.S. Kilberg, Specificity of the system y^+ transporter for arginine analogs: transplant of nitric oxide synthase inhibitors, *FASEB J.* 6:A1255 (1992).

57. K. Schmidt, P. Klatt and B. Mayer, Characterization of endothelial cell amino acid transport systems involved in the actions of nitric oxide synthase, *Mol. Pharm.* 44:615 (1993).

58. E. Nava, R.M.J. Palmer and S. Moncada, The role of nitric oxide in endotoxic shock: effects of N^G-monomethyl-L-arginine, *J. Cardiovasc. Pharm.* 20:S132 (1992).

59. C.E. Wright, D.D. Rees and S. Moncada, Protective and pathological roles of nitric oxide in endotoxin shock, *Cardiovasc. Res.* 26:48 (1992).

60. T.R. Billiar, R.D. Curran, B.G. Harbrecht, D.J. Stuehr, A.J. Demetris and R.L. Simmons, Modulation of nitrogen oxide synthesis *in vivo*: N^G-monomethyl-L-arginine inhibits endotoxin-induced nitrite/nitrate biosynthesis while promoting hepatic damage, *J. Leukoc.Biol.* 48:565 (1990).

61. R.C. Bone, The pathogenesis of sepsis, *Ann. Int. Med.* 115:457 (1991).

BIOSYNTHESIS OF NITRIC OXIDE

Bernd Mayer

Institut für Pharmakologie und Toxikologie
Universität Graz
Universitätsplatz 2
Graz, Austria

INTRODUCTION

In the past several years, the L-arginine/NO pathway has been recognized as part of a wide-spread signal transducing system, involved in a variety of biological processes. NO is generated in a Ca^{2+}-dependent enzymatic reaction from the amino acid L-arginine. As a potent activator of soluble guanylyl cyclase (sGC), NO exerts many of its effects through intracellular accumulation of the nucleotide cycic GMP (cGMP), which acts on multiple intracellular target proteins. In the the first part of this article, a brief synopsis will be given on enzymology of sGC related to its stimulation by NO, and in the second, more comprehensive part current knowledge about the mechanisms and regulation of NO biosynthesis will be reviewed.

SOLUBLE GUANYLYL CYCLASE

In various mammalian cells accumulation of cyclic GMP (cGMP) is triggered by hormones and neurotransmitters that enhance intracellular concentrations of free Ca^{2+} (Waldman and Murad, 1987). Cyclic GMP mediates the intracellular response to these extracellular signals and contributes to the regulation of various biologic processes, such as smooth muscle relaxation, platelet inhibition, and perhaps also to the regulation of neurotransmitter release in the brain. The molecular targets of cGMP, including cGMP-stimulated protein kinases which phosphorylate specific substrates, cGMP-regulated ion channels and phosphodiesterases were reviewed recently (Walter, 1989; Butt et al., 1993; Schmidt et al., 1993). Formation of cGMP from Mg^{2+}-GTP is catalyzed by a family of guanylyl cyclases which exist in two major forms, the membrane-bound and the soluble guanylyl cyclases. Both forms have been purified, cloned, sequenced, and expressed as functionally intact enzymes. The membrane-bound guanylyl cyclases consist of a membrane-spanning region, an extracellular domain for binding of natriuretic peptides, and an intracellular catalytic domain. Soluble guanylyl cyclase (sGC) represents the receptor for NO and is predominantly found in cytoplasmic fractions (Koesling et al., 1991).

Biochemical, Pharmacological, and Clinical Aspects of Nitric Oxide
Edited by B. A. Weissman *et al.*, Plenum Press, New York, 1995

37

The soluble enzyme is stimulated several hundred-fold by NO and its progenitors, e.g. sodium nitroprusside, sydnonimines like SIN-1, or organic nitrates. These drugs have been used to treat coronary artery disease since more than 100 years and exert their potent vasodilator activities through NO-mediated activation of sGC (Feelisch and Noack, 1987). It has been demonstrated that sGC purified from bovine lung contains stoichiometrical amounts of heme (Gerzer et al., 1981; Humbert et al., 1990), and since NO exhibits high affinity to heme iron, it has been speculated that stimulation of sGC by NO may be due to binding of the NO radical to the prosthetic heme group. This hypothesis was recently confirmed by constructing a heme-deficient mutant of sGC that had unaffected basal cGMP forming activity but was completely insensitive to stimulation by NO (Wedel et al., 1994). Purification and molecular cloning of sGC revealed that it represents a heterodimeric protein with a native molecular mass of 150 kDa. The C-terminal parts of the two different subunits show similarities to the intracellular domains of the membrane-bound guanylyl and adenylyl cyclases, indicating that these regions may be involved in catalytic function (Koesling et al., 1991). Structural diversity of each of the two subunits (Yuen et al., 1990; Harteneck et al., 1991) suggests that different sGC heterodimers may be expressed in a tissue-specific manner (Ujiie et al., 1993). Possible, as yet unknown differences in the regulation of the various isoforms of sGC may help to understand the physiological consequences of these findings.

ENDOGENOUS NITRIC OXIDE

Physiological activation of sGC remained elusive until the discovery of endothelium-dependent relaxation by Furchgott and Zawadzki (1980). They showed that acetylcholine-stimulated vascular endothelial cells release a diffusible substance with vasorelaxing properties (endothelium-derived relaxing factor; EDRF). EDRF was later demonstrated to be a direct activator of sGC (Förstermann et al., 1986; Ignarro et al., 1986). In 1987, two groups have identified EDRF as NO or a labile NO-containing compound (Ignarro et al., 1987; Palmer et al., 1987). Identification was predominantly based on the detection of nitrite ions in the effluent of hormone-stimulated endothelial cells and on chemical similarities between EDRF and NO, e.g. short half-life in the superfusate and inactivation by superoxide.

Today we know that biosynthesis of NO is not confined to the endothelium but occurs in many other tissues, too. NO is produced in response to a variety of autacoids which increase intracellular Ca^{2+}. In the brain, NO is released from distinct populations of neurons upon activation of the NMDA subtype of glutamate receptors (Garthwaite et al., 1988; Bredt et al., 1991a; Garthwaite, 1991). In the peripheral nervous system, NO-producing (nitrergic) fibers innervate many tissues, including most smooth muscles, heart, intestine, kidney, and pancreas. Finally, bone marrow-derived blood cells produce large amounts of NO upon synergistic activation by cytokines and LPS. This is apparently part of host-defense mechanisms in unspecific immune response, since NO has been identified as a mediator of macrophage cytotoxicity (Nathan and Hibbs, 1991). Unlike the actions of NO as cellular messenger, NO cytotoxicity is not mediated by sGC. Instead, inhibition of several non-heme iron and iron sulfur proteins (Drapier and Hibbs, 1988; Kwon et al., 1991; Lepoivre et al., 1991), chemical modification of DNA (Wink et al., 1991; Nguyen et al., 1992), and covalent modification of glyceraldehyde-3-phosphate dehydrogenase (Dimmeler et al., 1992) are some of the putative cytotoxic actions of NO and/or its oxygen metabolites (Henry et al., 1993). Taken together, most of the molecular actions of NO appear to result from its chemical reactions with molecular oxygen, superoxide, and iron-containing proteins. Thus, biology of NO may be largely determined by the cellular availability of these target molecules.

NITRIC OXIDE SYNTHASES

Subsequent to demonstration of NO biosynthesis by mammalian cells, the terminal guanidino group of the amino acid L-arginine has been identified as the physiological precursor of NO (Palmer et al., 1988; Sakuma et al., 1988; Schmidt et al., 1988). Enzymatic NO formation was first described by Marletta et al. (1988), who found that soluble fractions of cytokine-activated macrophages metabolize L-arginine to L-citrulline and NO in the presence of NADPH. The role of NADPH as essential cofactor in NO formation was soon confirmed in broken cell preparations of endothelial cells (Mayer et al., 1989; Förstermann et al., 1991), brain (Knowles et al., 1989), lung (Mayer and Böhme, 1989), adrenal gland (Palacios et al., 1989), and blood platelets (Radomski et al., 1990). Cytokine-inducible NO formation in macrophages was found to be independent of Ca^{2+}, whereas constitutive NO synthesis e.g. in endothelium and brain required micromolar concentrations of Ca^{2+}, suggesting that differently regulated isoforms of NO synthase (NOS) may be expressed in different cells.

In fact, purification and characterization of NOS revealed the existence of three isozymes: i) a cytosolic, Ca^{2+}-dependent enzyme constitutively expressed in neuronal cells (Bredt and Snyder, 1990; Mayer et al., 1990; Schmidt et al., 1991), a membrane-associated, also Ca^{2+}-dependent NOS in vascular endothelial cells (Pollock et al., 1991), and iii) a cytokine-inducible, Ca^{2+}-independent enzyme in macrophages (Hevel et al., 1991; Stuehr et al., 1991; Yui et al., 1991). The isolated proteins appear as single bands with apparent molecular masses of approximately 160 kDa (brain NOS) and 130 kDa (endothelial and macrophage NOS) on SDS gels, whereas the native brain and macrophage enzymes may be homodimers in their active state (Schmidt et al., 1991; Baek et al., 1993). Molecular cloning of NOS from various sources revealed considerable sequence similarities between the different isoforms (Bredt et al., 1991b; Lamas et al., 1992; Lyons et al., 1992; Marsden et al., 1992; Sessa et al., 1992; Xie et al., 1992; Geller et al., 1993), and they apparently represent products of distinct genes which each being localized on a different chromosome (Kishimoto et al., 1992; Sessa et al., 1993).

It has been shown that brain (Bredt and Snyder, 1990) and endothelial (Busse and Mülsch, 1990) NOS are calmodulin requiring enzymes, explaining their regulation via intracellular Ca^{2+}. However, not only neuronal (Bredt et al., 1991b) but also Ca^{2+}-independent, inducible NOS contains a consensus sequence for calmodulin binding (Xie et al., 1992). Biochemical analysis of the purified macrophage enzyme showed that it contained calmodulin as a subunit, indicating that the inducible isoforms bind calmodulin at resting Ca^{2+}-concentrations, whereas the constitutively expressed isoforms, like most other calmodulin-dependent enzymes, need micromolar Ca^{2+} for calmodulin binding (Cho et al., 1992).

Initial studies indicated that the different NOS isozymes are cytosolic proteins (Marletta et al., 1988; Knowles et al., 1989; Mayer et al., 1989; Busse and Mülsch, 1990), but more recent work showed that endothelial NOS is predominantly (>80 %) localized in particulate fractions (Förstermann et al., 1991; Pollock et al., 1991; Mayer et al., 1993b). Membrane association of the endothelial isoform is most likely due to post-translational myristoylation, since modification of the putative N-terminal myristoylation domain by site-directed mutagenesis resulted in the expression of a soluble mutant of the enzyme (Busconi and Michel, 1993). Albeit brain and macrophage NOS have no consensus sequence for myristoylation, these isoforms may also - at least partially - be associated with membranes, as shown by means of biochemical (Förstermann et al., 1992; Hiki et al., 1992; Schmidt et al., 1992b) and histochemical techniques (Wolf et al., 1992). These enzymes may be loosely attached to membranes through hydrophobic interactions and are easily solubilized upon homogenization of the tissue.

MECHANISMS OF NO SYNTHESIS

Although NOS isozymes are differently regulated and apparently found at different subcellular sites, they exhibit similar biochemical properties. Biosynthesis of NO involves 5 electron oxidation of one of the chemically equivalent N^G-nitrogens of L-arginine leading to the concomitant production of L-citrulline (Marletta et al., 1988). This reaction is accompanied by an NADPH-dependent reduction of molecular oxygen (Mayer et al., 1991), which is incorporated into both NO and L-citrulline (Kwon et al., 1990; Leone et al., 1991), suggesting a mono- or dioxygenase-like reaction. Stoichiometrical data show that 1.5 mol of NADPH are utilized for the formation of 1.0 mol of L-citrulline (Mayer et al., 1991; Stuehr et al., 1991). Two of the three NADPH-derived reducing equivalents seem to be utilized for the initial hydroxylation of L-arginine into N^G-hydroxy-L-arginine, and oxidative cleavage of this intermediate to NO and L-citrulline may require an additional electron (Stuehr et al., 1991b; Klatt et al., 1993). Substrate oxidation in the catalytic center of the enzyme is catalyzed by a cytochrome P_{450}-like heme iron (Klatt et al., 1992a; McMillan et al., 1992; Stuehr and Ikeda-Saito, 1992; White and Marletta, 1992), and the shuttle of electrons from NADPH to the heme is apparently mediated by the reduced flavins FAD and FMN (Hevel et al., 1991; Mayer et al., 1991; Stuehr et al., 1991a).

Thus NOS isozymes seem to represent self-sufficient cytochromes P_{450}, consisting of a flavin-containing reductase domain and a heme iron-containing catalytic oxygenase domain. In fact, the C-terminal half of NOS shows considerable sequence similarities to cytochrome P_{450} reductase (Bredt et al., 1991b) and exhibits similar catalytic activities (Klatt et al., 1992b). For brain NOS it has been clearly established that the flavin-mediated electron shuttle, which is responsible for the observed reductase activity, is the calmodulin-dependent step of NO formation (Klatt et al., 1992b; Abu-Soud and Stuehr, 1993). Besides exogenously added cytochrome c or rat liver cytochrome P_{450}, the artificial low molecular mass electron acceptor nitro blue tetrazolium is also enzymatically reduced by NOS (Klatt et al., 1992b), allowing simple histochemical localization of the neuronal enzyme in tissue slices by so-called NADPH diaphorase staining (Hope et al., 1991).

When the neuronal enzyme is activated by Ca^{2+}/calmodulin in the presence of subsaturating concentrations of L-arginine (or tetrahydrobiopterin; see below), NADPH-dependent oxygen activation uncouples from substrate metabolism, leading to the generation of superoxide anions and hydrogen peroxide (Mayer et al., 1991; Heinzel et al., 1992; Pou et al., 1992). At low intracellular concentrations of L-arginine, Ca^{2+}-activated NOS may therefore generate superoxide anions along with NO. These species could combine to form peroxynitrite (Beckman et al., 1990) and contribute to toxic processes involved in neurodegenerative diseases (Halliwell, 1992; Coyle and Puttfarcken, 1993; Lipton et al., 1993). N^G-Methyl-L-arginine (L-NMA) does not block this substrate-independent oxygen reduction, while N^G-nitro-L-arginine (L-NNA) turned out as a potent inhibitor of this reaction (Heinzel et al., 1992; Pou et al., 1992; Klatt et al., 1993). This unexpected effect of L-NNA is presumably due to reversible inactivation of neuronal and endothelial NOS (Mayer et al., 1993b; Klatt et al., 1994a). Macrophage NOS appears to down-regulate its uncoupled reduction of oxygen, as it consumes only small quantities of NADPH in the absence of L-arginine (Abu-Soud and Stuehr, 1993). However, it generates significant amounts of hydrogen peroxide in the presence of the substrate analog L-NMA (Olken and Marletta, 1993), indicating that inducible NOS, in contrast to the brain enzyme, requires a ligand bound to its substrate site for reduction of molecular oxygen to occur. These results suggest structural differences in the catalytic sites of constitutive and inducible NOS, and this may be of considerable interest for the development of isoform-specific inhibitors of NOS.

ROLE OF TETRAHYDROBIOPTERIN IN NO BIOSYNTHESIS

Tetrahydrobiopterin (H4biopterin) has been known for decades as cofactor of enzymes which hydroxylate the aromatic amino acids phenylalanine, tyrosine, and tryptophan (Nichol et al., 1985). Amino acid hydroxylases are non-heme iron proteins and use H4biopterin as donor of electrons for activation of molecular oxygen. Accordingly, H4biopterin is co-oxidized with the substrates. The quinoid form of H2biopterin (q-H2biopterin) is produced as initial oxidation product, its intramolecular rearrangement yields H2biopterin. In intact cells or crude preparations, these oxidation products are cycled back to H4biopterin at the expense of NAD(P)H by dihydropteridine (q-H2biopterin) or dihydrofolate (H2biopterin) reductases.

H4Biopterin stimulates all NOS isozymes known so far (Kwon et al., 1989; Tayeh and Marletta, 1989; Mayer et al., 1990; Pollock et al., 1991). The pteridine seems to be obligatory for NO synthesis, since basal enzyme activities observed in the absence of exogenously added H4biopterin correlate well with the amount of biopterins bound to NOS (Mayer et al., 1991; Hevel and Marletta, 1992; Schmidt et al., 1992a). It may depend on homogenization and purification techniques how much of H4biopterin remains tightly bound to the purified enzymes, perhaps accounting for the variable degrees of NOS stimulation by added H4biopterin reported by different groups (Dwyer et al., 1991; Giovanelli et al., 1991; Schmidt and Murad, 1991; Evans et al., 1992; Klatt et al., 1992c).

Identification of H4biopterin as cofactor of NOS's prompted several researchers to suggest that the pteridine may have a function in NO formation similar to its role in aromatic amino acid hydroxylation and catalyze the initial N-oxygenation of L-arginine. However, it was not possible to assign the activity of H4biopterin to a distinct step of L-arginine oxidation (Stuehr et al., 1991; Klatt et al., 1993), and the pteridine is apparently not involved directly in the NOS-catalyzed, L-arginine-independent reduction of molecular oxygen (Heinzel et al., 1992). Moreover, H4biopterin seems to be active as cofactor in NO synthesis at much lower than stoichiometric concentrations, since one molecule of the cofactor was found to be sufficient for the formation of up to 20 molecules of product (Giovanelli et al., 1991; Mayer et al., 1991). Accordingly, redox-activity of H4biopterin would implicate its continuous recycling at the cost of NADPH during NO synthesis, but in spite of several attempts we obtained no experimental evidence to support redox-cycling of H4biopterin (Werner, E.R. and Mayer, B., unpublished observations). However, the methods which are currently available test for redox-cycling of free H4biopterin only and therefore do not exclude the possibility that the enzyme-bound cofactor is redox-active.

Negative results similar to ours led Giovanelli and coworkers to propose that H4biopterin is not a reactant in NO synthesis but rather acts as an allosteric effector of the enzyme (Giovanelli et al., 1991). In support of this hypothesis, it was shown that H4biopterin is required to keep macrophage NOS in its active dimeric state and that dissociated inactive monomers only re-associate when heme, H4biopterin and L-arginine are present at the same time (Baek et al., 1993). Although neuronal NOS seems to behave differently and remains a dimer under conditions that would induce dissociation of macrophage NOS (Schmidt et al., 1991; Klatt et al., 1994a), some kind of synergistic interaction between L-arginine and H4biopterin binding sites may also occur in the course of constitutive NO synthesis. In a recent study it was found that L-arginine decreased the K_D of brain NOS for H4biopterin from about 200 nM to 30 nM and that pteridine binding to the enzyme converted the substrate site of NOS in an high affinity state, indicating an allosteric interaction between the two binding domains (Klatt et al., 1994b). However, the role of the pteridine may not be confined to its effect on NOS conformation, since the oxidized derivative H2biopterin bound to the pteridine site of brain NOS with a fairly high affinity of about 2 μM but was inactive as a cofactor in NO synthesis (Klatt et al., 1994b). These results may indicate a dual role of H4biopterin in NO synthesis: binding of the pteridine may convert NOS into an active conformational state, and the bound cofactor may participate in a redox-active manner in the oxidation of L-arginine.

REGULATION OF THE NO/cGMP SYSTEM

Regulation of the NO/cGMP signal transducing system may be complex and is only partially understood. Soluble GC seems to be predominantly activated by NO, but polyunsaturated fatty acids and/or their hydroperoxy derivatives, superoxide and hydroxyl radicals, thiols, carbon monoxide (CO) and several other species also may contribute to regulation of enzyme activity (Waldman and Murad, 1987; Schmidt, 1992). Especially activation of sGC by CO has attracted much attention recently, because inhibitors of heme oxygenase, an enzyme that produces CO from protoporphyrin IX (Maines et al., 1993), were found to block long-term potentiation in the hippocampus (Zhuo et al., 1993) and odorant-induced accumulation of cGMP in olfactory neurons (Verma et al., 1993). However, so far no appropriate mechanisms for regulation of heme oxygenase have been identified, and CO-induced stimulation of purified sGC is only around 5 % of that produced by NO (Mayer, B., unpublished results). Thus, alternate pathways for CO biosynthesis and sensitive molecular targets need to be discovered before CO can be considered as a novel neurotransmitter.

In addition to the formation of cGMP, breakdown of the cyclic nucleotide is also a tightly controlled process, and several different phosphodiesterase (PDE) isozymes may limit intracellular cGMP accumulation (Beavo and Reifsnyder, 1990). Thus, regulation of cGMP hydrolysis may depend on the pattern of PDE isoforms expressed in a given tissue. The brain, for instance, contains substantial amounts of Ca^{2+}/calmodulin-stimulated (type I) PDE's with high affinities for cGMP (Wu et al., 1992). These enzymes may rapidly hydrolyze cGMP in Ca^{2+}-activated neurons, resulting in a predominantly paracrine function of NO in synaptic transmission (Mayer et al., 1992; Mayer et al., 1993a).

Although regulation of NO formation occurs primarily through intracellular Ca^{2+}, there is convincing evidence that several additional mechanisms contribute to the modulation of NO synthesis. Thus, NOS activities may be affected by phosphorylation (Brüne and Lapetina, 1991; Nakane et al., 1991; Bredt et al., 1992; Marin et al., 1992; Michel et al., 1993), as well as by the intracellular availability of L-arginine (Rosenblum et al., 1992; Schott et al., 1993), H_4biopterin (Werner et al., 1993) or molecular oxygen (Rengasamy and Johns, 1991). Of note, limited L-arginine or H_4biopterin availability would not only reduce rates of NO formation but additionally induce uncoupling of NOS-catalyzed oxygen reduction and, therefore, result in the generation of superoxide, which may combine with NO to peroxynitrite and thus contribute to cytotoxicity (see above).

NO is a potent inhibitor of rat liver microsomal cytochrome P_{450} (Wink et al., 1993), and NOS isozymes have been identified as cytochromes P_{450} (Klatt et al., 1992a; McMillan et al., 1992; Stuehr and Ikeda-Saito, 1992; White and Marletta, 1992). Thus, it is conceivable that binding of NO to the prosthetic heme group of NOS could block NO formation. Indeed, several reports indicate that NOS is inhibited by its reaction product NO (Rogers and Ignarro, 1992; Assreuy et al., 1993; Buga et al., 1993; Rengasamy and Johns, 1993). Unfortunately, these previous studies were carried out with rather complex systems such as crude enzyme preparations or intact cells. To settle the biochemical mechanisms underlying the inhibitory effects of NO we have therefore investigated feedback inhibition of NOS with purified brain NOS. However, initial experiments showed that the isolated enzyme was neither inhibited by high concentrations of NO donors nor stimulated by oxyhemoglobin, a scavenger of endogenously produced NO (Mayer et al., 1994). More recently we have measured concentrations of free NO in the reaction mixtures by means of an NO-sensitive electrode. Intriguingly, we did not detect any formation of NO by purified NOS unless high amounts of superoxide dismutase (SOD) were present. Thus, NO appears to be efficiently inactivated by superoxide generated during in vitro incubation of NOS. Further studies showed that SOD (5,000 U/ml) markedly inhibited formation of L-citrulline by purified NOS and that the effect of SOD was antagonized by oxyhemoglobin (Mayer, B., Klatt, P., Werner, E.R., and Schmidt, K., submitted for publication). Together with the previous findings described above, these results indicate that enzymatically produced NO blocks its own synthesis and that cells may contain sufficient SOD and/or other mechanisms to prevent superoxide-mediated inactivation of NO. The steady state concentrations of NO that are required for NOS inhibition are not precisely known but may be in the range of 0.1 - 1 μM, suggesting that negative feedback regulation of NOS may become physiologically relevant under some circumstances. Moreover, these data may be of considerable clinical interest, because high levels of NO may occur during infusion of organic nitrates or NO inhalation (Ahlner et al., 1991; Geggel, 1993; Rossaint et al., 1993),

Acknowledgments

Experimental work in my laboratory was supported by grant P 8836 of the Fonds zur Förderung der Wissenschaftlichen Forschung in Österreich.

REFERENCES

Abu-Soud, H.M. and D.J. Stuehr, 1993, Nitric oxide synthases reveal a novel role for calmodulin in controlling electron transfer, Proc. Natl. Acad. Sci. USA 90, 10769-10772.

Ahlner, J., R.G.G. Andersson, K. Torfgard and K.L. Axelsson, 1991, Organic nitrate esters - clinical use and mechanisms of actions, Pharmacol. Rev. 43, 351-423.

Assreuy, J., F.Q. Cunha, F.Y. Liew and S. Moncada, 1993, Feedback inhibition of nitric oxide synthase activity by nitric oxide, Br. J. Pharmacol. 108, 833-837.

Baek, K.J., B.A. Thiel, S. Lucas and D.J. Stuehr, 1993, Macrophage nitric oxide synthase subunits purification, characterization, and role of prosthetic groups and substrate in regulating their association into a dimeric enzyme, J. Biol. Chem. 268, 21120-21129.

Beavo, J.A. and D.H. Reifsnyder, 1990, Primary sequence of cyclic nucleotide phosphodiesterase isoenzymes and the design of selective inhibitors, Trends Pharmacol. Sci. 11, 150-155.

Beckman, J.S., T.W. Beckman, J. Chen, P.A. Marshall and B.A. Freeman, 1990, Apparent hydroxyl radical production by peroxynitrite: implications for endothelial injury from nitric oxide and superoxide, Proc. Natl. Acad. Sci. USA 87, 1620-1624.

Bredt, D.S. and S.H. Snyder, 1990, Isolation of nitric oxide synthetase, a calmodulin-requiring enzyme, Proc. Natl. Acad. Sci. USA 87, 682-685.

Bredt, D.S., C.E. Glatt, P.M. Hwang, M. Fotuhi, T.M. Dawson and S.H. Snyder, 1991a, Nitric oxide synthase protein and messenger RNA are discretely localized in neuronal populations of the mammalian CNS together with NADPH diaphorase, Neuron 7, 615-624.

Bredt, D.S., P.M. Hwang, C.E. Glatt, C. Lowenstein, R.R. Reed and S.H. Snyder, 1991b, Cloned and expressed nitric oxide synthase structurally resembles cytochrome P-450 reductase, Nature 351, 714-718.

Bredt, D.S., C.D. Ferris and S.H. Snyder, 1992, Nitric oxide synthase regulatory sites - phosphorylation by cyclic AMP-dependent protein kinase, protein kinase-C, and calcium/calmodulin protein kinase identification of flavin and calmodulin binding sites, J. Biol. Chem. 267, 10976-10981.

Brüne, B. and E.G. Lapetina, 1991, Phosphorylation of nitric oxide synthase by protein kinase-A, Biochem. Biophys. Res. Commun. 181, 921-926.

Buga, G.M., J.M. Griscavage, N.E. Rogers and L.J. Ignarro, 1993, Negative feedback regulation of endothelial cell function by nitric oxide, Circ. Res. 73, 808-812.

Busconi, L. and T. Michel, 1993, Endothelial nitric oxide synthase - N-terminal myristoylation determines subcellular localization, J. Biol. Chem. 268, 8410-8413.

Busse, R. and A. Mülsch, 1990, Calcium-dependent nitric oxide synthesis in endothelial cytosol is mediated by calmodulin, FEBS Lett. 265, 133-136.

Butt, E., J. Geiger, T. Jarchau, S.M. Lohmann and U. Walter, 1993, The cGMP-dependent protein kinase - gene, protein, and function, Neurochem. Res. 18, 27-42.

Cho, H.J., Q.W. Xie, J. Calaycay, R.A. Mumford, K.M. Swiderek, T.D. Lee and C. Nathan, 1992,

Calmodulin is a subunit of nitric oxide synthase from macrophages, J. Exp. Med. 176, 599-604.

Coyle, J.T. and P. Puttfarcken, 1993, Oxidative stress, glutamate, and neurodegenerative disorders, Science 262, 689-695.

Dimmeler, S., F. Lottspeich and B. Brüne, 1992, Nitric oxide causes ADP-ribosylation and inhibition of glyceraldehyde-3-phosphate dehydrogenase, J. Biol. Chem. 267, 16771-16774.

Drapier, J.C. and J.B.J. Hibbs, 1988, Differentiation of murine macrophages to express nonspecific cytotoxicity for tumor cells results in L-arginine-dependent inhibition of mitochondrial iron-sulfur enzymes in the macrophage effector cells., J. Immunol. 140, 2829-2838.

Dwyer, M.A., D.S. Bredt and S.H. Snyder, 1991, Nitric oxide synthase - irreversible inhibition by L-NG-nitroarginine in brain invitro and invivo, Biochem. Biophys. Res. Commun. 176, 1136-1141.

Evans, T., A. Carpenter and J. Cohen, 1992, Purification of a distinctive form of endotoxin-induced nitric oxide synthase from rat liver, Proc. Natl. Acad. Sci. USA 89, 5361-5365.

Feelisch, M. and E.A. Noack, 1987, Correlation between nitric oxide formation during degradation of organic nitrates and activation of guanylate cyclase, Eur. J. Pharmacol. 139, 19-13.

Förstermann, U., A. Mülsch, E. Böhme and R. Busse, 1986, Stimulation of soluble guanylate cyclase by an acetylcholine induced endothelium derived factor from rabbit and canine arteries, Circ. Res. 58, 531-538.

Förstermann, U., J.S. Pollock, H.H.H.W. Schmidt, M. Heller and F. Murad, 1991, Calmodulin-dependent endothelium-derived relaxing factor nitric oxide synthase activity is present in the particulate and cytosolic fractions of bovine aortic endothelial cells, Proc. Natl. Acad. Sci. USA 88, 1788-1792.

Förstermann, U., H.H.H.W. Schmidt, K.L. Kohlhaas and F. Murad, 1992, Induced RAW-264.7 macrophages express soluble and particulate nitric oxide synthase - inhibition by transforming growth factor-beta, Eur. J. Pharmacol. 225, 161-165.

Furchgott, R.F. and J.V. Zawadzki, 1980, The obligatory role of endothelial cells in the relaxation of arterial smooth muscle by acetylcholine, Nature 288, 373-376.

Garthwaite, J., 1991, Glutamate, nitric oxide and cell-cell signalling in the nervous system, Trends Neurosci. 14, 60-67.

Garthwaite, J., S.L. Charles and R. Chess-Williams, 1988, Endothelium-derived relaxing factor release on activation of NMDA receptors suggests role as intercellular messenger in the brain, Nature 336, 385-388.

Geggel, R.L., 1993, Inhalational nitric oxide - a selective pulmonary vasodilator for treatment of persistent pulmonary hypertension of the newborn, J. Pediatr. 123, 76-79.

Geller, D.A., C.J. Lowenstein, R.A. Shapiro, A.K. Nussler, M. Disilvio, S.C. Wang, D.K. Nakayama, R.L. Simmons, S.H. Snyder and T.R. Billiar, 1993, Molecular cloning and expression of inducible nitric oxide synthase from human hepatocytes, Proc. Natl. Acad. Sci. USA 90, 3491-3495.

Gerzer, R., E. Böhme, F. Hofmann and G. Schultz, 1981, Soluble guanylate cyclase purified from bovine lung contains heme and copper, FEBS Lett. 132, 71-74.

Giovanelli, J., K.L. Campos and S. Kaufman, 1991, Tetrahydrobiopterin, a cofactor for rat cerebellar nitric oxide synthase, does not function as a reactant in the oxygenation of arginine, Proc. Natl. Acad. Sci. USA 88, 7091-7095.

Halliwell, B., 1992, Reactive oxygen species and the central nervous system, J. Neurochem. 59, 1609-1623.

Harteneck, C., B. Wedel, D. Koesling, J. Malkewitz, E. Böhme and G. Schultz, 1991, Molecular cloning and expression of a new alpha-subunit of soluble guanylyl cyclase - interchangeability of the alpha-subunits of the enzyme, FEBS Lett. 292, 217-222.

Heinzel, B., M. John, P. Klatt, E. Böhme and B. Mayer, 1992, Ca^{2+}/calmodulin-dependent formation of hydrogen peroxide by brain nitric oxide synthase, Biochem. J. 281, 627-630.

Henry, Y., M. Lepoivre, J.-C. Drapier, C. Ducrocq, J.-L. Boucher and A. Guissani, 1993, EPR characterization of molecular targets for NO in mammalian cells and organelles, FASEB J. 7, 1124-1134.

Hevel, J.M. and M.A. Marletta, 1992, Macrophage nitric oxide synthase - relationship between enzyme-bound tetrahydrobiopterin and synthase activity, Biochemistry 31, 7160-7165.

Hevel, J.M., K.A. White and M.A. Marletta, 1991, Purification of the inducible murine macrophage nitric oxide synthase - identification as a flavoprotein, J. Biol. Chem. 266, 22789-22791.

Hiki, K., R. Hattori, C. Kawai and Y. Yui, 1992, Purification of insoluble nitric oxide synthase from rat cerebellum, J. Biochem. 111, 556-558.

Hope, B., G. Michael, K. Knigge and S. Vincent, 1991, Neuronal NADPH diaphorase is a nitric oxide synthase, Proc. Natl. Acad. Sci. USA 88, 2811-2814.

Humbert, P., F. Niroomand, G. Fischer, B. Mayer, D. Koesling, K.-D. Hinsch, H. Gausepohl, R. Frank, G. Schultz and E. Böhme, 1990, Purification of soluble guanylyl cyclase from bovine lung by a new immunoaffinity chromatographic method, Eur. J. Biochem. 190, 273-278.

Ignarro, L.J., R.G. Harbison, K.S. Wood and P. Kadowitz, 1986, Activation of purified soluble guanylate cyclase by endothelium-derived relaxing factor from intrapulmonary artery and vein: stimulation by acetylcholine, bradykinin and arachidonic acid, J. Pharmacol. Exp. Ther. 237, 893-900.

Ignarro, L.J., G.M. Buga, K.S. Wood, R.E. Byrns and G. Chaudhuri, 1987, Endothelium-derived relaxing factor produced and released from artery and vein is nitric oxide, Proc. Natl. Acad. Sci. USA 84, 9265-9269.

Kishimoto, J., N. Spurr, M. Liao, L. Lizhi, P. Emson and W.M. Xu, 1992, Localization of brain nitric oxide synthase (NOS) to human chromosome-12, Genomics 14, 802-804.

Klatt, P., K. Schmidt and B. Mayer, 1992a, Brain nitric oxide synthase is a haemoprotein, Biochem. J. 288, 15-17.

Klatt, P., B. Heinzel, M. John, M. Kastner, E. Böhme and B. Mayer, 1992b, Ca^{2+}/calmodulin-dependent cytochrome c reductase activity of brain nitric oxide synthase, J. Biol. Chem. 267, 11374-11378.

Klatt, P., B. Heinzel, B. Mayer, E. Ambach, G. Werner-Felmayer, H. Wachter and E.R. Werner, 1992c, Stimulation of human nitric oxide synthase by tetrahydrobiopterin and selective binding of the cofactor, FEBS Lett. 305, 160-162.

Klatt, P., K. Schmidt, G. Uray and B. Mayer, 1993, Multiple catalytic functions of brain nitric oxide synthase. Biochemical characterization, cofactor-requirement and role of N^G-hydroxy-L-arginine as an intermediate, J. Biol. Chem. 268, 14781-14787.

Klatt, P., K. Schmidt, F. Brunner and B. Mayer, 1994a, Inhibitors of brain nitric oxide synthase. Binding kinetics, metabolism, and enzyme inactivation, J. Biol. Chem. 269, 1674-1680.

Klatt, P., M. Schmid, E. Leopold, K. Schmidt, E.R. Werner and B. Mayer, 1994b, The pteridine binding site of brain nitric oxide synthase. Kinetics of tetrahydrobiopterin binding, specificity, and allosteric interaction with the substrate domain, J. Biol. Chem. (in press).

Knowles, R.G., M. Palacios, R.M.J. Palmer and S. Moncada, 1989, Formation of nitric oxide from L-arginine in the central nervous system: a transduction mechanism for stimulation of the soluble guanylate cyclase, Proc. Natl. Acad. Sci. USA 86, 5159-5162.

Koesling, D., E. Böhme and G. Schultz, 1991, Guanylyl cyclases, a growing family of signal transducing enzymes, FASEB J. 5, 2785-2791.

Kwon, N.S., C.F. Nathan and D.J. Stuehr, 1989, Reduced biopterin as a cofactor in the generation of nitrogen oxides by murine macrophages, J. Biol. Chem. 264, 20496-20501.

Kwon, N.S., C.F. Nathan, C. Gilker, O.W. Griffith, D.E. Matthews and D.J. Stuehr, 1990, L-citrulline production from L-arginine by macrophage nitric oxide synthase. The ureido oxygen derives from dioxygen, J. Biol. Chem. 265, 13442-13445.

Kwon, N.S., D.J. Stuehr and C.F. Nathan, 1991, Inhibition of tumor cell ribonucleotide reductase by macrophage-derived nitric oxide, J. Exp. Med. 174, 761-767.

Lamas, S., P.A. Marsden, G.K. Li, P. Tempst and T. Michel, 1992, Endothelial nitric oxide synthase - molecular cloning and characterization of a distinct constitutive enzyme isoform, Proc. Natl. Acad. Sci. USA 89, 6348-6352.

Leone, A.M., R.M.J. Palmer, R.G. Knowles, P.L. Francis, D.S. Ashton and S. Moncada, 1991, Constitutive and inducible nitric oxide synthases incorporate molecular oxygen into both nitric oxide and citrulline, J. Biol. Chem. 266, 23790-23795.

Lepoivre, M., F. Fieschi, J. Coves, L. Thelander and M. Fontecave, 1991, Inactivation of ribonucleotide reductase by nitric oxide, Biochem. Biophys. Res. Commun. 179, 442-448.

Lipton, S.A., Y.B. Choi, Z.H. Pan, S.Z.Z. Lei, H.S.V. Chen, N.J. Sucher, J. Loscalzo, D.J. Singel and J.S. Stamler, 1993, A redox-based mechanism for the neuroprotective and neurodestructive effects of nitric oxide and related nitroso-compounds, Nature 364, 626-632.

Lyons, C.R., G.J. Orloff and J.M. Cunningham, 1992, Molecular cloning and functional expression of an inducible nitric oxide synthase from a murine macrophage cell line, J. Biol. Chem. 267, 6370-6374.

Maines, M.D., J.A. Mark and J.F. Ewing, 1993, Heme oxygenase, a likely regulator of cGMP production in the brain - induction invivo of HO-1 compensates for depression in NO synthase activity, Mol. Cell. Neurosci. 4, 398-405.

Marin, P., M. Lafoncazal and J. Bockaert, 1992, A nitric oxide synthase activity selectively stimulated by NMDA receptors depends on protein kinase-C activation in mouse striatal neurons, Eur. J. Neurosci. 4, 425-432.

Marletta, M.A., P.S. Yoon, R. Iyengar, C.D. Leaf and J.S. Wishnok, 1988, Macrophage oxidation of L-arginine to nitrite and nitrate: nitric oxide is an intermediate, Biochemistry 27, 8706-8711.

Marsden, P.A., K.T. Schappert, H.S. Chen, M. Flowers, C.L. Sundell, J.N. Wilcox, S. Lamas and T. Michel, 1992, Molecular cloning and characterization of human endothelial nitric oxide synthase, FEBS Lett. 307, 287-293.

Mayer, B. and E. Böhme, 1989, Ca^{2+}-dependent formation of an L-arginine-derived activator of soluble guanylyl cyclase in bovine lung, FEBS Lett. 256, 211-214.

Mayer, B., K. Schmidt, P. Humbert and E. Böhme, 1989, Biosynthesis of endothelium-derived relaxing factor: a cytosolic enzyme in porcine aortic endothelial cells Ca^{2+}-dependently converts L-arginine into an activator of soluble guanylyl cyclase, Biochem. Biophys. Res. Commun. 164, 678-685.

Mayer, B., M. John and E. Böhme, 1990, Purification of a Ca^{2+}/calmodulin-dependent nitric oxide synthase from porcine cerebellum. Cofactor-role of tetrahydrobiopterin, FEBS Lett. 277, 215-219.

Mayer, B., M. John, B. Heinzel, E.R. Werner, H. Wachter, G. Schultz and E. Böhme, 1991, Brain nitric oxide synthase is a biopterin- and flavin-containing multi-functional oxido-reductase, FEBS Lett. 288, 187-191.

Mayer, B., P. Klatt, E. Böhme and K. Schmidt, 1992, Regulation of neuronal nitric oxide and cyclic GMP formation by Ca^{2+}, J. Neurochem. 59, 2024-2029.

Mayer, B., D. Koesling and E. Böhme, 1993a, Characterization of nitric oxide synthase, soluble guanylyl cyclase, and Ca^{2+}/calmodulin-stimulated cGMP phosphodiesterase as components of neuronal signal transduction, Adv. Second Messenger Phosphoprotein Res. 28, 111-119.

Mayer, B., M. Schmid, P. Klatt and K. Schmidt, 1993b, Reversible inactivation of endothelial nitric oxide synthase by NG-nitro-L-arginine, FEBS Lett. 333, 203-206.

Mayer, B., E.R. Werner, E. Leopold, P. Klatt and K. Schmidt, 1994, In "Biology of Nitric Oxide" (eds M. Feelisch, R. Busse, and S. Moncada), Portland Press, Colchester (in press).

McMillan, K., D.S. Bredt, D.J. Hirsch, S.H. Snyder, J.E. Clark and B.S.S. Masters, 1992, Cloned, expressed rat cerebellar nitric oxide synthase contains stoichiometric amounts of heme, which binds carbon monoxide, Proc. Natl. Acad. Sci. USA 89, 11141-11145.

Michel, T., G.K. Li and L. Busconi, 1993, Phosphorylation and subcellular translocation of endothelial nitric oxide synthase, Proc. Natl. Acad. Sci. USA 90, 6252-6256.

Nakane, M., J. Mitchell, U. Förstermann and F. Murad, 1991, Phosphorylation by calcium calmodulin-dependent protein kinase-II and protein kinase-C modulates the activity of nitric oxide synthase, Biochem. Biophys. Res. Commun. 180, 1396-1402.

Nathan, C.F. and J.B. Hibbs, 1991, Role of nitric oxide synthesis in macrophage antimicrobial activity, Curr. Opin. Immunol. 3, 65-70.

Nguyen, T., D. Brunson, C.L. Crespi, B.W. Penman, J.S. Wishnok and S.R. Tannenbaum, 1992, DNA damage and mutation in human cells exposed to nitric oxide invitro, Proc. Natl. Acad. Sci. USA 89, 3030-3034.

Nichol, C.A., G.K. Smith and D.S. Duch, 1985, Biosynthesis and metabolism of tetrahydrobiopterin and molybdopterin, Annu. Rev. Biochem. 54, 729-764.

Olken, N.M. and M.A. Marletta, 1993, NG-Methyl-L-arginine functions as an alternate substrate and mechanism-based inhibitor of nitric oxide synthase, Biochemistry 32, 9677-9685.

Palacios, M., R.G. Knowles, R.M. Palmer and S. Moncada, 1989, Nitric oxide from L-arginine stimulates the soluble guanylate cyclase in adrenal glands, Biochem. Biophys. Res. Commun. 165, 802-9.

Palmer, R.M.J., D.S. Ashton and S. Moncada, 1988, Vascular endothelial cells synthesize nitric oxide from L-arginine, Nature 333, 664-666.

Palmer, R.M.J., A.G. Ferrige and S. Moncada, 1987, Nitric oxide release accounts for the biological activity of endothelium-derived relaxing factor, Nature 327, 524-526.

Pollock, J.S., U. Förstermann, J.A. Mitchell, T.D. Warner, H.H.H.W. Schmidt, M. Nakane and F. Murad, 1991, Purification and characterization of particulate endothelium-derived relaxing factor synthase from cultured and native bovine aortic endothelial cells, Proc. Natl. Acad. Sci. USA 88, 10480-10484.

Pou, S., W.S. Pou, D.S. Bredt, S.H. Snyder and G.M. Rosen, 1992, Generation of superoxide by purified brain nitric oxide synthase, J. Biol. Chem. 267, 24173-24176.

Radomski, M.W., R.M. Palmer and S. Moncada, 1990, An L-arginine/nitric oxide pathway present in human platelets regulates aggregation, Proc. Natl. Acad. Sci. USA 87, 5193-5197.

Rengasamy, A. and R.A. Johns, 1991, Characterization of endothelium-derived relaxing factor/nitric oxide synthase from bovine cerebellum and mechanism of modulation by high and low oxygen tensions, J. Pharmacol. Exp. Ther. 259, 310-316.

Rengasamy, A. and R.A. Johns, 1993, Regulation of nitric oxide synthase by nitric oxide, Mol. Pharmacol. 44, 124-128.

Rogers, N.E. and L.J. Ignarro, 1992, Constitutive nitric oxide synthase from cerebellum is reversibly inhibited by nitric oxide formed from L-arginine, Biochem. Biophys. Res. Commun. 189, 242-249.

Rosenblum, W.I., G.H. Nelson and T. Shimizu, 1992, L-arginine suffusion restores response to acetylcholine in brain arterioles with damaged endothelium, Am. J. Physiol. 262, H961-H964.

Rossaint, R., K.J. Falke, F. Lopez, K. Slama, U. Pison and W.M. Zapol, 1993, Inhaled nitric oxide for the adult respiratory distress syndrome, New Engl. J. Med. 328, 399-405.

Sakuma, I., D.J. Stuehr, S.S. Gross, C. Nathan and R. Levi, 1988, Identification of arginine as a precursor of endothelium-derived relaxing factor, Proc. Natl. Acad. Sci. USA 85, 8664-8667.

Schmidt, H.H.H.W., 1992, NO, CO and OH - endogenous soluble guanylyl cyclase-activating factors, FEBS Lett. 307, 102-107.

Schmidt, H.H.H.W., H. Nau, W. Wittfoht, J. Gerlach, K.-E. Prescher, M.M. Klein, F. Niroomand and E. Böhme, 1988, Arginine is a physiological precursor of endothelium-derived nitric oxide, Eur. J. Pharmacol. 154, 213-216.

Schmidt, H.H.H.W. and F. Murad, 1991, Purification and characterization of a human NO synthase, Biochem. Biophys. Res. Commun. 181, 1372-1377.

Schmidt, H.H.H.W., J.S. Pollock, M. Nakane, L.D. Gorsky, U. Förstermann and F. Murad, 1991, Purification of a soluble isoform of guanylyl cyclase-activating-factor synthase, Proc. Natl. Acad. Sci. USA 88, 365-369.

Schmidt, H.H.H.W., R.M. Smith, M. Nakane and F. Murad, 1992a, Ca^{2+}/calmodulin-dependent NO synthase type-I - A biopteroflavoprotein with Ca^{2+}/calmodulin-independent diaphorase and reductase activities, Biochemistry 31, 3243-3249.

Schmidt, H.H.H.W., T.D. Warner, M. Nakane, U. Förstermann and F. Murad, 1992b, Regulation and subcellular location of nitrogen oxide synthases in RAW264.7 macrophages, Mol. Pharmacol. 41, 615-624.

Schmidt, H.H.H.W., S.M. Lohmann and U. Walter, 1993, The nitric oxide and cGMP signal transduction system - regulation and mechanism of action, Biochim. Biophys. Acta 1178, 153-175.

Schott, C.A., G.A. Gray and J.C. Stoclet, 1993, Dependence of endotoxin-induced vascular hyporeactivity on extracellular L-arginine, Br. J. Pharmacol. 108, 38-43.

Sessa, W.C., J.K. Harrison, C.M. Barber, D. Zeng, M.E. Durieux, D.D. Dangelo, K.R. Lynch and M.J. Peach, 1992, Molecular cloning and expression of a cDNA encoding endothelial cell nitric oxide synthase, J. Biol. Chem. 267, 15274-15276.

Sessa, W.C., J.K. Harrison, D.R. Luthin, J.S. Pollock and K.R. Lynch, 1993, Genomic analysis and expression patterns reveal distinct genes for endothelial and brain nitric oxide synthase, Hypertension 21, 934-938.

Stuehr, D.J., H.J. Cho, N.S. Kwon, M.F. Weise and C.F. Nathan, 1991a, Purification and characterization of the cytokine-induced macrophage nitric oxide synthase: an FAD- and FMN-containing flavoprotein, Proc. Natl. Acad. Sci. USA 88, 7773-7777.

Stuehr, D.J., N.S. Kwon, C.F. Nathan, O.W. Griffith, P.L. Feldman and J. Wiseman, 1991b, N omega-hydroxy-L-arginine is an intermediate in the biosynthesis of nitric oxide from L-arginine, J. Biol. Chem. 266, 6259-6263.

Stuehr, D.J. and M. Ikeda-Saito, 1992, Spectral characterization of brain and macrophage nitric oxide synthases

- cytochrome-P-450-like hemeproteins that contain a flavin semiquinone radical, J. Biol. Chem. 267, 20547-20550.

Tayeh, M.A. and M.A. Marletta, 1989, Macrophage oxidation of L-arginine to nitric oxide, nitrite, and nitrate. Tetrahydrobiopterin is required as a cofactor, J. Biol. Chem. 264, 19654-19658.

Ujiie, K., J.G. Drewett, P.S.T. Yuen and R.A. Star, 1993, Differential expression of mRNA for guanylyl cyclase-linked endothelium-derived relaxing factor receptor subunits in rat kidney, J. Clin. Invest. 91, 730-734.

Verma, A., D.J. Hirsch, C.E. Glatt, G.V. Ronnett and S.H. Snyder, 1993, Carbon monoxide - a putative neural messenger, Science 259, 381-384.

Waldman, S. and F. Murad, 1987, Cyclic GMP synthesis and function, Pharmacol. Rev. 39, 163-195.

Walter, U., 1989, Physiological role of cGMP and cGMP-dependent protein kinase in the cardiovascular system, Rev. Physiol. Biochem. Pharmacol. 113, 42-88.

Wedel, B., P. Humbert, C. Harteneck, J. Foerster, J. Malkewitz, E. Böhme, G. Schultz and D. Koesling, 1994, Mutation of His-105 of the b1-subunit yields a nitric oxide-insensitive form of soluble guanylyl cyclase, Proc. Natl. Acad. Sci. USA 91, 2592-2596.

Werner, E.R., G. Werner-Felmayer and H. Wachter, 1993, Tetrahydrobiopterin and cytokines, Proc. Soc. Exp. Biol. Med. 203, 1-12.

White, K.A. and M.A. Marletta, 1992, Nitric oxide synthase is a cytochrome-P-450 type hemoprotein, Biochemistry 31, 6627-6631.

Wink, D.A., K.S. Kasprzak, C.M. Maragos, R.K. Elespuru, M. Misra, T.M. Dunams, T.A. Cebula, W.H. Koch, A.W. Andrews, J.S. Allen and L.K. Keefer, 1991, DNA deaminating ability and genotoxicity of nitric oxide and its progenitors, Science 254, 1001-1003.

Wink, D.A., Y. Osawa, J.F. Darbyshire, C.R. Jones, S.C. Eshenaur and R.W. Nims, 1993, Inhibition of cytochromes-P450 by nitric oxide and a nitric oxide-releasing agent, Arch. Biochem. Biophys. 300, 115-123.

Wolf, G., S. Würdig and G. Schunzel, 1992, Nitric oxide synthase in rat brain is
predominantly located at neuronal endoplasmic reticulum - an electron microscopic demonstration of NADPH-diaphorase activity, Neurosci. Lett. 147, 63-66.

Wu, Z., R.K. Sharma and J.H. Wang, 1992, Catalytic and regulatory properties of calmodulin-stimulated phosphodiesterase isozymes, Adv. Second Messenger Phosphoprotein Res. 25, 29-43.

Xie, Q.W., H.J. Cho, J. Calaycay, R.A. Mumford, K.M. Swiderek, T.D. Lee, A.H. Ding, T. Troso and C. Nathan, 1992, Cloning and characterization of inducible nitric oxide synthase from mouse macrophages, Science 256, 225-228.

Yuen, P.S.T., L.R. Potter and D.L. Garbers, 1990, A new form of guanylyl cyclase is preferentially expressed in rat kidney, Biochemistry 29, 10872-10878.

Yui, Y., R. Hattori, K. Kosuga, K. Eizawa, K. Hiki and C. Kawai, 1991, Purification of nitric oxide synthase from rat macrophages, J. Biol. Chem. 266, 12544-12547.

Zhuo, M., S.A. Small, E.R. Kandel and R.D. Hawkins, 1993, Nitric oxide and carbon monoxide produce activity-dependent long-term synaptic enhancement in hippocampus, Science 260, 1946-1950.

MECHANISMS OF SHEAR STRESS-DEPENDENT ENDOTHELIAL NITRIC OXIDE RELEASE: CARDIOVASCULAR IMPLICATIONS

Markus Hecker, Ingrid Fleming, Kazuhide Ayajiki, and Rudi Busse
Centre of Physiology
Johann Wolfgang Goethe University Clinic
Theodor-Stern-Kai 7
D-60590 Frankfurt/Main
Germany

SUMMARY

Endothelial cells produce a variety of factors involved in the control of vascular tone, platelet activation and cell growth, one of the most important being nitric oxide (NO). Although continuously produced in small amounts by the endothelium, various physical and humoral stimuli greatly enhance the release of NO. The physiologically most important stimulus for the release of NO from these cells is considered to be the shear stress (or viscous drag) exerted on the luminal surface of the endothelium by the streaming blood. This stimulus does not only affect NO production acutely, but may also be required to maintain endothelial NO synthase expression. This brief overview resumes current knowledge on the potential mechanisms involved both in the acute and long-term effects of shear stress on endothelial NO formation.

FACTORS DETERMINING SHEAR STRESS

The shear stress (τ) exerted on the luminal surface of the endothelium can be estimated, under the assumption of a constant laminar flow, according to the following equation, where η is the viscosity, Q the flow rate and r the inner radius of the artery:

$$r = \frac{4\eta Q}{r^3 \tau}$$

From this equation it becomes apparent that vicosity and flow are linearly related to the shear stress which, on the other hand, is inversely related to the third power of the vessel radius. It follows therefore that narrowing of the arterial lumen by, e.g. 50%, will

Biochemical, Pharmacological, and Clinical Aspects of Nitric Oxide
Edited by B. A. Weissman *et al.*, Plenum Press, New York, 1995

49

result in a 4-fold greater increase in shear stress than the same percentage increase in flow or viscosity.

ACUTE EFFECTS OF ELEVATED SHEAR STRESS ON ENDOTHELIAL NITRIC OXIDE FORMATION

An increase in shear stress, generated either by an increase in flow at constant diameter or by a vasoconstriction at constant flow (Fig. 1), enhances the release of NO from endothelial cells *in situ* (e.g. luminally perfused, endothelium-intact segments of small conduit arteries), and this release is maintained during the period in which shear stress remains elevated (Hecker et al., 1993). Moreover, the level of shear stress and the release of NO elicited by altering either diameter or flow are positively correlated, suggesting that local changes in tone (e.g. neurogenic or myogenic vasoconstriction), may be as important as changes in flow for the regulation of endothelial NO release *in vivo* (Pohl et al., 1991; Busse et al., 1993; Griffith and Edwards, 1990). A similar relationship between endothelial NO production and hemodynamic variables determining shear stress, including rhythmic deformation of the endothelium, can also be demonstrated in the isolated perfused rabbit heart (Lamontagne et al., 1992). Increasing fluid viscosity, e.g. by adding dextran or polyethylene glycol to the perfusate, has also been shown to enhance

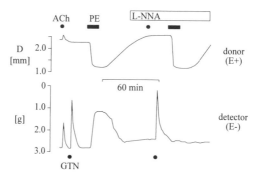

Figure 1: Release of NO from an isolated perfused, endothelium-intact segment of the rabbit iliac artery, as detected by the dilator response (shown in g of induced tone) of an endothelium-denuded ring segment of rabbit femoral artery superfused with the luminal effluate from the donor segment. The dilator response of the detector was calibrated by comparison with the response to the endothelium-independent vasodilator, glyceryl trinitrate (GTN, 100 pmol bolus). Bolus application of the endothelium-dependent vasodilator, acetylcholine (ACh, 10 nmol), caused a transient dilator response, while short-term administration of phenylephrine (PE,10^{-5}M, 10 min) elicited not only a profound constriction of the donor segment (determined microscopically as decrease in diameter, mm), but also a marked relaxation of the detector which was sustained as long as the tone of the donor segment remained elevated. Note that treatment of the donor segment with the NO synthase inhibitor, N^G-nitro-L-arginine (L-NNA, 10^{-4}M), completely abolished these dilator responses, demonstrating that they were mediated by the release of NO.

SHEAR STRESS-DEPENDENT SIGNAL TRANSDUCTION MECHANISMS

Changes in intracellular Ca^{2+}

It has long been suspected that the endothelial response to increased shear stress is associated with an increase in the intracellular concentration of free calcium (Ca^{2+}_i), although in the past somewhat conflicting data have been reported (Mo et al., 1991).

More recently, however, several studies performed with cultured endothelial cells indeed imply that an increase in shear stress is associated with an increase in Ca^{2+}_i (Schwarz et al., 1992; Shen et al., 1992; Geiger et al., 1992). This Ca^{2+} increase bears a certain resemblance to the endothelial response to receptor-dependent agonists and presumably involves both the mobilisation of Ca^{2+} from intracellular stores and the influx of extracellular Ca^{2+}. Indeed, following an increase in shear stress both an activation of phospholipase C (Bhagyalakshmi et al., 1992) and a rapid increase in inositol-1,4,5-trisphosphate (IP_3) levels have been detected in cultured endothelial cells (Nollert et al., 1990; Prasad et al., 1993). Evidence for Ca^{2+} influx has been obtained with arteriolar endothelial cells *in situ*, which respond with a sustained increase in Ca^{2+}_i to elevated shear stress (Falcone et al., 1993). The question remains, however, as to how endothelial cells are able to sense a change in shear stress and initiate the signal transduction pathway leading to phospholipase C activation and Ca^{2+} influx.

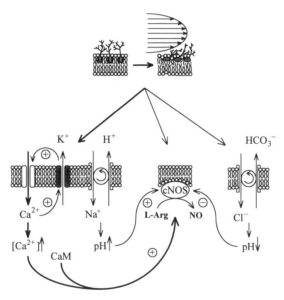

Figure 2: Putative signal transduction mechanisms involved in shear stress-dependent endothelial NO release. Changes in membrane fluidity associated with a distortion of the glycocalyx may lead to a direct activation of the membrane-bound NO synthase. They also cause an increase in pH_i via activation of the Na^+/H^+ exchanger, hence reinforcing the stimulation of the pH-sensitive enzyme. Even though an IP_3-mediated mobilisation of intracellular Ca^{2+} does play a role (not depicted here), the influx of extracellullar Ca^{2+} is likely to be mainly responsible for the sustained increase in NO synthase activity during periods of elevated shear stress. The driving force for extracellular Ca^{2+} entry is augmented by the concomitant shear stress-induced activation of Ca^{2+}-dependent K^+ channels which remain open due to the increase in intracellular Ca^{2+}. Note that activation of the Na^+/bicarbonate exchanger by elevated shear may lower pH_i and thus NO synthase activity.

No matter how the Ca^{2+} response to shear stress is brought about, an increase in Ca^{2+}_i will lead to an activation of the Ca^{2+}/calmodulin-dependent endothelial NO synthase. Indeed, the shear stress-dependent release of NO from both cultured (Macarthur et al., 1993) and native endothelial cells (Cooke et al., 1991) is mainly dependent on the presence of extracellular Ca^{2+}.

Alterations in intracellular pH

Another mechanism possibly contributing to the shear stress-dependent activation of NO synthase in endothelial cells is a change in intracellular pH (pH_i). Under a variety of circumstances cellular deformation not only results in an activation (or inactivation) of stretch-sensitive ion channels, but also stimulates the Na^+/H^+ exchanger. Several structural components of the cytoskeleton, such as actin filaments, are thought to play a role in transducing the physical s(shear stress or stretch) to the Na^+/H^+ exchanger (Watson, 1991). Of note in this context is that an increase in pH_i subsequent to activation of the Na^+/H^+ antiporter in endothelial cells seems to be associated with the sustained phase of NO release following stimulation with a receptor-dependent agonist, such as bradykinin (Fleming et al., 1994). Since the activity of the endothelial NO synthase is also strongly pH-sensitive in the physiological range (Hecker et al., 1994), alterations in pH_i may indeed represent an important mechanism for the regulation of NO biosynthesis in endothelial cells by both humoral and physical stimuli (Fig. 2). However, it must be emphasised that alterations in pH_i are likely to affect Ca^{2+} entry into endothelial cells, and that the potential involvement of other ion transport mechanisms, such as the Na^+/Ca^{2+} exchanger, cannot be excluded. Moreover, concomitant activation of the Na^+/bicarbonate exchanger following exposure to elevated shear stress results in an intracellular acidification (Ziegelstein et al., 1992) which may offset the stimulatory effect of an activation of the Na^+/H^+ exchanger on endothelial NO formation.

Role of the membrane potential

The activation of K^+ channels represents another signal transduction mechanism involved in the shear stress-dependent release of NO from the endothelium (Fig. 2). Mechanical deformation of endothelial cells, for example, is known to activate an inwardly rectifying K^+ channel (Olesen et al., 1988), and the subsequent membrane hyperpolarization augments the driving force for Ca^{2+} entry (Lückhoff and Busse, 1990). Moreover, iberiotoxin and charybdotoxin, inhibitors of Ca^{2+}-activated K^+ channels (Cooke et al., 1991), but not glybenclamide (Hecker et al., 1993; Cooke et al., 1991), an inhibitor of the ATP-dependent K^+ channel, inhibit the shear stress-dependent release of NO from native endothelial cells *in situ*. These findings suggest that activation of Ca^{2+}-dependent K^+ channels plays an important modulatory role in the shear stress-dependent formation of NO.

THE SHEAR STRESS SENSOR

The viscous drag caused by the streaming blood (fluid) is likely to be sensed by structures located at the outer leaflet of the endothelial cell membrane which are coupled to ion channels, the cytoskeleton or membrane-attached Ca^{2+} stores. The glycocalyx, i.e. membrane glycoproteins and glycolipids forming a network of anastomosing strands on the luminal surface of the endothelium, is the most likely candidate for such as shear stress-sensing structure. It is conceivable that a distortion of the glycocalyx may cause a change in the fluidity of the plasma membrane, and since the endothelial NO synthase appears to be predominantly localised to this membrane (Hecker et al., 1994), a change in membrane fluidity may directly modulate NO synthase activity (Fig. 2). This hypothesis is supported by the finding that removal of sialic acid residues from the glycocalyx by pre-treatment with neuraminidase selectively attenuates the shear stress-dependent release of NO from native endothelial cells *in situ* (Hecker et al., 1993).

EFFECTS OF ELEVATED SHEAR STRESS ON NITRIC OXIDE SYNTHASE EXPRESSION IN ENDOTHELIAL CELLS

Comparison of the NO synthase activity present in cultured cells with that of freshly isolated endothelial cells or native endothelial cells *in situ* reveals a striking difference regardless of the species or type of vessels from which the cells have been isolated (Fig. 3) such that NO synthase activity decreases with time in culture. This difference is reflected in the NO-producing capacity of these cells under basal conditions, their NO synthase content (determined by immunoblot analysis) and the level of mRNA encoding the enzyme (Hecker et al., 1994). It would therefore appear that NO synthase expression *in vivo* is maintained by, or as a consequence of, the continuous exposure of the endothelium to certain stimuli. One likely candidate for such a stimulus is the shear stress to which the cells are continuously exposed to *in vivo*, but which is absent in culture. This hypothesis was supported by the finding that exposure of cultured endothelial cells to physiological levels of shear stress for several hours results in a significant increase in NO synthase activity and content as well as NO synthase mRNA levels (Busse et al., 1994; Nishida et al., 1992). Moreover, the functional relevance for such a shear stress-dependent change in NO synthase expression *in vitro* has recently been shown *in vivo* by the demonstration of a marked upregulation of NO synthase expression in the aortic endothelium from chronically exercised dogs (Sessa et al., 1994).

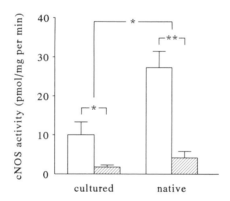

Figure 3: Comparison of the NO synthase activity present in the cytosolic (open columns) and microsomal (hatched columns) fraction obtained from cultured (3-4 days) and freshly isolated (native) bovine aortic endothelial cells. Enzyme activity was determined by monitoring the N^G-nitro-L-arginine-sensitive conversion of L-[3H]arginine to L-[3H]citrulline (mean SEM, $n=3$; *$P<0.05$, **$P<=0.01$ as indicated).

The signal transduction mechanism involved in the long-term effects of shear stress on NO synthase expression in endothelial cells is currently unknown, but may involve changes in pH_i and/or Ca^{2+}_i and the induction of immediate early genes (IEGs), such as members of the *fos* and *jun* family (Nollert et al., 1992). Activation of either cAMP-dependent protein kinases or protein kinase C may also lead to the expression of these IEGs (Nollert et al., 1992), although there is no convincing evidence implicating these kinases in the response to shear stress. Indeed, inhibition of protein kinase C is without effect on the shear stress-dependent NO synthase expression in cultured endothelial cells (Uematsu et al., 1993). More recently, this subject gained a new perspective following the identification of a shear stress-responsive element in the promotor region of the endothelial NO synthase gene (Nadaud et al., 1994). How changes in shear stress are conveyed to this DNA sequence and which nuclear transcription factor(s) is involved therein, remains to be elucidated.

CARDIOVASCULAR IMPLICATIONS

Under physiological conditions, the maintenance of an adequate vascular tone depends on the delicate balance between vasodilator and vasoconstrictor influences. In the coronary and forearm circulation of healthy subjects, endothelium-dependent dilator responses caused by increasing blood flow or by infusing receptor-dependent agonists, such as acetylcholine or bradykinin, has been repeatedly documented. The reduction or loss of these endothelium-dependent dilator responses is a common characteristic reflecting endothelial dysfunction in a number of pathophysiological states, such as atherosclerosis, hypertension, hypercholesterolaemia, diabetes and heart failure (Kubo et al., 1991; Creager et al., 1990; Linder et al., 1990; Vita et al., 1989; Zeiher et al., 1991). In the absence of a vasoconstricting principle, this endothelial dysfunction may lead simply to an attenuation of endothelium-dependent responses, as demonstrated by impaired flow-mediated coronary dilation in patients with atherosclerosis. However, in patients with ischemic heart disease or hypercholesterolaemia, intracoronary infusion of either acetylcholine or serotonin, both of which have direct vasoconstrictor effects on vascular smooth muscle, led to a constriction of the epicardial coronary arteries (Zeiher et al., 1991; Golino et al., 1991). This inadequate vasomotor response is mainly related to the impairment of endothelial NO production, since in healthy subjects a dilation is observed by virtue of the simultaneous release of NO from the endothelium. Consequently, the prevention or reversal of the functional and morphological alterations of the endothelium associated with the aforementioned diseases represents an obvious therapeutic goal. A better understanding othe principal mechanisms involved in the continuous shear stress-dependent endothelial release of NO may help not only to elucidate the nature of these dysfunctions, but also to design novel approaches towards their therapy.

Acknowledgements

The work described from our laboratory was supported by the Deutsche Forschungsgemeinschaft (Bu 436/4-3, He 1587/4-1), the Commission of the European Union (BMH1-CT92-1893), the Deutsche Gesellschaft für Herz- und Kreislaufforschung (I.F.) and the Japanese Ministry of Education, Science and Culture (K.A.).

REFERENCES

Bhagyalakshmi, A., F. Berthiaume, K.M. Reich and J.A. Frangos, 1992. Fluid shear stress stimulates membrane phospholipid metabolism in cultured human endothelial cells, J. Vasc. Res. 29, 443.

Busse, R., A. Mülsch, I. Fleming and M. Hecker, 1993. Mechanisms of nitric oxide release from the vascular endothelium. Circulation 87, V18.

Busse, R., M. Hecker and I. Fleming, 1994. Control of nitric oxide and prostacyclin synthesis in endothelial cells. Arzneim. Forsch./Drug Res. 44, 392.

Creager, M.A., J.P. Cooke, M.E. Mendelsohn, S.J. Gallagher, S.M. Coleman, J. Loscalzo and V.H. Dzau, 1990. Impaired vasodilation of forearm resistance vessels in hypercholesterolemic humans, J. Clin. Invest. 86, 228.

Cooke, J. P., E. Rossitch, N. A. Andon, J. Loscalzo and V. J. Dzau, 1991. Flow activates an endothelial potassium channel to release an endogenous nitrovasodilator, J. Clin. Invest. 88, 1663.

Falcone, J.C., L. Kuo and G.A. Meininger, 1993. Endothelial cell calcium increases during flow-induced dilation in isolated arterioles. Am. J. Physiol. 264, H653.

Fleming, I., M. Hecker and R. Busse, 1994. Intracellular alkalinisation induced by bradykinin sustains activation of the constitutive nitric oxide synthase in endothelial cells. Circ. Res., in press.

Geiger, R. V., B. C. Berk, R. W. Alexander and R. M. Nerem, 1992. Flow-induced calcium transients in single endothelial cells: spatial and temporal analysis, Am. J. Physiol. 262, C1411.

Golino, P., F. Piscione, J.T. Willerson, M. Cappellibigazzi, A. Focaccio, B. Villari, C. Indolfi, E. Russolillo, M. Condorelli and M. Chiarello, 1991. Divergent effects of serotonin on coronary artery dimensions and blood flow in patients with coronary atherosclerosis and control patients, N. Engl. J. Med. 324, 641.

Griffith, T. M. and D. H. Edwards, 1990. Myogenic autoregulation of flow may be inversely related to endothelium-derived relaxing factor activity, Am. J. Physiol. 258, H1171.

Hecker, M., A. Mülsch, E. Bassenge and R. Busse, 1993. Vasoconstriction and increased flow: Two principal mechanisms of shear stress-dependent endothelial autacoid release. Am. J. Physiol. 265, H828.

Hecker, M., A. Mülsch, E. Bassenge, U. Forstermann and R. Busse, 1994. Subcellular localisation and characterization of nitric oxide synthase(s) in endothelial cells - physiologic implications. Biochem. J. 299, 247.

Kubo, S.H., T.S. Rector, A.J. Bank, R.E. Williams and S.M. Heifetz, 1991. Endothelium-dependent vasodilation is attenuated in patients with heart failure, Circulation 84, 1589.

Lamontagne, D., U. Pohl and R. Busse, 1992. Mechanical deformation of vessel wall and shear stress determine the basal EDRF release in the intact coronary vascular bed, Circ. Res. 70, 123.

Linder, L. W. Kiowski, F.R. Bühler and T.F. Lüscher, 1990. Indirect evidence for release of endothelium-derived relaxing factor in human forearm circulation *in vivo* - blunted response in essential hypertension, Circulation 81, 1762.

Lückhoff, A. and R. Busse, 1990. Activators of potassium channels enhance calcium influx into endothelial cells as a consequence of potassium currents, Naunyn-Schmiedebeg's Arch. Pharmacol. 342, 94.

Macarthur, H., M. Hecker, R. Busse and J.R. Vane, 1993. Selective inhibition of agonist-induced but not shear stress-dependent endothelial autacoid release by thapsigargin. Br. J. Pharmacol. 108, 100.

Melkumyants, A.M., S.A. Balashov and V.M. Khayutin, 1989. Endothelium dependent control of arterial diameter by blood viscosity, Cardiovasc. Res. 23, 741.

Mo, M., S. G. Eskin and W. P. Schilling, 1991. Flow-induced changes in Ca^{2+} signaling of vascular endothelial cells - effect of shear stress and ATP, Am. J. Physiol. 260, H1698.

Nadaud, S., A. Bonnardeaux, M. Lathrop and F. Soubrier, 1994. Gene structure, polymorphism and mapping of the human endothelial nitric oxide synthase gene, Biochem. Biophys. Res. Commun. 198, 1027.

Nishida, K., D.G. Harrison, J.P. Navas, A.A, Fisher, S.P. Dockery, M. Uematsu, R.M. Nerem, R.W. Alexander and T.J. Murphy, 1992. Molecular cloning and characterization of the constitutive bovine aortic endothelial cell nitric oxide synthase, J. Clin. Invest. 90, 2092.

Nollert, M.U., S.G. Eskin and L.V. McIntyre, 1990. Shear stress increases inositol trisphosphate levels in human endothelial cells, Biochem. Biophys. Res. Commun. 170, 281.

Nollert, M.U., N.J. Panaro and L.V. McIntire, 1992. Regulation of genetic expression in shear stress-stimulated endothelial cells, Ann. N. Y. Acad. Sci. 665, 94.

Olesen, S. P., D. E. Clapham and P. F. Davies, 1988. Haemodynamic shear stress activates a K^+ current in vascular endothelial cells, Nature 331, 168.

Pohl, U., K. Herlan, A. Huang and E. Bassenge, 1991. EDRF-mediated shear-induced dilation opposes myogenic vasoconstriction in small rabbit arteries, Am. J. Physiol. 261, H2016.

Prasad, A.R.S., S.A. Logan, R.M. Nerem, C.J. Schwartz and E.A. Sprague, 1993. Flow-related responses of intracellular inositol phosphate levels in cultured aortic endothelial cells, Circ. Res. 72, 827.

Schwarz, G., G. Callewaert, G. Droogmans and B. Nilius, 1992. Shear stress induced calcium transients in endothelial cells from human umbilical cord veins, J. Physiol. (Lond.) 458, 527.

Sessa, W.C., K. Pritchard, N. Seyedi, J. Wang and T.H. Hintze, 1994. Chronic exercise in dogs increases coronary vascular nitric oxide production and endothelial cell nitric oxide synthase gene expression, Circ. Res. 74, 349.

Shen, J., F. W. Luscinskas, A. Connolly, C. F. Dewey and M. A. Gimbrone, 1992. Fluid shear stress modulates cytosolic free calcium in vascular endothelial cells, Am. J. Physiol. 262, C384.

Uematsu, , M., J.P. Navas, K. Nishida, Y. Ohara, T.J. Murphy, R.W. Alexander, R.M. Nerem and D.G. Harrison, 1993. Mechanisms of endothelial cell NO synthase induction by shear stress, Circulation 88, I-184.

Vita, J.A., C.B. Treasure, P. Ganz, D.A. Fox, R.D. Fish and A.P. Selwyn, 1989. Control of shear stress in the epicardial coronary arteries of humans - impairment by atherosclerosis, J. Am. Coll. Cardiol. 14, 1193.

Watson, P.A., 1991. Function follows form: generation of intracellular signals by cell deformation, FASEB J. 5, 2013.

Zeiher, A.M., H. Drexler, H. Wollschlager and H. Just, 1991. Modulation of coronary vasomotor tone in humans - progressive endothelial dysfunction with different early stages of coronary atherosclerosis, Circulation 83, 391.

Ziegelstein, R.C., L. Cheng and M.C. Capogrossi, 1992. Flow-dependent cytosolic acidification of vascular endothelial cells, Science 258, 656.

DETERMINATION OF NITRIC OXIDE LEVELS BY FLUORESCENCE SPECTROSCOPY

G. Gabor and N. Allon

Israel Institute for Biological Research
Ness Ziona, 70450
    Israel

INTRODUCTION

Nitric Oxide (NO), a short lived radical molecule (Kelm and Schrader, 1990), was considered as an environmental pollutant, as an ozon scavenger. The important role of NO in diverse biological processes such as brain ischemia, immune regulation, neurotansmission and penile erection, was recently reported (Kelm and Schrader, 1990; Stuehr and Marletta, 1985; Palmer et al., 1986), invokes the need for an accurate, specific method for the determination of this species. Ultimately, the method should enable in situ measurements, therefore it must be nondestructive to tissue.

The common analytical methods for the determination of NO or nitrite in aqueous solutions or in the gas phase are potentionmetric (Choi and Fung, 1980) - employing a specific electrode for pH, with the suitable media and membranes or polarography. Electrochemical microprobes employed for physiological measurements were also reported (Shibuki, 1990; Malinski and Taha, 1992). To differentiate between the nitrite ion and various NO compounds, specific membranes were designed (O'Reilly, et al., 1991). These sensors lack the specificity for NO. According to Hassan and Tadros (1982) the sensor does not detect NO levels below 10^{-2}M, and its response reflect, mainly, the NO_2 level. Another disavantage of electrochemical sensors is that local currents, like in the CNS cause perturbations that distort the results.

NO_x determination by the highly sensitive chemiluminescent method is based on the oxidation of NO under severe conditions (by O_3) yielding NO_2^* in the excited state. NO_2^* can be determined quantitatively, either by its own chemiluminescence (Fontijn, et al., 1970) or by luminol chemiluminescence. This method has been used for environmental detection of NO_x, but, obviously, a) is unable to differentiate between the various NO_x species; and b) it cannot be applied for in situ physiological detection.

Optical sensors, utilizing reactions that (1) proceed under mild conditions (2) do not require an aqueous media, and (3) are not influenced by local currents, are advantageous.

Biochemical, Pharmacological, and Clinical Aspects of Nitric Oxide
Edited by B. A. Weissman *et al.*, Plenum Press, New York, 1995

57

It should be noted that Freeman et al. (1992) reported the measurement of NO_x by an optical sensor, based on changes in the absorption of corrin.

To differentiate between NO and other nitrogen oxides, we introduced a selective reaction for NO, yielding a measurable optical signal. Such a reaction is the formation of nitrosothiols, (Williams, 1985; Stamler, et al., 1992) according to reaction la

$$\text{a} \qquad\qquad \text{b}$$
$$(1)\ NO + RSH \longrightarrow RSNO \longrightarrow RSSR + NO$$

A pink product is obtained absorbing at 544 nm and 334 nm.

This is a second order reaction, that depends on the concentrations of the reactants (eq 2). The rate constant (k) also depends indirectly on the hydrogen ion concentration when HNO is used as the source for NO since the pKa of HNO_2 between 2 and 3 determines the availability of NO.(Gomes and Borges, 1993).

$$(2)\ rate = k\ [RSH]\ [NO]$$

The nitrosothiol decomposes by homolysis of the S-N bond yielding the disulfide and NO (Oae, et al., 1978) (eq lb). The decomposition is a slow process with cysteine and even slower with its N-acetyl derivative or with glutathione in aqueous solutions, at room temperature (Gabor and Allon, to be published). However, it is fast with dithiothreitol (DTT), in which the ring closure probably supplies the driving force.

To detect NO via its nitrosothiol derivative(s), seems very attractive, since these compounds were also suggested as the possible active species in biological processes (Stamler, et al., 1992, Kowaluk and Fung, 1990, Gaston et al., 1993). To apply the absorption of nitrosothiols would yield rather high limits of detection, since the extremely low absorption coefficients at 334 nm and at 544 nm, $890M^{-1}$ and $16M^{-1}$ would enable detection of 1.1×10^{-5} M and 6.2×10^{-4} M respectively (Kowaluk and Fung, 1990). As this is not satisfactory, we introduced the Inner Filter Effect (Walt et al., 1993) (IFE), that utilizes fluorescence spectrosopy and enables determination of $10^{-4} - 5 \times 10^{-7}$ M NO.

The IFE, basically the perturbation of the fluorescence of a fluorescent compound, by a non-fluorescent analyte, enables its determination by the highly sensitive fluorescence measurements (Gabor and Walt, 1991; Walt et al., 1993). Since the absorption of quinine sulfate overlaps the absorption of the analyte (Fig. l), it was selected as the fluorescer.

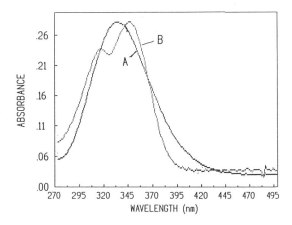

Figure l: Absorption specta of aqueous solutions at pH l of a) nitrosothiol and b) quinine.

For concentrations of NO below 5×10^{-7} M, we also utilized the production of nitrosothiols (eq. 1) thus providing specificity, but we applied the thiols (RSH) in excess, and determined the excess thiol by the well known fluorescent thiol reagent, CPM (Parvari et al., 1983) (eq. 3).

$$(3) \ CPM + RS- \ (excess) --> CPMRS$$

Reaction 3, which is basicly a condensation of the CPM reagent with a thiol, involves the opening of the maleimide double bond, and as a result, the slightly fluorescent reagent (CPM) yields a highly fluorecent condensation product (Parvari et al., 1983).

CPM has been used previously for a) thiol detection in polyacrylamid gels (Yamamoto et al., 1977), b) the determination of cellular and non protein thiols (Ayers,et al., 1986), c) hystological preparations (Sippel, 1981) and d) structural studies of proteins (Odom et al., 1983).

The physiological concentration of NO (10^{-8} - 10^{-10} M) - will easily be detected by the previously reported limit of detection of the CPM reaction (0.01 nmole, Parvari et al., 1983). The instability of the nitrosothiol has no interference as its decomposition yields disulfides (Williams, 1985) (eq. lb) (and no reduced thiols) in addition to NO.

MATERIALS AND METHODS

N-acetylcysteine (NAC) and glutathione (GLU) were from Sigma, USA. CPM was from Molecular Probes, USA. Sodium phosphates - mono and dibasic - and sodiumnitrite were from Merck, Germany. HCl, H_2SO_4, isopropanol (IP), dimethyl formamide (DMFA) of Analar grade were used without further purification.

Absorption was recorded on an HP8452A Diode Array Spectrophotometer. An SLM 500, equipped with an IBM PC, was used for fluorescence measurements.

Preparation of Nitrosothiols

Saturated aqueous solution of NO (28 mM), was obtained by bubbling NO gas into an aqueous solution of O.I N HCl (pH l). The instantaneous formation of the nitrosothiol (NACNO or GLUNO) from stoichiometric quantities of the reagents in eq. 1 was followed by monitoring either the absorption spectra of the product (Fig. l, curve A); or the absorption at 334 nm and 544 nm (Fig. 2).

Rats were decapitated and brains were removed and placed in 1 ml ice-cold O.1 M phosphate buffer. Brains were homogenated utilizing a polyton at maximal speed (30 s). The homogenates were kept at O°C. Prior to the measurements, they were diluted by O.lN HCl.

Fluorescence measurements

A) With quinine: Nitrosothiol levels of $5x10^{-7}$ - 10^{-4} M

Calibration curves for NACNO (or GLUNO) were prepared by adding given quantities of nitrite or aqueous O.lN HCl NO solution to a NAC solution(Fig. 3). Twenty µl of each solution were added to 2 ml H_2SO_4 containing the suitable quantity of quinine sulfate, and the fluorescence intensity - excited at 334 nm - was monitored at 453 nm (I[334/453]) (Fig. 3).

The introduction of brain homogenates did not change the calibration curves (fig. 4). The calibration curve at pH 7.4 (Fig. 5) was obtained by diluting 20 µl of various concentrations of nitrosothiols, prepared at pH l, into 2 ml phosphate buffer O.l M, pH

7.4. At this pH the quinine is not protonated, therefore the fluorescence excited at 334 nm was recorded at 385 nm.

B) With CPM: levels of 10^{-10} - 10^{-7} M

Nitrosothiols were prepared with an excess of the thiol reagent (RSH). This was followed by the determination of the excess thiol with CPM by monitoring the fluorescenc

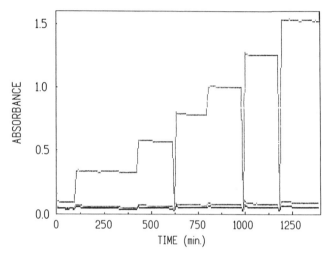

Figure 2: Typical production of Nitrosothiol at pH 1 in 0.1 N HCl monitored by the absorption at 334 nm and 544 nm. [NAC] = 1.6×10^{-3} M. Twenty μl portions of 2.8×10^{-4} M HNO_2 in 0.1 N HCl solution were added, 5 times. The last portion contained 5.6×10^{-4} M in order to saturate all the NAC present.

intensity - I(390/487). This is an accurate measure of the [NO] present, provided that the initial (overall) concentration of the thiol is known.

The concentration of the NACNO stock solution was 10^{-3} M. CPM stock solution was prepared by dissolving the solid in a mixture of IP/DMFA 6:1. The precipitate was discarded. The solution was diluted 1:10 with IP and the absorption spectrum recorded (Fig. 6).

The concentration was calculated applying the reported absorption coefficients of ε (390) = 23250 and ε(390) = 25000 of unreacted CPM and cysteine bound CPM, respectively (He et al., 1993). The condensation of the CPM-thiol (product of reaction 3) was followed by monitoring the fluorescence, excited at 390 nm, at 487 nm versus time (fig. 7).

Sampling the fluorescence intensities at given time periods and plotting them versus the concentrations yielded straight lines, with excellent correlation coefficients (R), that is, fluorescence intensity [I(390/487)] is a linear function of NO concentrations. We have prepared calibration curves in the biological/environmental NO concentration ranges (Figs 8 & 9), i.e. in the 10^{-8} - 10^{-10} M range. In a series of measurements we maintained the thiol concentration (in excess) constant, while the NO concentration was varied.

Statistics

Experimental results were treated by a linear regression software. Correlation coefficients (R), reported in the captions to figures, establish linearity.

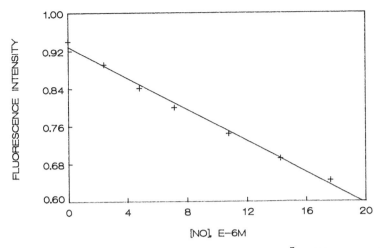

Figure 3: Calibration curve for NO at pH 1, in 0.1 N H_2SO_4. $[Q] = 4 \times 10^{-7}$ M. NO concentration range: 1-20 $\times 10^{-6}$ M. Fluorescence excited at 334 nm (λx) monitored at 453 nm (λm) R = 0.9971.

RESULTS AND DISCUSSION

A) Detection of Nitrosothiols levels at 5×10^{-7} - 10^{-7} M: Selection of fluorescer

To exploit the IFE for the determination of a non-fluorescent compound the analyte a fluorescer is introduced. A fluorescer is a highly fluorescent compound. Its absorption or fluorescence band, for employing the primary or secondary IFE, respectively, must overlap the   fluorescer, since its absorption band has an excellent overlap with that of nitrosothiols (Fig. 1). Since both compounds follow the Beer Lambert law, the relative quantities of the light absorbed by each of them is determined by the ratio of their absorption coefficients at 334 nm. Thus, the light absorbed by the   given wavelength fluorescer and concomitantly the emitted light intensity are modulated. This modulation is a linear function of the modulator. The IFE was recently introduced to enhance the sensitivity of pH and CO_2 sensors and was also applied for K+ determination (Gabor and Walt, 1991; Walt et al., 1993).

Preparation of calibration curves

For the NO concentration range of 10^{-3} - 10^{-4} M it is preferable to apply the more effective secondary IFE, i.e. to use a fluorescer whose emission band overlaps the absorption of the analyte. However our ultimate goal is to determine concentrations in the 10^{-6} - 10^{-8} M range. We, therefore, employed the primary IFE, providing a rather small modulation (Gabor, to be published), thus improving the limit of detection by two orders of magnitude only.

By applying N-acetylated thiols in excess, a stable nitrosothiol is formed, that releases NO only after 24-48 hrs at a very slow rate (Gabor and Allon, to be published). The difference in the rates of reactions la and lb guarantees that only negligible quantities of NO are realeased during the analysis. Excess NO would either react with the excess thiol present or catalize the decomposition of the nitrosothiols (Gabor and Allon, to be published), and thus interfere with the analysis.

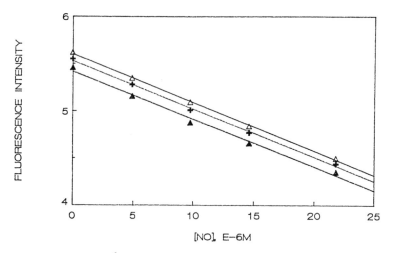

Figure 4: As above [Q] = 2 x 10^{-6} M (Δ), R = 0.9995, with brain homogenates (0.5 gr. rat brain in 2.5 ml 0.1 M phosphate buffer diluted x10 (+) R=0.9989,and x100,). (▲) R= 0.9960 by HCl 0.lN. NO concentration range: 1-25 x 10^{-6} M.

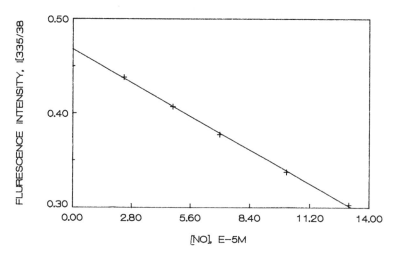

Figure 5: Calibration curve for NO at pH 7.4 in 0.1 M phosphate buffer, λx= 334nm, λm = 385nm, R = 0.9997.

Freshly prepared NACNO at pH 1 was stable for at least 24 hours at room temperature, before it started to decompose according to eq lb. This delay provides sufficient time for a) the preparation of diluted NACNO - quinine mixtures, and b) the determination of the fluorescent intensities of each solution, prior to the release of NO from the nitrosothiols. Calibration curves at pH 1 and pH 7 - fluorescence intensity versus NO concentration are linear (Fig. 3, 5). Considering the dependence of the generation rate of the nitrosothiols on the pH, according to eq. 2, all the nitrosothiols used were prepared at pH 1, and then diluted by 0.1 N HCl (pH 1), or 0.1 M phosphate buffer to obtain pH 7.4.

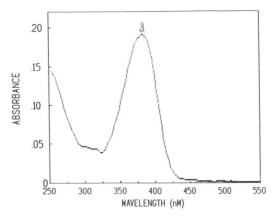

Figure 6: Absorption spectrum of CPM reagent in aqeous solution (7.9 x 10^{-6} M).

For highest sensitivity, optimal fluorescer concentrations were determined. (Table 1). A good correlation (R = 0.9950) is shown between the fluorescence and absorption measurements (Fig. 10).

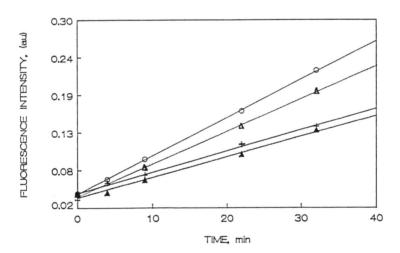

Figure 7: Condensation of CPM with the excess of thiol as recorded by fluorescence at 487nm (excited at 390nm). (+) generation of fluorescence by thermal decomposition of 7.25 x 10^{-7} M CPM at pH 7.0; with (a) [NAC] = [NO] = 10^{-7} M (▲); (b) [NAC] as in (a), [NO] = 2.5 x 10^{-8} M (o); (c) [NAC] as in (a), [NO] = $5x10^{-8}$ M (Δ).

Since the production of the nitrosothiols is a quantitative reaction, linear versus both NO and thiol concentrations, it may be applied also for GLU or GLUNO determinations in tissue and body fluids. The presence of GLUNO in biological systems was recently pointed out by Stamler et al. (1993)

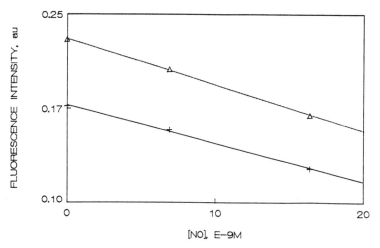

Figure 8: orescence was excited at 390nm and recorded at 487nm. Sampling at 40 min (+) and 57 min
(Δ) after mixing the solutions. NO concentration range: 0.5 - 2.5 x 10^{-8} M.

B) Nitrosothiol levels of 10^{-10} - 10^{-8}M (Biological and atmospheric levels).

For the in situ monitoring of NO levels in biological or atmospheric samples, the more
sensitive "excess thiol back titration" is applied. This back titration must have a resolution
of the order of magnitude of the biological NO levels. The CPM-thiol condensation has
been shown to be a highly accurate method for the quantitative determination of thiols
(Parvari et al., 1983; Yamamoto et al., 1977; Ayers et al., 1986; Sippel, 1981; Odom et
al., 1983). Good resolution in the 0.01-3 nmol concentration range, well below the
biological NO concentrations, were reported.

The fluorescence of the condensation product originates in a coumarin-maleimidyl
derivative that lost the maleimidyl double bond as a result of the condensation process.
However, the loss of this double bound occurs also in a much slower thermal process.
Therefore, the actual fluorescence intensity measured at 487, and excited at 390 nm,
originates in two processes. Fig 7 shows the thermal (+) and the thiol induced generation
of the fluorescent species. When equimolar quantities of NO and thiol are used (o,Δ), i.e.,
in the absence of excess thiol in reaction 1, only the thermal process was observed (Δ).
Considering that nitrosothiol is the possible active species in biological systems
(Kowalukand Fung, 1990; Ignarro et al., 1981; Gaston et al., 1993; Stamler et al., 1992),
this method is superior to the recently published NO detection by chemiluminescence that
has the disadvantages of a) being perturbed by hemoglobin, and b) not having the
necessary sensitivity.

NO determination by applying nitrosothiols is advantageous for the following
reasons: a) the formation of nitrosothiols is not influenced by oxygen, b) it is selective,
only NO among all NO_x compounds reacts with thiols, and c) its generation at
physiological pH values (pH 7.4) occurs from NO only, and not from the nitrite ion
(Gomes and Borges, 1993). The only prerequisite for the present method is the
knowledge of the overall thiol concentration. This, however, is easily determined by the
vast quantity of thiol specific reagents, including CPM (Haughland, 1992-1993).

Both methods are presently applied in our laboratory to various biological systems..
Ultimately, since only two reagents are involved in the process, they will be immobilized
at the tip of an optical fiber, to enable in situ measurements.

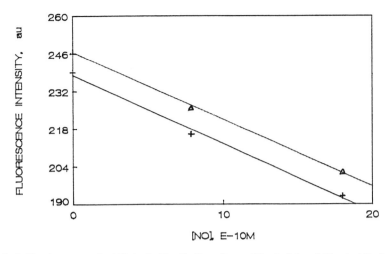

Figure 9: Calibration curves for NO (as in Fig. 8). Sampling at 29 min (+) and 38 min (Δ) after mixing the solutions. NO concentration range: 0 - 25 x 10^{-10} M.

Table 1: Optimal quinine concentrations (Co) for NO determination in various ranges.

Range of NO Conc.		Co
1-10 x 10^{-5} M	1.2 x 10^{-5} M
7.5 x 10^{-7} - 10^{-5} M	0.4- 2 x 10^{-6} M

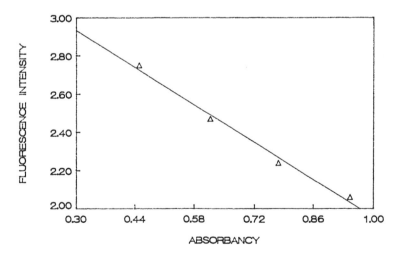

Figure 10: Correlation of fluorescence, excited at 334nm and recorded at 453nm, and absorption at 334nm of the respective stock solutions, R = 0.9950.

REFERENCES

Ayers, F.C., Warner, G.L., Smith, K.L. and Lawrence, D.A., 1986, Fluorometric quantitation of cellular and nonprotein thiols, Anal. Biochem. 154:186-193.

Choi, K.K. and Fung, K.W., 1980, Determination of nitrate and nitrite in meat products by using a nitrate ion-selective electrode, Analyst 105:241-245.

Fontijn, A., Sabadell, J., and Ronco, R.J., 1970, Homogeneous chemiluminescent measurement of nitric oxide with ozone, Anal. Chem. 42:575-579.

Freeman, M.K. and Bachas, L.G., 1992, Fiber optic sensor for NO_x, Anal. Chim. Acta. 256:269-275.

Gabor, G. and Walt, D.R., 1991, Sensitivity enhancement of fluorescent pH indicators by inner filter effects, Anal. Chem. 63:793-796 .

Gaston, B., Reilley, J., Drazen, J.M., Fackler, J., Ramdev, P., Arnelle, D., Mullins, M.E., Sugarbaker, D.J., Chee, C., Singel, D.J., Loscalzo, J., and Stamler, J.S., 1993, Endogenous nitrogen oxides and bronchodilator S-nitrosothiols in human airways. Proc. Nat. Acad. Sci. 90:10957-10961 and ref. quoted therein.

Gomes, M.G. and Borges, S.S., 1993, UV-visible spectrum of nitrous acid in solution: pK_a determination and analytical applications, Anal. Chem. Acta. 282:81-85 and references quoted therein.

Hassan, S.S.M. and Tadros, F.S., 1985, Performance characteristics and some applications of the nitrogen oxide gas sensor, Anal. Chem. 57:162-166.

Haughland, R.P. Molecular Probes 1992-1993

He, H., Li, H., Mohr, G., Kovacs, B., Werner, T., and Wolfbeis, O.S., 1993, Novel type of ion-selective fluorosensor based on inner filter effect: An optrode for potassium, Anal. Chem. 65:123-127.

Ignarro, L.J., Lippton, H., Edwards, J.C., Baricos, W.H., Hyman, A.L., Kadowitz, P.J., and Gruetter, L.A., 1981, Mechanism of vascular smooth muscle relaxation by organic nitrates, nitroprosside and nitric oxide: Evidence for the involvement of S-nitrosothiols as active intermediates, J. Pharmcol. Exp. Ther. 218:739-749.

Kelm, M.A. and Schrader, J., 1990, Control of coronary vascular tone by nitric oxide, Circ. Res. 66:1561-1575.

Kikuchi, K., Nagano, T., Hayakawa, H., Hirata, Y., and Hirobe, M., 1993, Detection of nitric oxide production from a perfused organ by luminol-H_2O_2 system, Anal. Chem. 65:1794-1799.

Kowaluk, E.A. and Fung, H.L.J., 1990, Spontaneous liberation of nitric oxide cannot account for in vivo vascular relaxation by S-nitrosothiols, J. Pharmcol. Exp. Ther. 255:1256-1264.

Maeda, M., Aoki, K., and Munemori, M., 1980, Chemiluminescence method for determination of nitrogen dioxide, Anal. Chem. 52:307-311.

Malinski, T. and Taha, Z., 1992, Nitric oxide release from a single cell measured in situ by a porphyrinic-based microsensor, Nature 358:676.

O'Reilly, S.A., Daunert, S., and Bachas, L.G., 1991, nitrogen oxide gas sensor based on a nitrite-selective electrode, Anal. Chem. 63:1278-1281.

Oae, S., Kim, Y.H., Fukushima, D., and Shinhama, K., 1978, New syntheses of thionitrites and their chemical reactivities, J.C.S. Perkin Trans. I. pp 913-917.

Odom, O.W., Yeng, H., Subramanian, A.R., and Hardesty, B., 1984, Relaxation time, interthiol distance, and mechanism of action of ribosomal protein S1, Arch. Biochem. Biophys. 230:178-193.

Palmer, R.M.J, Ferrige, A.G., and Moncada, S., 1987, Nitric oxide release accounts for the biological activity of endothelium-derived relaxing factor, Nature 327:524-526.

Parvari, R., Pecht, I., and Soreq, H. 1983, A microfluorometric assay for cholinesterases, suitable for multiple kinetic determinations of picomoles of released thiocoline, Anal. Biochem. 133:450-456 and ref. quoted therein.

Shibuki, K., 1990, An electrochemical microprobe for detecting nitric oxide release in brain tissue, Neurosci. Res. 9:69-76.

Sippel, T.O., 1981, New fluorochromes for thiols: Maleimide and iodoacetamide derivatives of a 3-phenylcoumarin fluorophore, J. Histochem. Cytochem. 29:314-316.

Stamler, J.S., Singel, D.J., and Loscalzo, J., 1992, Biochemistry of nitric oxide and its radox-activated forms, Science 258:1898-1902 and references quoted therein .

Stamler, J.S., Simon, D.I., Osborne, S.A., Mullins, M.E., Jaraki, 0., Michel, T., Singel, D.J., and Loscalzo, J., 1992, S-nitrosylation of proteins with nitric oxide: synthesis and characterization of novel biologically active compound, Proc. Natl. Acad. Sci. 89:444-448.

Stuehr, D.J. and Marletta, M.A., 1985, Mammalian nitrate biosynthesis: Mouse macrophages produce nitrite and nitrate in response to Eschrichia coli polypolysachride, Proc. Natl. Acad. Sci. 82:7738-7742.

Walt, D.R., Gabor, G., and Goyet C. 1993, Multiple-indicator fiber-optic sensor for high-resolution pCO_2 sea water measurements, Anal. Chim. Acta . 274 : 47-52

Williams, D.L.H., 1985, S-nitrosation and the reactions of S-nitroso compounds, Chem. Soc. Rev. 14:171-196 and ref. quoted therein.

Yamamoto, K., Sekine, T., and Kanaoka, Y., 1977, Fluorescent thiol reagents, Anal. Biochem, 79:83-94

66

S-NITROSOTHIOLS: CORRELATION OF BIOLOGICAL CHEMISTRY WITH PHYSIOLOGICAL ACTIONS

Jonathan S. Stamler,

Divisions of Respiratory Medicine and Cardiovascular Medicine,
Duke University Medical Center
Durham, NC 27710, USA.

INTRODUCTION

The reactivity of thionitritrites (RS-NOs) has been well-appreciated by synthetic organic chemists since the turn of the twentieth century (1). These compounds have more recently captured the attention of biologists in several different lines of research: the study of the antimicrobial effects of nitrites (2), the biotransformation of organic nitrates (3), and the identification of endothelium derived relaxing factor (EDRF)(4). In each of these areas, S-nitrosothiols have been proposed as biological mediators; yet there is little consensus on their functions. Moreover, the importance of RS-NO in the metabolism of organic nitrates, their role in the prevention of organic nitrate tolerance, and the contribution of RS-NOs to the biological activities of EDRF, remain issues engendering active controversy. Unfortunately, many of these disputes are provoked by erroneous dogma on the mechanism(s) of synthesis, action and decomposition of various RS-NO. These problems are further compounded by extrapolation from the pharmacological effects of exemplary RS-NO such as S-nitroso-cysteine, to the molecular RS-NO class in general.

One way to understand the limitation of such generalizations is to appreciate that thiol containing peptides and proteins can also serve as substrates for S-nitrosylation (5), and thus as major components of the NO-responsive signalling circuitry (6). Indeed, Snitrosylation reactions may serve in the transduction of an NO signal through modulation of signal lifetime or via direct effects on protein function. In this perspective, I review some of the basic chemistry of RS-NO pertinent to biological systems, and present some examples of how this may impact on regulation of NO signal transduction in different systems. In the broadest sense, S-nitrosylation of amino acids, peptides and proteins should be viewed as an integral aspect of redox signalling in cells, a concept which has been addressed in detail elsewhere (6,7).

Biochemical, Pharmacological, and Clinical Aspects of Nitric Oxide
Edited by B. A. Weissman *et al.*, Plenum Press, New York, 1995

67

Stability

RS-NO have been regarded as very short-lived species. Early studies on benzene thionitrite describe an extremely unstable compound (8). Later reports on S-nitroso-cysteine revealed similar instability under physiological conditions (4). Taken together, these data have led to the notion that RS-NO are uniformly unstable. Unfortunately, these exemplary RS-NO are exceptional cases. For example, the short lifetime of S-nitroso-cysteine is an artifact of *in vitro* systems: S-nitroso-cysteine is unusually susceptible to trace metals present in physiological buffers, which facilitate homolytic cleavage of the S-N bond (9,10). This mechanism of decomposition is not operative under more physiological conditions due to the presence of thiols which serve to scavenge trace metals (10). Whereas free copper and iron are in the nanomolar range in many buffers, levels range between 10-12 M and 10-17 M in biological systems. To further confuse matters, buffer constituents influence the lifetime of RS-NO. Thus, half-life determinations may vary quite dramatically in different physiological buffers. In Table 1, I summarize the important factors influencing the stability of RS-NO.

Table 1. Factors Influencing RS-NO Lifetime

1) Transition metals (Cu/Fe)
2) Light
3) Temperature
4) Buffer composition
5) O_2 tension
6) Nucleophiles (i.e. thiols; amines)
7) Redox reactants (i.e. ascorbate)
8) Concentration (of RS-NO)
9) Structure of R group

In Table 2, I provide the half-lives of several commonly used RS-NO under a given set of physiological conditions.

Table 2. Lifetimes of Exemplary RS-NO

RS-NO	SEC-MIN	MIN-HOURS	HOURS-DAYS
S-NO-cysteinylglycine	+		
S-NO-cysteine	+		
S-NO-cysteamine	+		
S-NO-lipoic acid	+		
S-NO-dithiothreitol	+		
S-NO-glutathione		+	
S-NO-penicillamine		+	
S-NO-N-acetyl-penicillamine			+
S-NO-N-acetylcysteine			+
S-NO-albumin			+
S-NO-tissue plasminogen activator	+		
S-NO-cathepsin B	+		

Results apply to most physiologic buffers in the absence of added metal chelators (e.g. EDTA).

Absolute values are less important than the relative lifetimes as compared to other RS-NO under the same conditions. Note that lifetimes range from seconds to many hours.

Decomposition

The contention in the literature is that RS-NO decompose homolytically to yield nitric oxide (NO•) and disulfide

$$2RS\text{-}NO \rightarrow 2NO^\bullet + RSSR$$

However, there is essentially no evidence for the above stoichiometry under physiological conditions. RS-NO can liberate nitric oxide; however, this requires one electron reduction $((NO^+(N^{+3}) \rightarrow NO^\bullet (N^{+2}))$. In physiological systems, candidate one electron reductants include superoxide (O_2^-) and ascorbate; there is also evidence for enzymatic reduction (11,12). The reaction of RS-NO with superoxide is probably not of physiological relevance, since RS-NO coexist with NO• which exibits greater reactivity. Thus, reactions in vivo must be viewed in the context of the relative reactivities of NO•, O_2^- and RS-NO• with other available substrates.

The importance of heterolytic mechanisms of RS-NO decomposition has been underestimated (10). Specifically, RS-NO can decompose either through transfer of the NO group (as NO^+) to other nucleophilic centers, or by liberation NO^- in the specific case of vicinal thiol groups (13). For example, S-nitroso-N-acetyl-penicillamine - a relatively long lived compound - transfers its NO group to glutathione (as NO^+) essentially instantaneously under most physiological conditions.

| Glutathione | S-nitroso-N-acetyl penicillamine | S-nitroso-glutathione | N-acetyl penicillamine |

It can be inferred that an. equilibrium will exist between thiols and S-nitrosothiols in biological systems. The equilibrium will be dictated by thiol concentration and reactivity, the latter a function of thiol pKa. The relationship is somewhat complex. Thiols with higher pKa's tend to be more reactive; however, nitrosation is sustained by the thiolate anion (RS^-). It is therefore difficult empirically to predict the equilibrium between a given RSH and R'SNO in a biological millieu.

The mechanism of decomposition of S-nitroso-dithiols is dictated by thiol proximity (13). Where thiols are in close proximity (1,4 or less), the respective thionitrites are very unstable:

disulfide formation is accelerated due to the high effective thiol molarity. This is rationalized by the existence of a thionitrite resonance form in which the sulfur is positively charged making it susceptible to nucleophilic attack by adjacent thiolate ($RSN=O \Leftrightarrow RS^+-N-O^-$)(6). NO^- is liberated in the process. Interestingly, many proteins depend on reversible oxidation-reduction of vicinal thiols for control of function. Examples of such regulation through S-nitrosylation are given below. It should be implicit from these data that caution is warrented before attributing the effects of RS-NO to nitric oxide itself.

Transport

The notion of a transport function for RS-NO arises from the finding that S-nitroso-albumin is prevalent plasma (14,15). My own interpretation of these data is that albumin, the predominant source of thiol in plasma (~ 600 μM), serves a buffer-like function in regulating steady levels of NO and amino acid RS-NO in the nanomolar range. Thus, while S-nitroso-albumin exists as a circulating pool, it is unlikely to play a major role in transport of NO from one site in the body to another. However, with local changes in redox state or availability of reactants, as may occur in organ disease, albumin might well modulate the local NO response. Specifically, levels of several redox factors - O_2^-, ascobate and thiols in particular - are tightly coupled to RS-NO liftime. It follows that RS-NO may be more reactive than free nitric oxide in the face of challenge by ambient nucleophiles and/or related redox active species.

S-nitroso-albumin has provided additional insights into the intermediary metabolism of NO in vivo. The obvious question that arises is how a large impermeable macromolecule causes vasorelaxation and platelet inhibition when this requires activation of intracellular guanylate cyclase. Answers to this apparent paradox can be gleaned from in vitro mechanisms of RS-NO decomposition. These studies indicate that heterolytic transfer of NO^+ from albumin to low molecular weight thiols is easily accomplished (14,16). Evidence for such NO group transfer from albumin to cysteine and to other nucleophilic centers on the the plasma membrane of cells has been recently demonstrated *in vitro* and *in vivo*. (17,18,19). Whether NO is then transported into the cell or is releasesd at the cell surface through reductive activation of RS-NO, remains to be determined. Either pathway would allow for activation of guanylate c,vclase. Signalling by RS-NO can also be initiated at the level of the cell membrane (6,7,18).

Targeting

Nitric oxide reacts in biological systems with oxygen (O_2), superoxide and transition metals (6,20). In the broadest sense, these are the biological targets of nitric oxide. In contrast, RS-NO tend to react with nucleophiles (10). The most abundant and reactive nucleophile in biological systems is thiolate anion (RS^-), hence the propensity for RS-NO to target thiol centers (6). Nevertheless, RS-NO have the added capability of targeting transition metals, as $NO^\bullet$ can be released in physiologic systems. Thus, homolytic fission of RS-NO facilitates reactions with metal centers, whereas heterolytic mechanisms of decomposition facilitate interactions with thiols. Accordingly, RS-NO responsive targets contain either metals or thiols strategically located at either allosteric or active sites. In some biologic responses, interactions with both metal and thiol targets act in concert to support the NO mediated response. For example, smooth muscle relaxation by NO/RSNO is mediated by interactions with both the heme center of guanylate cyclase and a thiol domain of a calcium dependent potassium channel (21). In this context, it is important to appreciate that NO- itself does not interact with -hence cannot control - thiol-dependent systems. Thus, low molecular weight thiols and thiol-containing proteins function in appropriate channeling of the NO group, and thereby serve as integral components of NO-responsive signalling pathways.

Protection

Nitric oxide is highly susceptible to inactivation by O_2 and superoxide. Moreover, the products of these reactions - NO_x and peroxynitrite ($OONO^-$) - are believed to account for much of the toxicity of $NO^\bullet$ in cellular systems. Studies indicate that RS-NO are relatively resistant to reactions with O_2 and O_2^- At the same time, these compounds retain NO-like bioactivity. Thus, the formation of RS-NO may be viewed as part of the homeostatic mechanism designed to maintain NO -responsive control in states of oxidant stress.

We have observed that O_2^- may interact with RS-NO, yielding $NO^\bullet$. Since $NO^\bullet$ reacts rapidly with superoxide, peroxynitrite is formed in the process. The question arises whether this reaction, and the potential toxicological implications of peroxynitrite production (22), have physiological relevance. Counter-arguments to this assertion have been alluded to. In particular, one must view this reaction in the context of relative reactivities of NO, O_2^- and RS-NO. When compared with nitric oxide, RS-NO are less reactive Furthermore, the reaction mechanism predicts the rate law to be second order in $[O_2^-]$ for RS-NO, and first order in $[O_2^-]$ with nitric oxide.

Matters are made all the more complex by competing reactions of thiol with superoxide, related reactive oxygen intermediates and $OONO^-$ itself. Furthermore, reactions of $OONO^-$ with thiol may represent an important route of RS-NO formation in biological systems (23,24). Studies *in vivo* support this contention: oxidant stress favors formation of RS-NO (25) suggesting that this pathway is an important component of the cell's antioxidant arsenal.

Regulation

Covalent attachment of the NO group to sulfhydryl residues on proteins can modulate protein function through several discrete mechanisms (6): 1) by conferring novel NO-like bioactivities to the protein; 2) by inducing structural changes that serve as a switching mechanism; 3) by blockade of active site thiols resulting in functional attenuation; and 4) by conferring new reactivit,v to the protein. I will provide a few representative examples of proteins for which some aspects of the effects of S-nitrosylation on structure and biological function are known.

1. Conferred NO-like activity

S-nitrosylation endows proteins with extended NO-like activities: the ability to relax blood vessels, dilate airways, attenuate microbial growth and inhibit platelet aggregation (5,10,17,19). These conferred activities may have a variety of physiological functions. For example, the antiplatelet properties of the S-nitrosoalbumin reservoir in plasma may participate in the normal antithrombotic hemostatic mechanism that serves to maintain vessel patency. Alternatively, the accumulation of S-nitroso-proteins in the airways of patients with bronchopneumonia (25), due to the impairment of alveolar-capillary membrane integrity, may serve to limit the airway hyperresponsiveness incurred with inflammation. RS-NO may also function to attentuate the local inflammatory process by virtue of their antioxidant and antimicrobial properties (25,26). The effects of other S-nitrosoproteins can be quite selective. For example, the formation of S-nitroso-tissue plasminogen activator (SNO-t-PA) may provide a mechanism of selectively delivering and concentrating NO in areas of thrombus formation, at which sites a deficit of EDRF is likely to exist. Specifically, endogenous thrombolysis is achieved through endothelial elaboration of t-PA (fibrinolysis) and NO (platelet dispersal), under which conditions S-nitrosylation of t-PA is readily achieved. Because of its relative fibrin specificity, i.e. t-PA exhibits greatly enhanced enzymatic activity in the presence of fibrin, the actions of S-NO-tPA are localized to the fibrin clot (27). Notwithstanding the importance of this targeting mechanism, S-nitrosylation also modestly enhances the catalytic activity of the enzyme and confers on t-PA potentially important vasodilatory and antiplatelet properties (27). Thus, S-nitrosylation of proteins may contribute to a diversity of control mechanisms that function in achieving system-specific homeostasis.

2. *Conformational changes*

S-nitrosylation of proteins can increase protein activity, and/or serve as part of a functional switching mechanism (26). Analogy to phosphorylation is noteworthy: structural changes in proteins are induced by covalent attachment of a chemical group. The molecular basis for conformational changes induced by S-nitrosylation (NO group attachment) may result from one of several mechanisms: disruption of hydrogen bonding, interference with intramolecular ionic interactions of the SH group, or the potentiation of disulfide formation (6). The last mechanism is operative in the case of vicinal thiols: the high effective molarity of adjacent thiols drives the formation of disulfide, an effect which is in large part entropic (see above discussion) (6,13). Thus, the formation of disulfide serves as the switching mechanism. Systems or biochemical processes known to be regulated by NO in this manner include excitatory neurotransmission through the NMDA subtype of glutamate receptor (18), protein kinase signalling in cytokine-activated macrophages (28), type I adenylate cyclase activation in hippocampal tissues (29) and endothelium dependent relaxations mediated through a calcium dependent potassium channel (21).

S-nitrosylation of isolated thiols on proteins such as t-PA, G proteins and p21[ras], induces an activation-associated conformational change that is best rationalized by disruption of intramolecular thiol interactions (6). The ramifications for t-PA include a modest increase in enzymatic (amidolytic) activity, without alterations in fibrin(ogen) binding affinity or the Ki of its cognate serine protease inhibitor, plaminogen activator inhibitor-1 (27). S-nitrosylation-stimulated increases in enzymatic activity are most evident at low substrate concentrations in the presence of fibrin(ogen), suggesting that NO induces a structural change in either t-PA or the t-PA/fibrin complex, that promotes the interaction with plasminogen.

G proteins are fundemental components of cell signalling networks and p21[ras] is a key protein in biochemical pathways triggered by ligand bound cell surface receptor tyrosine kinases. Their activation by NO (30) may therefore have diverse physiological consequences. S-nitrosylation increases the rate limiting step in G protein activation, namely, GTP-GDP exchange (Lander, personal communication). Thus NO (NO^+) appears to mimic the actions of guanine nucleotide exchange factors.

3. *Functional inhibition*

When proteins contain thiols at their active sites, S-nitrosylation indiscriminately inhibits their activities. This has been demonstrated for numerous proteins of different classes (6,10). The reason for inactivation by S-nitrosylation is that the NO group tends to decrease the nucleophilicity of the sulfur: The order of sulfhydryl reactivity is $S^- > SH > S-NO$. Thus, NO-for-proton exchange may be viewed as a reversible mechanism of thiol deactivation .

4. Altered reactivity

S-Nitrosothiols have been shown recently to support reactions with nucleotides (23,31). This had been first interpreted as an ADP-ribosylation reaction: a covalent modification in which the ADP-ribose moiety of NAD is transferred to a cysteine residue. The presumtion being that the NO group is displaced in the process. More recent data indicate that this reaction is neither a true ADP-ribosylation nor supported by NAD^+. Rather, it is NADH that is probably involved in this modification (6). The reduced nicotinamide is susceptible to nitrosative attack, thereby activating the ring. This in turn facilitates thiolation. Accordingly, where NAD^+/NADH binding sites on proteins are present in close proximit,v to active site RS-NO (as in the prototypic enzyme glyceraldehyde-3-phosphate dehydrogenase) the ring becomes susceptible to nucleophilic attack by active site thiolate. This leads to a linkage between the thiolate and nicotinamide ring.

Noteably, NAD^+ appears to support the reaction, albeit less effeciently. This is likely explained by the requirement for added thiol, which can react with nicotinamide (attack at C4) to give the dihydro (NADH) eqivalent.

An alternative mechanism, in which thioate attack occurs on the C-1 position of the ribose (of NADH), may also be operative in certain proteins if steric constraints are not limiting. This reaction could be viewed as an ADP-ribosylation.

NADH

Toxicity

There are three physiological systems in which evidence supports a protective function for RS-NO against nitric oxide-related toxicity: The gastrointestinal tract in which the acidic pH is uniquely conducive to formation of carcinogenic nitrosoamines; the lung, where NO has been viewed as an atmospheric pollutant and toxic contaminant of cigarette smoke; and the cardiovascular system, where RS-NO may attenuate the atherogenic potential of aminothiols cysteine and homocysteine.

G.I. tract. The mutagenicity of nitrosoamines and related deamination reactions of DNA have resulted in active efforts by the food industry to establish mechanisms of limiting their production. Several groups, active during the 70's and 80's, reported on the protective effects of thiols (reviewed in 20, reference 32). The greater reactivity (and natural abundence) of thiol over amine allow it to compete well in nitrosation reactions (20). RSNO form in the process. More recent studies demonstrate that thiols such as glutathione attenuate N-nitrosation reactions in cell systems challenged by inflammatory cytokines (32).

Lung. An extensive literature implicates nitric oxide, nitrogen dioxide (NO_2) and peroxynitrite in lung injury (33). There is additional concern that the metabolism of NO in the oxgen rich millieu of the lung, may lead to the formation of nitrosamines. Indeed, animal studies reveal that certain NO_x promote growth of lung tumors (33). Most recently, Mercer and colleagues, showed that low levels of nitric oxide administered over several weeks cause atrophic interstitial changes in the lung, characteristic of early emphysema (34). Moreover, the more reactive NO_2 species has a distinct injury profile, causing pulmonary fibrosis (34). Taken with studies showing that the NO_x content of smoke correlates well with its cytotoxicity, the histopathology of individual NO_x appear to provide insight into a diversity of lung diseases (35).

Since most cells in the lung have the capacity to produce NO (33) - the airway epithelium being one of the most productive cells identified to date - the relevant issue becomes one of understanding how cells take measures to defend against NO• mediated injury. Analysis of airway lining fluid from normal subjects indicate that RS-NO, largely the adduct with glutathione, are present at high nanomolar concentrations (25). Levels of RSNO increase significantly in patients with inflammatory lung disease and form in very high concentrations upon administration of NO-gas (25). Lavage concentrations of NO_2^-, and other metal-nitrosyl complexes do not correlate well with the presence of lung disease (25). Taken with the findings that RS-NO• are more potent and long-lived relaxants of human airways than NO•, these observations suggest a central role for RS-NO in regulation of airway luminal homeostasis. An attractive and unifying concept is that RS-NO serve to preserve the bioactivity of NO• while simultaneously limiting its potential oxygen-dependent toxicity.

Cardiovascular. The formation of RS-NO has been proposed as a mechanism of limiting the adverse vascular effects of homocysteine (35). Elevated levels of homocysteine are an independent risk factor for atherosclerosis and are also associated with a wide variety of thrombotic complications. Oxidized products of homocysteine (homocystine, homocysteine thiolactone and homocysteic acid, cumulatively referred to as homocyst(e)ine) may further increase the homocysteine-related burden (36). Notwithstanding, the diversity of mechanisms by which homocysteine may exert its atherothrombotic potential, the reactivity of the SH group is believed to be of central importance (35). Thiol-mediated production of H_2O_2 results in endothelial damage, in turn leading to a prothrombotic and atherogenic diathesis (37).

Atherogenic effects of homocysteine can take many years to manifest. It is therefore of interest that short exposures of homocysteine to endothelial cells results in formation of S-nitroso-homocysteine. The biological actions and metabolism of this compound are remarkably different from those of the free thiol. Specifically, S-NO-homocysteine is a potent antiplatelet agent and vasodilator (35). Moreover, S-NO-homocysteine does not generate H_2O_2 species or undergo oxidative conversion to homocysteine disulfide and homocysteine thiolactone. These data then suggest that NO can modulate the pathogenicity of homocysteine through attenuation of thiol reactivity.

The notion that an NO-to-free thiol index may provide a more accurate measure of the pathogenic potential of homocysteine than the absolute level of thiol excess deserves consideration. Defined as such, hypohomocystenemia may indicate a relative deficiency of NO (as a result of endothelial injury)(35). The mechanism of hyperhomocysteneimia, notwithstanding, the resultant endothelial damage would predictably embarrasse. NO production and consequently, set a cycle in motion in which the antithrombotic cytoprotective mechanisms of S-nitrosation are increasingly compromised at the expense of a predisposition to atherosclerosis and thrombosis (35). One may further speculate that the cytoprotective mechanism of S-nitrosation may play a more general role in modulating the atherogenicity of other sulfur-containing amino acids. In particular, evidence has accumulated implicating cysteine in the oxidation of LDL, which enhances its uptake via the scavenger receptor (38). This pathway represents the molecular correlate of foam cell formation. S-nitroso-cysteine may be 'risk adverse' since nitrosation attenuates its oxidant potential (J.S.S. unpublished observations). In this context, it is interesting to note the controversy over the identity of EDRF, which centers around S-nitroso-cysteine (4). As discussed below, several S-nitrosothiols - S-NO-homocysteine included - likely contribute to this activity.

Physiology

EDRF (exemplary of bioactivty in physiological systems; reference 39 contains certain original aspects of this discussion).

There has been a fair amount of controversy over the identity of EDRF. Much of this dispute is centered on the question of whether EDRF is NO itself or a closely related adduct thereof such as a nitrosothiol. Reflection on these studies suggests that the apparent controversy may be largely explained by differences in methodology, as the identity of EDRF appears to be critically dependent on assay conditions. This can be understood best by appreciating that one of the most distinctive features of NO• is its chemical reactivity. Indeed, it is the intrinsic reactivity of NO•, resulting in formation of surrogates possessing similar bioactivity, which has lead to this dispute. Thus, many contradictory results can be explained by the availability of reactants: in systems where thiol is limiting (e.g. in vitro bioassays) the bioactivity of the system exists mainly in the form of free NO•. However, when thiol is present at physiological concentrations the activity of EDRF is potentiated through formation of RS-NO (40-42). Since biological systems contain millimolar concentrations of thiol there is a natural predisposition for RS-NO to form. One may therefore conclude, that an equilibrium likely exists between NO• and RS-NO in biological systems that will be influenced by redox state.

Most studies on the identity of EDRF have relied largely on pharmacological tools rather than true chemical identification of species. The limited understanding of the biometabolism of RS-NO has further confused matters. For example, lifetime determinations, as assessed by bioactivity of molecular candidates (NO•, X-NO), are often compared with that of authentic EDRF. However, such comparisons assume that EDRF is generally resistant to minor changes in redox state and availability of reactants. Unfortunately, this is not the case: artifactual contamination of systems with redox metals, and dramatic changes in the lifetime of selected RS-NO with very minor changes in pH or buffer composition, make such comparisons almost impossible to interpret. Notwithstanding such limitations, recent evidence strongly indicates that the bioactivity of EDRF cannot be accounted for solely by nitric oxide. First, NO• is relatively impotent at relaxing resistence arterioles, the major site at which EDRF exerts its action (43), and second, EDRF has been shown to activate a potassium channel through interactions with a thiol containing domain (21). Because reactions with thiol groups involve an NO^+ moiety (or some higher oxide of nitrogen) this activity cannot be attributed to NO•. In contrast, RS-NO are excellent candidates for such regulation through sulfhydryl centers. Other plausible explanations for these data include: 1) reaction of NO• with superoxide at the membrane to form OONO, which in turn modifies the channel's thiol; or alternatively, 2) the presence of a high steady state level of NO• in the membrane which facilitates an otherwise slow reaction with oxygen. NO_x that form in the membrane could then nitrosylate the potassium channel.

One may conclude that RS-NO are likely to play an important role in control of vasomotor tone by EDRF. The reasoning used here, morever, can be extrapolated to other physiological systems. Thus, bioactivity in physiological systems will exist in the form of NO• and its related adducts, the equilibrium dictated by both availability of reactants (thiol and metals) as well as ambient redox state.

Acknowledgment: JSS is a Pew Scholar in the Biomedical Sciences and the recipient of a Clinical Investigator Award from the National Institutes of Health (HL 02582-01). This work is also funded by a grant from the NIH (HL52529)

REFERENCE

1. Oae S, Shinhama K (1983) Organic thionitrites and related substances. Organic Preparations and Procedures 15:165-198.
2. Morris SL, Hansen JN (1981) Inhibition of Bacillus cereus spore outgrowth by covalent modifications of a sulfhydryl group by nitrosothiol and iodoacetate. J Bacteriol 148:465-471.
3. Ignarro LJ, Lippton H, Edwards JC, Baricos WH, Hyman AL, Kadowitz PH, Gruetter CA (1981) Mechanism of vascular smooth muscle relaxation by organic nitrates, nitrites, nitroprusside and nitric oxide: Evidence for the involvement of S-nitrosothiols as active intermediates. J Pharm Exp Ther 218:739-749.
4. Myers PR, Minor RL, Guerra R, Bates JN, Harrison DG (1990) Vasorelaxant properties of the endothelium-derived relaxing factor more closely resemble Snitrosocysteine than nitric oxide. Nature; 345:161-163.
5. Stamler JS, Simon DI, Osborne JA, Mullins ME, Jaraki O, Michel T, Singel DJ, Loscalzo J (1992) S-nitrosylation of proteins with nitric oxide: Synthesis and characterization of biologically active compounds. Proc Natl Acad Sci USA 89:444-448.
6. Stamler JS (1994) Redox signalling: nitrosylation and related target interactions of nitric oxide. Cell 78:14-20.
7. Crapo J, Stamler JS (1994) Signalling by non-receptor surface-mediated redox-active biomolecules. J Clin Invest 93:2304.

8. Tasker HS, Jones HQ (1909) The action of mercaptans on acid chlorides Part II. The acid chlorides of phosphorous, sulfur and nitrogen. J Chem Soc 95:1910.

9. McNainly J, Williams DLH (1993) Fate of nitric oxide from the decomposition of S-nitrosothiols. Endothelium, 1:141A.

10. Stamler JS (1994) S-nitrosothiols and the bioregulatory actions of nitrogen oxides through reactions with sulfhydryl groups. Current Topics in Microbiology and Immunology (in press).

11. Kowaluk EA, Fung HL (1990) Spontaneous liberation of nitric oxide cannot account for in vitro vascular relaxation by S-nitrosothiols. J Pharmacol Exp Ther 255:1256-1264.

12. Radomski MW, Rees DD, Durta A, Moncada S (1993) S-nitroso-glutathione inhibits platelet activation in vitro and in vivo. Br J Pharmacol 107:745-749.

13. Arnelle DP, Stamler JS (1994) Liberation of NO^+, $NO^{\bullet}$ and NO^- from thionitrites: Implications for regulation of physiological functions by S-nitrosylation and acceleration of disulfide formation. Archiv Biochem Biophys (submitted).

14. Stamler JS, Jaraki O, Osborne, J, Simon DI, Keaney J, Vita J, Singel D, Valeria RC (1992) Nitric oxide circulates in mammalian plasma primarily as an S-nitroso adduct of serum albumin. Proc Natl Acad Sci USA 89:7674-7677.

15. Stamler JS, Loh E, Roddy MA, Currie KE, Creager MA (1993) Nitric oxide regulates basal systemic and pulmonary vascular resistance in healthy humans. Circulation 89: 2035-2040.

16. Scharfstein JS, Kearney JF, Slivka A, Welch GN, Vita JA, Stamler JS, Loscalzo J (1994) In vivo transfer of NO between a plasma protein-bound reservoir and low-molecular-weight thiol. J Clin Invest (in press).

17. Simon DI, Stamler JS, Jaraki O, Keaney J, Osborne JA, Francis SA, Singel DJ, Loscalzo J (1993) Antiplatelet properties of protein S-nitrosothiols derived from nitric oxide and endothelium-derived relaxing factor. Arterioscler and Thrombosis 13:791-799.

18. Lipton SA, Choi YB, Pan ZH, Lei SZ, Vincent Chen HS, Sucher NJ, Loscalzo J, Singel DJ, Stamler JS (1993) A redox-based mechanism for the neuroprotective and neurodestructive effects of nitric oxide and related nitroso-compounds. Nature 364:626-632.

19. Gaston B, Drazen JM, Jansen A, Sugarbaker DJ, Loscalzo J, Richards W, Stamler JS (1994) Relaxation of human bronchial smooth muscle by S-nitrosothiols in vitro. J Pharm Exp Ther. 268:976-984.

20. Stamler JS, Singel D, Loscalzo J (1992) Biochemistry of nitric oxide and its redox activated forms. Science 258:1898-1902.

21. Bolotina VM, Najibi S, Palacino JJ, Pagano PJ, and Cohen RA (1994) Nitric oxide directly activates calcium-dependent potassium channels in vascular smooth muscle. Nature 368, 850-853.

22. Beckman JS, Beckman TW, Chen J, Marshall PA, Freeman BA (1990) Apparent hydroxyl radical production by peroxynitrite: implications for endothelial injury from nitric oxide and superoxide. Proc Natl Acad Sci, USA 87:1620-1624.

23. Mohr S, Stamler JS, and Brune B (1994) Mechanism of covalent modification of glyceraldehyde-3-phosphate dehydrogenase at its active site thiol by nitric oxide, peroxynitrite and related nitrosating agents. FEBS Lett. 348, 223-227.

24. Wu M, Kaminski PM, Fayngersh RP, Groszek LL, Pritchard KA, Kintze TH, Stemerman MB, Wolin MS (1994) Peroxynitrite induces vascular relaxation vai nitric oxide. Am J. Physiol 35: H2108-H2113.

25. Gaston B, Reilly J, Drazen JM, Fackler J, Ramdev P, Arnelle D, Mullins ME, Sugarbaker DJ, Chee C, Singel DJ, Loscalzo J, and Stamler JS (1993) Endogenous bronchodilator S-nitrosothiols in human air~vays. Proc Natl Acad Sci USA 90, 1095710961.

26. Rockett KA, Auburn MM, Lowden WB, Clark IA (1991). Killing of plasmodium falciparum in vivo by nitric oxide derivatives. Infection and Immunity 59: 3280-3283.

27. Stamler JS, Simon DI, Jaraki O, Osborne JA, Francis S, Mullins M, Singel D, and Loscalzo J (1992) S-nitrosylation of tissue-type plasminogen activator confers vasodilatory and antiplatelet properties on the enzyme. Proc Natl Acad Sci USA 89: 8087-8091.

28. Gopalakrishna R, Chen ZH, and Gundimeda V (1993) Nitric oxide and nitric oxidegenerating agents induce a reversible inactivation of protein kinase C activity and phorbol ester binding. J Biol Chem 268, 27180-27185.

29. Duhe RJ, Nielsen MD, Dittman AH, Villacres EC, Chol EJ, and Storm JR (1994). Oxidation of critical cysteine residues of type I adenylyl cyclase by o-Iodosobenzoate or nitric oxide reversibly inhibits stimulation by calcium and calmodulin. J Biol Chem 269: 7290-7296.

30. Lander HM, Sehajpal PK, and Novogrodsyk A. (1993) Nitric oxide signaling: a possible role for G proteins. Immunology 151: 7182-7187.

31. Brune B., Dimmler S, Molina y Vedia L, and Lapatina EG (1994) Nitric oxide: a signal for ADP ribosylation of proteins. Life Sci. 54, 61-70.

32. Grisham MB, Ware K, Gilleland HE, Gilleland LB, Abell CL, Yamada T. (1992) Neutrophil-mediated nitrosamine formation: Role of nitric oxide in rats. Gastroenterology: 103: 1260-1266.
33. Gaston B, Drazen JM, Loscalzo J, Stamler JS (1994) The biology of nitrogen oxides in the airways. State-of-the-Art. Am J Resp Critical Care Med Dis, 149:538-551.
34. Mercer RR, Costa DL, Crapo JD (1993). Alveolar septal injury from low level exposures to nitric oxide (abstract) Am Rev Respir Dis 147:A385.
35. Stamler JS, Osborne JA, Jaraki O, Rabbani LE, Mullins M, Singel D, Loscalzo J (1993) Adverse effects of homocysteine are modulated by endothelium-derived relaxing factor and related oxides of nitrogen. J Clin Invest 1:308-318.
36. Malino MR (1990) Hyperhomocyst(e)iremia: a common and easily reversible risk factor for occlusive atherosclerosis. Circulation 81:2004-2006.
37. Starkebaum G and Harlan JM (1986) Endothelial cell injury due to copper-catalyzed hydrogen peroxide generation from homocysteine. J Clin Invest 77:1370-1376.
38. Heinecke J, Rosen WH, Suzuki LA, Chait A (1987) The role of sulfur-containing aninocaids in superoxide production and modification of low density lipoprotein by arterial smooth muscle. J. Biol. Chem 262:10098-10103.
39. Stamler JS, Mendelsohn ME, Amarante P, Smick D, Andon N, Davies PF, Cooke JPl, and Loscalzo J (1989) N-acetylcysteine potentiates platelet inhibition by endotheliumderived relaxing factor. Circ Res 65:789-795.
40. Cooke JS, Stamler JS, Andon N, Davies PF, Loscalzo J (1990) Flow stimulates endothelial cells to release a nitrovasodilator that is potentiated by reduced thiol. Am J Physiol 28:H804-H812.
41. Feelisch M, TePoel M, Zamora R, Oeussen A, Moncada S (1994) Understanding the controversy over the identity of EDRF. Nature 368: 62-65.
42. Selke FW, Myers PR, Bates JN, Harrison DG (1990) Am J Physiol (Heart Circ Physiol) 258:H515-H520).

INITIAL CLINICAL EXPERIENCE WITH THE INTRACAVERNOUS APPLICATION OF THE NITRIC OXIDE DONOR SIN 1 IN THE TREATMENT OF PATIENTS WITH ERECTILE DYSFUNCTION

Michael C. Truss, Armin J. Becker, Christian G. Stief, and Udo Jonas

Department of Urology
Medizinische Hochschule Hannover
30623 Hannover, FRG

INTRODUCTION

Penile erection requires a series of events that includes cavernous and vascular smooth muscle relaxation, increased arterial inflow and subsequent venous outflow restriction. Recent work suggests that the initial step, cavernous and vascular smooth muscle relaxation, is mediated by the synthesis and release of nitric oxide from nerves innervating vascular and cavernous smooth muscles (Ignarro et al., 1990; Holmquist et al., 1991; Rajfer et al., 1992; Burnett et al., 1992). Therefore, the use of the L-arginine/nitric oxide pathway seems to be a possible approach in the treatment of erectile dysfunction. Linsidomine chlorhydrate (SIN-1, Corvasal intracoronaire®), the active hepatic metabolite of molsidomine (N-ethoxycarbomyl-3-morpholino- sydninimine), is believed to liberate nitric oxide nonenzymatically (nitric oxide donor). Theoretically, a nitric oxide donor may be superior to other vasoactive drugs because it may resemble more closely the physiologic sequence of events in penile erection. Our preliminary results with the intracavernous application of SIN-1 suggested a possible role in the treatment of patients with erectile dysfunction (Stief et al., 1992). We now report our extended follow up with SIN-1 in the diagnosis and treatment of patients with erectile dysfunction.

PATIENTS AND METHODS

All patients underwent a comprehensive and standardized work up for erectile dysfunction including a detailed case history, physical examination, sexual case history (questionaire), routine blood tests, pharmaco-Doppler ultrasound, corpus cavernosum electromyogram (Stief et al., 1990) and pharmacotesting. Where indicated, pharmacocavernosometry and -graphy was carried out (12 patients).

Biochemical, Pharmacological, and Clinical Aspects of Nitric Oxide
Edited by B. A. Weissman *et al.*, Plenum Press, New York, 1995

79

All 113 patients (8 patients with primary and 105 patients with secondary impotence) and 10 normal control subjects received 1 mg SIN-1 intracavernously. 71/113 patients (62.8%) received additional, at least 3, injections of a mixture of papaverine (15mg/ml) and phentolamine (0.5mg/ml) prior to pharmacotesting with SIN-1. Increasing doses of 0.25 - 2.0 ml were given according to the erectile response. All injections were given in a supine position. Responses to papaverine/phentolamine and SIN-1 were evaluated by a urologist after 10, 20 and 30 minutes by inspection and palpation and graded as follows: E 0 - no response, E 1 - slight tumescence, E 2 - medium tumescence, E 3 - full tumescence but no rigidity, E 4 - full tumescence with medium rigidity, sufficient for intercourse, E 5 - full rigid erection.

48 SIN- 1 responders entered an autoinjection program with SIN-1. All patients were seen as outpatients after the first 10 injections and thereafter following each series of 25 injections. At follow up visits a history and physical examination and routine blood tests were undertaken.

All patients as well as the normal control subjects were extensively informed of the study and the possible side effects (prolonged erections, cavernous fibrosis, infection, cavernous necrosis, systemic side effects such as hypotension). Written consent was obtained from all participants. The study was approved by the Ethics committee of the Medizinische Hochschule Hannover.

RESULTS

The mean patient age was 48.9 ± 11.9 years. Erectile dysfunction was prevalent since 56 ± 27.9 months. The mean age of the volunteers (control subjects with normal erectile function) was 34 ± 8.4 years. The patients past medical histories included nicotine abuse (25 patients), peripheral vascular disease (21 patients), hypertension (17 patients), diabetes (17 patients), hyperlipidemia (12 patients), pelvic trauma (9 patients) and alcohol abuse (6 patients). In 27 patients the medical history was not contributory.

Following intracavernous administration of SIN-1, all normal control subjects had full rigid erections (E 5) lasting 40-70 minutes which spontaneously resolved. No complications or side effects such as penile pain, hemmorrhage, infection or prolonged erections occurred. Of the patients with erectile dysfunction 40 had E 5, 38 E 4, 20 E 3, 14 E 2 and 1 E1 responses to intracavernous SIN-1 pharmacotesting. Again, no side effects were noted.

Electromyographic patterns in patients responding with E 4 and E 5 erections to SIN-1 (32 normal, 40 pathologic) did not differ significantly from patients responding with E 1 to E 3 erections (18 normal, 23 pathologic). With respect to risk factors no differences were found between responders and nonresponders except in patients following pelvic trauma and patients with primary erectile dysfunction. All 9 patients after pelvic trauma (mean age 30.8 ± 6.2 years) and all 8 patients with primary erectile dysfunction (mean age 35.6 ± 9.6 years) responded to SIN-1 with E 4 or E 5 erections. 9 of 12 patients (75%) who underwent pharmacocavernosomety and -graphy for suspected venous leakage, did not achieve erections sufficient for intercourse (E 1-3, mean age 56.3 ± 7.6 years).

71/113 patients (62.8%) also underwent pharmacotesting with increasing doses of a mixture of papaverine (15 mg/ml) and phentolamine (1 mg/ml). 64/71 patients (90.1%) had E 4 or E 5 erections, including all patients who showed adequate response to SIN-1 and 20/27 patients (74.1%) who failed. Mean doses of papaverine/phentolamine in responders and nonresponders to SIN-1 were 0.6 ± 0.3 ml and 1.5 ± 0.5 ml, respectively (p < 0.0001, student's t-test). 6/44 SIN-1 responders (13.6%) and 1/27 SIN-1 nonresponders (4%) experienced prolonged erections > 240 minutes with papaverine/phentolamine.

48 SIN-1 responders performed a total of 1160 self-injections (10-150 injections/patient, mean 24.1), no complications such as penile pain, fibrosis, infection or prolonged erections were noted. All patients with the exception of 3 (93.75%) were satisfied with their response to SIN-1. 3 patients withdrew from the study because the quality of the erectile responses to SIN-1 decreased.

DISCUSSION

Recently, nitric oxide has been identified as a mediator of cavernous smooth muscle relaxation and penile erection in vitro and in vivo (Ignarro et al., 1990; Holmquist et al., 1991; Rajfer et al., 1992; Burnett et al., 1992). Nitric oxide is synthesized from L-arginine by nitric oxide synthase (NOS); it acts on guanylate cyclase activation which subsequently leads to an intracellular increase of cyclic guanosine 3´, 5´monophosphate (cGMP) (Ignarro et al., 1990). The intracellular receptor for cGMP is cGMP dependent proteinkinase G (PKG) which is believed to phosphorylate ion channels causing intracellular calcium depletion and smooth muscle relaxation.

SIN-1 is a drug approved for the treatment of coronary spasms and for angiography of coronary arteries. It is believed to liberate nitric oxide nonenzymatically. The recommended dosage for angiography is 0.4 - 1 mg. Since our initial data showed a dose dependent response to SIN-1 with more favourable results with 1 mg (Stief et al., 1992), all subsequent patients received 1 mg.

In our present series 35 of 113 patients (31%) failed to respond with erections sufficient for intercourse. In our initial report (Stief et al., 1992) only 21 % failed, thus, our present data are somewhat less favourable. This may be attributed to the higher percentage of patients with assumed neurogenic erectile dysfunction in our first 63 patients, since patients with predominantly neurogenic impotence, i.e. diabetics and patients after pelvic trauma, tend to respond better to intracavernous pharmacotherapy (Jünemann 1991).

The fact that nonresponders to SIN-1 showed a tendency towards multiple risk factors and 20 of 27 nonresponders (74.1%) achieved erections sufficient for intercourse with papaverine/phentolamine indicates that papaverine/phentolamine may be preferable to SIN-1 in patients with a multifactorial origin of erectile dysfunction, i.e. patients with significant arterial vascular disease and diabetic neuropathy. The higher smooth muscle relaxing potential of papaverine/phentolamin is also reflected by the fact that SIN-1 nonresponders needed a significantly larger dosage of papaverine/phentolamine than nonresponders to induce an erection sufficient for intercourse (1.5 ± 0.5 vs. 0.6 ± 0.3 ml, p < 0.0001). Our observation that SIN-1 is not effective in the majority of patients with "venous leakage" is in accordance with the findings of others (Wegner and Knispel, 1993). If "venous leakage" is a symptom of incomplete cavernous relaxation (Carrier et al., 1993), further support is given on the assumption that SIN-1 causes submaximum cavernous relaxation. In contrast, SIN-1 gives excellent results in patients with (assumed) relatively intact cavernous tissue, i.e. younger patients with primary erectile dysfunction and erectile dysfunction due to pelvic trauma.

In 6 of 44 SIN-1 responders (13.6%) prolonged erections were seen with papaverine/phentolamine. In contrast, SIN-1 did not cause any prolonged erections, even in normal subjects and in patients who needed only minimum amounts of papaverine/phentolamine. Therefore, we consider SIN-1 the drug of choice the drug of choice in patients with proven or suspected increased sensitivity to other vasoactive agents. In addition, in the future SIN-1 may proove to be the drug of choice in other subgroups of patients (i.e. impotence after pelvic surgery, patients with diabetic neuropathy). If SIN-1 fails to induce a satisfactory erectile response, other agents, i.e. papaverine/phentolamine or prostaglandin E 1 should be administered. Possible explanations for the absent priapismogenic potential of SIN-1 may be a more physiological induction of erection and the rapid local metabolism of nitric oxide (Bush et al., 1992).

After up to 150 injections/patients no cavernous fibrosis was noted; with respect to local side effects such as intrapenile discomfort or pain, SIN-1 compares favourably to prostaglandin E 1 and the combination of papaverine and phentolamine. With prostaglandin E 1 20-40% of patients experience penile pain (Wetterauer, 1991) and with papaverine/phentolamine, although less intense, most patients report a slight burning sensation during administration. With SIN-1 no patients reported of such a discomfort, which may indicate that the substance is well tolerated by the cavernous tissue. This is also supported by the fact that no inflammatory or fibrous reactions were seen after multiple intracavernous injections in the rabbit model (Meyer et al., 1993).

Currently, all patients at our institution undergoing intracavernous pharmacotesting receive 1 mg SIN-1. In case of a satisfactory erectile response, all patients are counseled to enter a self injection program with SIN-1 for a maximum reduction of possible side effects. Patients not responding to SIN-1 are advised to undergo pharmacotesting with increasing doses of papaverine plus phentolamine. Responders continue with this regimen whereas non responders are offered a trial with intracavernous calcitonin gene-relate peptide plus prostaglandin E 1, since this combination was shown to be effective in the majority of papaverine/phentolamine nonresponders (Djamilian et al., 1993).

In conclusion, our data suggest that intracavernous SIN-1 is safe and efficacious in the majority of patients with erectile dysfunction, however, has a lower smooth muscle relaxing potential than a combination of papaverine and phentolamine. The fact that no prolonged erections were seen even in patients with a past history of priapisms may be explained by the more physiologic induction of erection with a nitric oxide donor and a rapid intracavernous decomposition of SIN-1.

REFERENCES

Burnett A.L., C.J. Lowenstein, D.S. Bredt, T.S.K. Chang, S.H. Snyder, 1992, Nitric oxide: a physiologic mediator of penile erection, Science 257, 401

Bush P.A., N.E. Gonzalez, L.J. Ignaro, 1992, Biosynthesis of nitric oxide and citrulline from L-arinine by constitutive nitric oxide synthase present in rabbit corpus cvernosum, Biochem. Biophys. Res.Comm, 186, 308

Carrier S., G. Brock, N.W. Kour, T.F. Lue, 1993, Pathophysiology of erectile dysfunction, Urology 42(4), 468

Djamilian M., C.G. Stief, M. Kuczyk, U. Jonas, 1993, Follow up results of a combination of calcitonin gene-related peptide and PGE1 in the treatment of erectile dysfunction, J. Urol. 149, 1296

Holmquist F., C.G. Stief, U. Jonas, K.E. Andersson KE, 1991, Effect of the nitric oxide synthase inhibitor NG-nitro-L-arginine on the erectile response to cavernous nerve stimulation in the rabbit, Acta Physiol. Scand, 143, 299

Ignarro L.J., P.A. Bush, G.M. Buga, K.S. Woods, J.M. Fukuto, J. Rajfer, 1990, Nitric oxide and cyclic GMP formation upon electrical field stimulation cause relaxation of corpus cavernosum smooth muscle Biochem. Biophys. Res. Comm. 170, 843

Jünemann K.P., 1991, Pharmacotesting in erectile dysfuncion, in: Erectile dysfunction, ed. U. Jonas, W.F. Thon, C.G. Stief (Springer Verlag, Berlin-Heidelberg-New York) p104

Meyer M.F., A. Taher, H. Krah, J. Staubesand, A.J. Becker, M. Kirchner, B. Mayer, U. Jonas, W.G. Forssmann, C.G. Stief, 1993, : Intracavernous application of SIN-1 in rabbit and man: Functional and toxicological results, Ann. Urol. 27, 79

Rajfer J, W.J. Aronson, P.A. Bush, F.J. Dorey, L.J. Ignarro, 1992, Nitric oxide as a mediator of relaxation of the corpus cavernosum in response to nonadrenergic, noncholinergic neurotransmission, N. Engl. J. Med, 326,90

Stief C.G., F. Holmquist, M. Djamilian, H. Krah, K.E. Andersson, U. Jonas, 1992, Preliminary results with the nitric oxide donor linsidomine choralhydrate in the treatment of human erectile dysfunction, J. Urol. 148, 1437

Stief C.G., M. Djamilian, F. Schaebsdau, M.C. Truss, R.W. Schlick, J.H. Abicht, E.P. Allhoff, U. Jonas, 1990, Single potential analysis of cavernous electric activity - a possible diagnosis of autonomic impotence?, World. J. Urol. 8, 75

Wegner H.E., H.H. Knispel, 1993, Effect of nitric oxide donor, Linsidomine chlorhydrate in treatment of human erectile dysfunction caused by venous leakage, Urology 42 (4), 409

Wetterauer U., 1991, Intracavernous pharmacotherapy for erectile dysfunction, in : Erectile dysfunction, ed. U. Jonas, W.F. Thon, C.G. Stief (Springer, Berlin-Heidelberg- New York) p 221

NITRIC OXIDE-INDUCED LYMPHOCYTE ACTIVATION: A ROLE FOR G PROTEINS

Harry M. Lander[1], Roberto Levi[1], and Abraham Novogrodsky[2]

[1]Department of Pharmacology, Cornell University Medical College,
New York, NY 10021, U.S.A.
[2]Felsenstein Medical Research Center, Beilinson Campus, Petah-Tikva and
Sackler School of Medicine, Tel Aviv University, Israel.

INTRODUCTION

Oxygen free radical generation has been implicated in mediating signal transmission initiated by a variety of stimuli (1-4). For example, Novogrodsky et al. (2) discovered that hydroxy radical scavengers blocked phorbol ester-induced mitogenesis in lymphocytes. Also, Schreck et al. (1) found that treating T lymphocytes with the free radical scavenger N-acetylcysteine, blocked activation of the nuclear transcription factor NF-κB by a variety of unrelated stimuli. We discovered various inductive effects which oxidants and other stress stimuli, such as Hg^{2+} and phenylarsine oxide, have on resting human peripheral blood mononuclear cells (PBMC) (5-9). We examined early parameters of cellular activation, including the rate of glucose uptake, $p56^{lck}$ protein tyrosine kinase activity and CD45 protein tyrosine phosphatase activity. The ability of hemin, Hg^{2+} and phenylarsine oxide to activate this signal transduction pathway led us to examine whether a more biologically relevant oxidant, nitric oxide, had similar effects (10).

The ability of reactive oxygen intermediates (ROI) to activate NF-κB (1) suggested to us that it was possible that Nitric Oxide (NO) had similar agonistic properties. Therefore, we examined the effect NO had on several parameters of cell activation in resting human PBMC.

MATERIALS AND METHODS

Isolation of PBMC

Human PBMC were isolated from healthy volunteers by Ficoll-Hypaque density gradient centrifugation as we previously described (5).

Biochemical, Pharmacological, and Clinical Aspects of Nitric Oxide
Edited by B. A. Weissman *et al.*, Plenum Press, New York, 1995

Preparation of NO Solutions and Compounds

NO solutions and SNAP were prepared as we previously described (10). Carbon monoxide solution was prepared in the same manner as we prepared the NO solution with a final concentration of 1 mM (11).

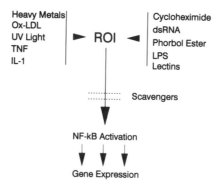

Figure 1. General scheme depicting the role of reactive oxygen intermediates (ROI) as mediators of NF-κB activation and gene expression by a variety of stimuli.

Electromobility Shift Assay

PBMC (40×10^6/ml) in 1 ml were treated for 4 h at 37°C in RPMI 1640 containing 5% heat inactivated fetal calf serum and the indicated treatments. Streptolysin-O and GTP-γ-S were purchased from Sigma Chemical Co. (St. Louis, MO). GDP-β-S was acquired from Biomol (Plymouth Meeting, PA). Cells were pelleted, washed once with cold PBS and resuspended in 250 μl of 10 mM HEPES, pH 7.9, 10 mM KCl, 1.5 mM $MgCl_2$, 1 mM EDTA, 0.5 mM DTT, 0.5 mM PMSF and 10% glycerol. Cells were left on ice for 10 min and NP-40 was added to a final concentration of 0.04%. After 5 min on ice, nuclear extracts were pelleted at 1,000 x g for 5 min. Supernatants were removed and 100 μl of 20 mM HEPES, pH 7.9, 200 mM KCl, 20% glycerol, 0.5 mM PMSF and 1 mM EDTA was added to the pellets. After another hour on ice, pellets were spun at 100,000×g for 20 min. Supernatants were stored at -70°C until ready for use. Protein concentrations were then determined. The NF-κB DNA probe used contained the -206 to -195 region of the IL-2 promoter (5'-CCAAGAGGGATTTCACCTAAATCC-3'). Approximately 10^4 cpm (0.2 ng) of 5'-end labeled DNA was added to 5 μg nuclear protein and 2 μg Poly(dIdC) in 20 μl of 10 mM Tris, pH 7.5, 50 mM NaCl, 1 mM EDTA, 1 mM DTT and 5% glycerol at room temperature for 20 min. Protein-DNA complexes were resolved on 4% polyacrylamide gels in 45 mM Tris, 45 mM borate and 1 mM EDTA pH 8.3 at 150V for 1.5 hr at room temperature. Gels were dried and exposed to X-ray film. The non-specific probe used contained the -93 to -69 region of the IL-2 promoter (5'TTACAAAA-TGTATAATGTGTATAA-3').

GTP/GTP p21^{ras} Ratio Assay

The assay to measure the GTP/GDP ratio on immunoprecipitated p21^{ras} was essentially that of Downard et al. (12). Jurkat T cells (4×10^6 cells/ml) were labeled in phosphate-free RPMI 1640 containing 200 μCi/ml ^{32}PO$_4^-$ for 16 hr. NO was added directly to 1 ml of sample for the indicated time after which cells were analyzed for the % of GTP - bound p21^{ras}. Anti-p21^{ras}-agarose (clone Y13-259, Santa Cruz Biotechnology, Santa Cruz, CA) was added for immunoprecipitation. After elution of guanine nucleotides, 5 μl of sample was spotted onto polyethylimine TLC plates, run for 3 hr in 0.75 M KH$_2$PO$_4$ (pH 3.4) and exposed to phosphor-imaging screens overnight. Spots migrating with the same Rf as GDP or GTP standards were quantified using a phosphorimager (Molecular Dynamics). The percent of GTP bound to p21^{ras} was calculated using the following formula which takes into account the extra phosphate on GTP as compared to GDP: (2/3 x GTP)/(GDP + 2/3 x GTP). Control samples had non-immune IgG + Protein A-agarose added rather than anti-p21^{ras} and no GDP or GTP spots were evident.

GTPase Assay

The GTPase assay was performed exactly as we previously described (13).

Circular Dichroism Spectral Analysis

Circular dichroism spectral analysis was performed at 22°C in 0.1 mm cuvettes in a JASCO 710 CD spectrophotometer. Samples were dissolved in 50 mM Tris buffer, pH 7.4, and measured with a 0.2 μm bandwidth, a 0.2 μm step scan and varying scan speeds of 60 - 200 μm/min. NO (50 μM) was added to p21^{ras} (17 μM) and spectral characteristics measured over varying time periods indicated that p21^{ras} and the p21^{ras}-NO complex remained stable for the duration of the data collection period. The spectra were analyzed using the LINCOMB program (Dr. G. D. Fasman, Brandeis University, Waltham, MA).

RESULTS

We examined whether nuclei isolated from resting human PBMC had enhanced NF-κB binding activity when the cells were exposed to NO. As seen in Figure 2, treatment with the NO-generating compounds sodium nitroprusside (SNP) or S-nitroso-N-acetyl-D,L-penicillamine (SNAP) for 4 hr led to the appearance of DNA-binding proteins specific for the NF-κB binding site in isolated nuclei. This binding activity was absent after 18 hr. In contrast, treatment of these cells with phytohemaglutinin (PHA) led to NF-κB binding activity which was sustained to 18 hr. It is possible that the short biological half-life of NO is reflected in its inability to provide long-term activation of NF-κB, as PHA does.

The activation of NF-κB by NO suggests that the cytokine TNF-α, whose expression is regulated by NF-κB, may be induced. We treated PBMC with NO, SNP or SNAP for 72 hr and assayed the cell culture supernatants for TNF-α levels. As seen in Table 1, TNF-α secretion was induced by each agent.

Activation of NF-κB by stimuli such as UV light and TNF-α has been shown to require activation of the G protein p21^{ras} (14). Therefore, we hypothesized that NO activation of NF-κB might also require the involvement of p21^{ras}. To test this, we permeabilized PBMC in the presence of the non-specific G protein inhibitor, GDP-,β-S, and examined the effect of NO on NF-κB activity. As seen in Figure 3, GDP-β-S blocked NO-induced NF-κB activation. Also, the G protein activator, GTP-γ-S, activated NF-κB binding activity (Figure 3).

These findings suggest that G proteins are involved in NO action, similar to what was found for UV light and TNF-α, where p21^{ras} was implicated (14). Therefore, we examined

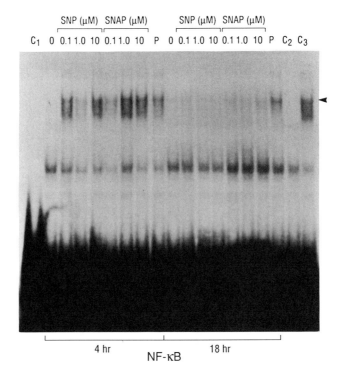

SNP (µM) SNAP (µM)   SNP (µM) SNAP (µM)

C_1 0 0.1 1.0 10 0.1 1.0 10 P   0 0.1 1.0 10 0.1 1.0 10 P C_2 C_3

4 hr   18 hr

NF-κB

Figure 2. Effect of SNP and SNAP on NF-κB binding activity in human PBMC. Human PBMC were treated for the indicated times with SNP or SNAP before isolation of nuclei and assay of NF-κB binding activity. P, cells treated with PHA (2 µg/ml). C_1, ^{32}P-DNA probe alone; C_2, nuclear extract from PHA-treated cells (4 hr) with 100-fold excess unlabeled DNA probe; C_3, the same sample as in C_2 but a nonspecific unlabeled DNA probe was added in excess. The arrowhead indicates the position of DNA-protein complexes.

Table 1. Effect of NO and NO-generating compounds on TNF-α ecretion from human PBMC treated for 72 hr.

Treatment	TNF-α (pg/ml)
0	0
SNP 1 µM	174
SNP 10 µM	160
SNAP 1 µM	0
SNAP 10 µM	166
NO 30 µM	121

whether NO activated p21^{ras} in T cells. p21^{ras}, a monomeric G protein, normally has GDP bound to it when in its resting (off) state. When activated, GDP is exchanged for GTP and therefore an increase in its associated GTP/GDP ratio is indicative of activation. We immunoprecipitated p21^{ras} from the human T cell line Jurkat which had its nucleotide pools preloaded with ^{32}PO$_4^-$ (Figure 4). Treatment with low concentrations of NO led to an increase in the GTP/GDP ratio on p21^{ras}, demonstrating an activating effect of NO on p21^{ras} in whole cells.

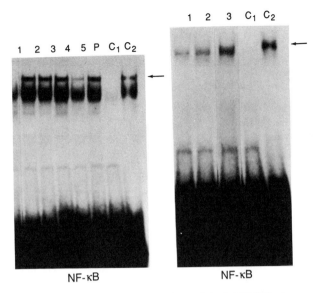

Figure 3. Effect of G protein modulators on NF-κB binding activity in PBMC in the presence or absence of NO. *Left Panel:* nuclei from PBMC treated with; *lane 1,* medium alone; *lane 2,* SNAP (10 μM); *lane 3,* streptolysin-O (SO, 0.4 U/ml) and SNAP; *lane 4,* SO, SNAP, and GTP-γ-S (1 mM); *lane 5, SO,* SNAP and GDP-β-S (1 mM). *Right Panel: lane 1,* medium alone; *lane 2, SO; lane 3,* SO and GTP-γ-S.

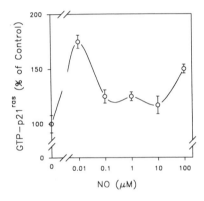

Figure 4. Effect of NO on GTP/GDP ratio on $p21^{ras}$ in T cells. The human Jurkat T cell line was stimulated with various amounts of NO for 10 min. Cells were washed, $p21^{ras}$ was immunoprecipitated and the bound nucleotides analyzed. Data are expressed as the percentage of GTP-bound $p21^{ras}$ of control. Control samples had a baseline value of $12.4 \pm 3.6\%$ GTP bound. Data represent the mean and standard deviation from 4 to 6 experiments.

Although it was believed that UV light and TNF-α activate $p21^{ras}$ by acting upstream of it, we tested whether NO could directly activate $p21^{ras}$. Therefore, we mixed NO with purified, recombinant $p21^{ras}$ *in vitro* and measured its intrinsic GTPase activity. As can be seen in Figure 5, NO, but not carbon monoxide, enhanced $p21^{ras}$ GTPase activity in a dose dependent manner.

This enhancement of GTPase activity, which could be reversed by addition of hemoglobin (data not shown), could either be due to enhanced GDP release (the rate limiting step in the hydrolytic cycle of G proteins) or be due to an increase in the intrinsic

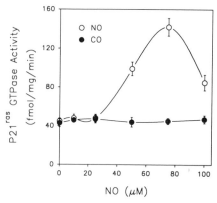

Figure 5. Effect of NO and carbon monoxide on p21^{ras} activity *in vitro*. Pure recombinant p21^{ras} was incubated with various concentrations of NO or CO for 10 min after which GTPase activity was measured.

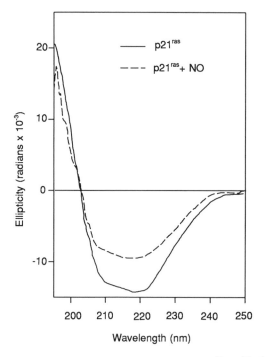

	% α-helix	% β-sheet	% residual (turns + random coil)
p21^{ras}	60	18	22
p21^{ras} + NO	36	44	20

Figure 6. Circular dichroism analysis of p21^{ras} in the presence and absence of NO. p21^{ras} (17 μM) in the presence and absence of NO (50 μM) was subjected to circular dichroism spectral analysis and the resultant changes in secondary structure calculated.

GTPase catalytic rate. The former case is characteristic of an activating event and the latter a de-activating event. We found that NO increased the GDP release from p21^{ras} preloaded with [^{3}H]GDP (data not shown) and therefore the observed increase in GTPase activity was due to activation of p21^{ras}. Finally, circular dichroism spectral analysis revealed profound conformational changes in the secondary structure of p21^{ras} induced by NO (Figure 6).

DISCUSSION

These studies have identified NO as a positive signaling molecule in the immune system. The generation of reactive nitrogen intermediates and initiation of its signaling mechanisms may therefore represent an analogous system to that described for reactive oxygen intermediates.

Our findings uncovering the ability of p21^{ras} to be directly activated by NO opens several new possible roles for NO. First, NO, which is generated at sites of local inflammation, may be acting as a positive feedback regulator by further activating local leukocytes. Second, activation of p21^{ras} or related monomeric G proteins may be a mechanism by which NO controls synaptic plasticity in the brain. Finally, the lymphokines produced by NO-activated lymphocytes may participate in many disease states including atherosclerosis, hypertension and rheumatoid arthritis. Hence, in addition to its known physiological roles, NO may initiate processes which are central to human pathology.

REFERENCES

1. Schreck, R., P. Rieber, and P. A. Baeuerle, 1991, Reactive oxygen intermediates as apparently widely used messengers in the activation of the NF-κB transcription factor and HIV-1. *Embo J.* 10, 2247.
2. Novogrodsky, A., A. Ravid, A. L. Rubin, and K. H. Stenzel, 1982, Hydroxyl radical scavengers inhibit lymphocyte mitogenesis. *Proc. Natl. Acad. Sci. USA.* 79, 1171.
3. Whitacre, C. M., and M. K. Cathcart, 1992, Oxygen free radical generation and regulation of proliferative activity of human mononuclear cells responding to different mitogens. *Cell. Immunol.* 144, 287.
4. Israel, N., M-A. Gougerot-Pocidalo, F. Aillet, and J-L. Verelizier, 1992, Redox status of cells influences constitutive or induced NF-κB translocation and HIV LTR activity in human and monocytic cell lines. *J. Immunol.* 149, 3386.
5. Lander, H. M., D. M. Levine, and A. Novogrodsky, 1992, Stress Stimuli-Induced Lymphocyte Activation. *Cell. Immunol.* 145, 146.
6. Lander, H. M., D. M. Levine, and A. Novogrodsky, 1993, Hemin Enhancement of Glucose Transport in Human Lymphocytes: Stimulationof Protein Tyrosine Phosphatase and Activation of p56^{lck} Tyrosine Kinase. *Biochem. J.* 291, 281.
7. Stenzel, K. H., A. L. Rubin, and A. Novogrodsky, 1981, The mitogenic and co-mitogenic properties of hemin. *J. Immunol.* 127, 2469.
8. Novogrodsky, A., M. Suthanthiran, and K. H. Stenzel, 1989, Immune stimulatory properties of metalloporphyrins. *J. Immunol.* 143, 3981.
9. Novogrodsky, A., M. Suthanthiran, and K. H. Stenzel, 1991, Ferro-mitogens: iron-containing compounds with lymphocyte-stimulatoryproperties. *Cell. Immunol.* 133, 295.
10. Lander, H. M., P. Sehajpal, D. M. Levine, and A. Novogrodsky, 1993, Activation of Human Peripheral Blood Mononuclear Cells by Nitric Oxide Generating Compounds. *J. Immunol.* 150, 1509.
11. Budavari, S, ed., 1989, *in:* The Merck Index, Merck & Co., Inc., Rahway, NJ, 1989, p. 275.
12. Downward, J., J. D. Graves, P. H. Warne, S. Rayter, and D. Cantrell, 1990, Stimulationof p21^{ras} upon T cell Activation. *Nature.* 346, 719.
13. Lander, H. M., P. K. Sehajpal, and A. Novogrodsky, 1993, Nitric Oxide Signaling: A Possible Role for G Proteins. *J. Immunol.* 151, 7182.
14. Devary, Y., C. Rosette, J. A. DiDonato, M. Karin, 1993, NF-κB Activation by Ultraviolet Light Not Dependent on a Nuclear Signal. *Science.* 261, 1442.

CORONARY HAEMODYNAMIC PROFILE OF THE NEW NITRO-ESTER DERIVATIVE ITF 296 IN THE CONSCIOUS DOG

Jacques Mizrahi[1], Robert J.Bache[2], Eberhard Bassenge[3],
Alain Berdeaux[4], Jean-Francois Giudicelli[4], Akira Ueno[5], Roberta
Cereda[1], Marco Sardina[1], Gianni Gromo[1], Mario Bergamaschi[1]

[1]Talfarmaco Research Center, Milano, Italy
[2]Dept. of Internal Medicine, University of Minnesota, Minneapolis,
  USA
[3]Inst. of Applied Physiology, University of Freiburg, Germany
[4]Dept.of Pharmacology, Faculty of Medicine, Universit› Paris-Sud,
  France
[5]Dept. of Pharmacology, Nagasaki University, School of Medicine,
  Japan

INTRODUCTION

The action of low doses of nitrovasodilators on coronary circulation is characterised by a selective dilatation of large conductance coronary arteries[1,2,3], which is accompanied by a minimal effect on small coronary resistance vessels[4,5,6,7]. This ability of nitroderivatives to dilate selectively large coronary arteries, becomes of major importance when the capability of the conduit epicardial coronary arteries to dilate in response to increases in blood flow is impaired, as it happens after removal of coronary endothelium with angioplasty[8] or in patients with atherosclerosis[9,10]. In those conditions, while the flow-dependent endothelium-mediated response is depressed, the endothelium-independent relaxing effect of nitravasodilators on large conduit coronary arteries remains effective. This has been confirmed in clinical studies, where the coronary vasospasm in anginal patients in which endothelium is likely not functional, has been effectively reversed by nitrovasodilators[11,12].

In addition to their effect on coronary circulation, low concentrations of nitrates have been shown to increase venous capacitance thereby reducing venous return, while higher doses are required to affect peripheral resistance vessels. The haemodynamic consequence of this selective effect is a near maximal dilatation of large coronary arteries, and an increase in venous capacitance at concentrations that have very little effect on peripheral vascular resistance[13]. However, the haemodynamic effects of nitrovasodilators are complex and after repeated administrations the primary vasodilator action of

Biochemical, Pharmacological, and Clinical Aspects of Nitric Oxide
Edited by B. A. Weissman *et al.*, Plenum Press, New York, 1995

93

nitroglycerin is subjected to counter regulatory reflex and neuro-hormonal influences that lead to attenuation of the therapeutic efficacy[14].

This paper reports on the results of experimental studies aimed to investigate the potential antianginal activity of a new nitrate-ester derivative ITF 296, [3-(2-Nitrooxyethyl)-3,4dihydro-2H-1,3-benzoxazin-4-one][15] in conscious dogs. This compound has been shown to induce concentration-related relaxation in different vascular preparations in vitro[16,17] which was not altered by removal of the endothelium, while it was markedly reduced by methylene blue or haemoglobin, suggesting NO and cGMP-mediated mechanisms[17].

Effects on coronary haemodynamics in conscious resting dogs[18,19]

The effects of ITF 296 on coronary and systemic haemodynamics have been investigated in conscious unrestrained dogs, chronically instrumented for the recording of the relevant parameters according to the following scheme: under general anaesthesia electromagnetic or pulsed Doppler flowmeter and pairs of piezo-electric crystals were applied to the left circumflex coronary artery, for the recording of coronary blood flow (CBF) and coronary artery diameter (CAD), respectively. Catheters were then introduced into the left ventricle and in the aorta for the measurement of left ventricular end-diastolic pressure (LVEDP), LVdP/dt, and arterial pressure. The haemodynamic effects of ITF 296 were compared with those of isosorbide dinitrate (ISDN), nitroglycerin (NTG) and nicorandil (NIC).

The intravenous injections of single doses of ITF 296, from 0.3 to 10 µg/kg i.v., selectively and dose-dependently increased CAD while leaving CBF and CVR almost unaffected (Figure 1). No major changes in heart rate (HR) and mean blood pressure (MBP) were recorded at these doses. CAD was further increased by $11.7 \pm 2.5\%$ and $14.1 \pm 0.7\%$ (p <0.01)[18], after the injection of ITF 296 100 and 125 µg/kg iv, this effect being accompanied by dose-related, significant changes in CBF, CVR, MBP and HR.

Like ITF 296, ISDN at low doses, increased the external diameter of the epicardial coronary arteries living CVR or CBF unaffected. However, doses of ISDN about ten fold higher than those of ITF 296 were required to provoke the same vasodilating effect (Figure 1). ISDN at 30 µg/kg induced also significant changes in HR and MBP.

At very low doses, 0.1 and 0.3 µg/kg i.v., NTG was about ten times more potent than ITF 296 in increasing selectively CAD, while the threshold dose influencing CVR to a significant extent was 1 µg/kg i.v. However, since the dose-response curve related to CAD for NTG and ITF 296 were not parallel, the difference in potency of the two drugs on large coronary vessels was progressively reduced with the dose, the two drugs being equipotent at 3 and 10 µg/kg i.v. Conversely, the difference in potency between NTG and ITF 296 on small resistance vessels (CVR) was maintained at all dose levels (Figure 1). NTG was also 30 times more potent than ITF 296 in reducing MBP and it provoked larger increases in HR.

The threshold dose of NIC which induced a significant increase in CAD $(4.2 \pm 0.5\%)$ without influencing CVR or CBF was found at 10 µg/kg. At higher doses, 50 and 250 µg/kg i.v., the effect of NIC on CAD was accompanied by significant changes in CVR and CBF. HR and MBP were also significantly modified by the same doses of NIC.

Tolerance development during long-term treatment[20]

Attenuation of the antianginal efficacy of NTG during prolonged exposure is well documented, and this results in a decrease of at least some of its therapeutic efficacy[3,14]. As dilatation of large compliant coronary arteries represents a clinically important parameter of nitrovasodilators action, the efficacy of nitrates on coronary vascular tone during long-term treatment, has been intensively investigated in patients and in experimental animals[21].

The possibility of the development of tolerance to ITF 296 has been investigated in a group of conscious dogs, chronically instrumented for the recording of left circumflex CAD, with piezo-electric crystals, ABP and HR. In these animals, ITF 296, 20 µg/kg/min, was continuously infused over 5 days through a chronically implanted pulmonary artery catheter. Dose-response curves relative to the large coronary vasodilating effect of ITF 296 (0.1 to 30 µg/kg/min), infused for 15 min., were performed the day before starting the 5-days infusion (day 0), and the day after infusion was stopped (day 6).

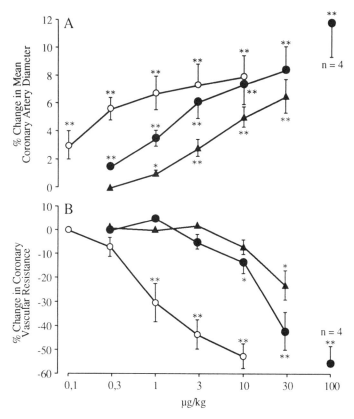

Figure 1. Maximal percent changes in *(A)* left circumflex coronary artery diameter and *(B)* coronary vascular resistance induced by ITF 296 (●), nitroglycerin (o) or isosorbide dinitrate (▲) after i.v. bolus injection in conscious dogs. Data are expressed as mean values ± SEM (n=6). *p<0,05; **p<0,01.

The intravenous infusion of ITF 296 at 20 µg/kg/min, resulted in a near maximal coronary dilator response, which was rather well maintained over the entire infusion period (Figure 2). The slight loss of coronary vasodilator activity recorded during the treatment, can be accounted for by the biological counter-regulation associated with the increase in renin-angiotensin system and sympathetic activity and/or the increase in venous capacitance caused by nitrovasodilators[14]. On the contrary, a substantial loss of nitroglycerin action on CAD, already at day 2-3 of infusion at 1.5 µg/kg/min, has been reported in a previous study done under the same experimental conditions, in the same animal preparation[3].

Effect of de-endothelialization on the vasodilator effect of ITF 296 on large coronary arteries[18]

In order to assess whether the vasodilator effect of ITF 296 on large coronary arteries is endothelium-dependent or independent, its action on coronary artery diameter has been investigated before and after de-endothelialization. The study was performed in a group of conscious dogs, chronically instrumented for the recording of CAD and CBF, with piezo-electric crystals and Doppler flowmeter, applied to the left circumflex coronary artery. De-endothelialization was performed by introducing a balloon angioplastic catheter into the left circumflex coronary artery in the area of the piezo-electric crystals.

Drugs were tested before and three days after endothelium removal, i.e. before any significant endothelial regeneration occurred[22].

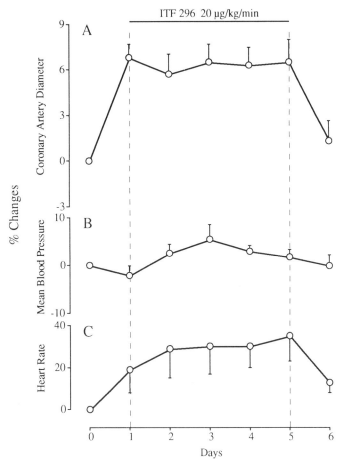

Figure 2. Maximal percent changes in *(A)* left circumflex coronary artery diameter, *(B)* mean arterial blood pressure and *(C)* heart rate during 5-days continuous infusion of ITF 296 (20 µg/kg/min) in conscious, chronically instrumented dogs. Data are expressed as mean values ± SEM (n=7).

The accomplishment of endothelium removal was assessed by testing the response of large coronary arteries to acetylcholine (Ach; endothelium-dependent vasodilatation) and to reactive hyperaemia test (RH; flow-dependent, endothelium-mediated dilatation). In these experiments the vasodilating response of large coronary arteries provoked by RH and Ach (0.3 µg/kg i.v.) was reduced by 86.7 ± 5.9 and 75.9 ± 8.6 % (P<0.01) respectively, after endothelium removal. On the contrary, the changes in CBF and CVR induced by either Ach or RH, were not altered by de-endothelialization.

The effect of ITF 296 (30 and 100 µg/kg iv) on large coronary artery diameter was slightly, but not significantly, reduced by removal of the endothelial lining. CVR and CBF were affected only slightly.

The results obtained with NTG, 1 µg/kg i.v., before and after de-endothelialization were qualitatively similar to those observed with ITF 296. The increase in CAD provoked by NTG did not undergo significant changes after endothelium removal, nor the effects on CVR or CBF.

In conclusion, either the flow-mediated endothelium-dependent dilatation of large coronary arteries evoked by RH or the endothelium-dependent vasodilatation evoked by Ach, were almost completely abolished after de-endothelialization. Conversely, the effect of ITF 296 and NTG on large coronary conductance arteries remained almost unaffected by endothelium removal, suggesting that the two drugs do not require endothelium integrity to exert their vasodilating action.

Effect on transmural coronary flow during treadmill exercise in conscious dogs with coronary stenosis[23]

Nitrovasodilators have been reported to improve myocardial perfusion distal to coronary artery stenosis by 1) dilating coronary stenosis, 2) decreasing LVEDP through venodilation and reduced venous return, and 3) dilating small coronary arteries which are beyond myocardial metabolic control[23].

In the presence of coronary artery disease with an occlusive component, angina pectoris may occur when myocardial metabolic demand exceed the ability of the diseased coronary vessels to deliver arterial inflow. The consequent myocardial ischaemia induces vasodilatation of the coronary resistance vessels; the resultant loss of vasomotor activity at the microvascular level and the subsequent decrease in coronary perfusion pressure distal to the stenotic region, lead to a reduction of the subendocardium perfusion[24,25]. Vasodilators, such as nitrates or calcium entry blockers, may exert a beneficial effect by reducing left ventricular systolic tension and thereby decreasing myocardial oxygen needs[26,27]. The ability of antianginal agents to increase blood delivery toward the ischaemic myocardium could be exerted either through an increase in collateral inflow to the ischaemic area or through a transmural redistribution of perfusion to favour blood flow toward the subendocardium where vulnerability to ischaemia is greatest[28].

In order to investigate whether ITF 296 could improve transmural coronary blood flow distal to a coronary stenosis, dogs were surgically instrumented for the recording of ABP, LVP and CBF. An hydraulic occluder was placed around the left anterior descending (LAD) coronary artery, distal to a Doppler velocity probe, and a silicone catheter was introduced into the LAD immediately distal to the hydraulic occluder, for the measurement of coronary pressure. Myocardial coronary blood flow was measured with labelled microspheres (15 µm in diameter). Myocardial wall thickening was measured by miniature piezo-electric crystals implanted in the area perfused by the LAD (ischaemic area) and by the left circumflex (LCX: control area) coronary arteries. Studies were performed with animal exercising on a motor-driven treadmill whose speed and grade were gradually increased until a heart rate of 200-220 beats/min. was obtained. As soon as the recorded haemodynamic variables reached the steady state, the occluder was progressively inflated to produce a coronary stenosis resulting in approximately 50% reduction of CBF and a distal coronary pressure of 45-65 mm Hg. Microspheres were then injected via a left atrial catheter. 90 sec. later the occluder was deflated and exercise discontinued. After 90 min rest, infusion of ITF 296 was started and the afore mentioned protocol was repeated at 90 min interval during infusion of ITF 296 or ISDN, at 20 µg/kg/min.

The infusion of ITF 296 had no effect on systemic haemodynamics at rest and during exercise with normal coronary flow or coronary artery stenosis. Coronary blood flow in the control area was not affected by ITF 296, while coronary blood flow distal to the coronary stenosis was markedly increased particularly in the innermost myocardial layers. As a consequence endo/epi ratio was increased from 0.33 ± 0.04 to 0.70 ± 0.1 (+112%) (Figure 3).

Similarly to ITF 296, ISDN had no effect on systemic haemodynamic parameters at rest or during exercise with normal coronary flow. During coronary stenosis, hypoperfusion in the LAD region was most pronounced in the subendocardium and this was reflected in the endo/epi ratio of 0.33 ± 0.05 as compared with 1.37 ± 0.07, in the control area supplied by LCX. Infusion of ISDN, 20 µg/kg/min, significantly increased coronary blood flow in the LAD region, particularly in the subendocardium, thus increasing endo/epi ratio to 0.56 ± 0.08 (p< 0.01). Remarkably, ITF 296 caused favourable redistribution of blood flow toward the subendocardium of the ischaemic region even in the absence of any major changes in systemic haemodynamics whereas ISDN decreases aortic and left ventricular systolic pressure, as well as left ventricular end diastolic pressure, likely as a result of systemic vasodilator effects.

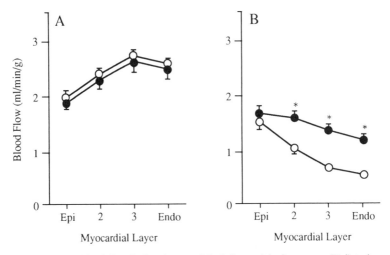

Figure 3. Myocardial blood flow in four layers of the left ventricle from outer (Epi) to inner (Endo) layer before (O) and during intravenous infusion of ITF 296, 20 ug/kg/min (●) in exercising dogs with a left anterior descending coronary artery stenosis. *(A):* myocardial blood flow in the normally perfused posterior wall. *(B):* myocardial blood flow in the anterior wall perfused by the stenotic left anterior descending coronary artery. Data are expressed as mean values ± SEM (n=6). *p<0.05 ITF 296 vs. Control.

Exercise caused significant increase in systolic wall thickening in the areas supplied by the two branches of the left coronary artery (20 ± 1 and 24 ± 3 %). During coronary stenosis, the increase in systolic wall thickening remained unchanged in the myocardial area supplied by LCX (control area) while it was dramatically decreased to $6 \pm 2\%$ in the area perfused by LAD (ischaemic area). Infusion of ITF 296 produced only a small but not significant increase in systolic thickening in the normally perfused LCX area during inflation of the occluder, whereas it significantly increased from 6 ± 2 to 13 ± 2 % in the area perfused by LAD. Like ITF 296, ISDN increased systolic wall thickening in the hypoperfused LAD area from 11 ± 4 to 15 ± 4 %, while no marked effect was observed on the systolic thickening of the normally perfused posterior wall .

CONCLUSIONS

The pharmacological profile of ITF 296 which arises from the data obtained in the reported experimental situations, in the conscious chronically instrumented dog, can be summarised as follows:

1) similarly to NTG and ISDN, the intravenous administration of low doses of ITF 296 either as bolus injections or as continuous infusion, led to a direct selective effect on the tone of the large conductance epicardial coronary arteries as the increase in CAD takes place in the absence of changes in CBF or CVR

2) although the rank order of vasodilating potency of the drugs used in these experiments, represented by their effect on CAD, is NTG > ITF 296 > ISDN >> NIC, the selectivity of action on the conductance versus the resistance segment of the coronary vasculature, as expressed by the ratio between the dose of each compound which exerts a significant threshold effect on CAD and CVR, is ITF 296 > ISDN > NTG > NIC.

3) the effect of ITF 296 on the diameter of epicardial coronary arteries is not affected by the removal of the endothelium, indicating that this drug, like nitrovasodilators studied for comparison, does not require endothelium integrity to exert its vasodilating action on large conductance coronary arteries. Therefore, ITF 296 should be classified as an endothelium-independent coronary dilator

4) the endothelium-independence of ITF 296 is similar to that of other nitrovasodilators, and clearly differentiates this drug from other coronary vasodilators, such as potassium channel openers and calcium entry blockers, which lose most of their vasodilating properties after endothelium removal[4]

5) the coronary dilator response elicited by ITF 296 is rather well maintained over long-term infusion (5 days), while tolerance develops quite rapidly during infusion with NTG[14]. This may indicate that attenuation of the effect might not develop in a marked manner, during long-term treatment with ITF 296

6) ITF 296 significantly increases myocardial blood flow distal to a coronary stenosis during exercise, thereby improving exercise-induced myocardial hypoperfusion and reduced myocardial function. The preferential increase in flow toward the subendocardium suggests that ITF 296 may also exert its anti-ischaemic action, through dilation of intramural penetrating arteries

7) the effect of ITF 296 on transmural coronary flow may predict a beneficial effect of this drug in patients with coronary artery diseases, by dilating large coronary conductance vessels and by vasodilating small penetrating arteries with abnormally high tone resulting from atherosclerosis or hyperlipidemia.

REFERENCES

1. R.L. Feldman, C.J. Pepine and R. Conyio, Magnitude of dilation of large and small coronary arteries by nitroglycerin, *Circulation* 64:324 (1981).
2. G.B. Brown, E. Bolson, R.B. Peterson, C.D. Pierce and H.T. Dodge, The mechanism of nitroglycerin action: stenosis vasodilatation as a major component of drug response, *Circulation* 64:1089 (1981).
3. D.J. Stewart, J. Holtz and E. Bassenge, Long-term nitroglycerin treatment: effect on direct and endothelium-mediated large coronary artery dilatation in conscious dogs, *Circulation* 75:847 (1987).
4. A. Berdeaux, C. Drieu La Rochelle, V. Richard and J.F. Giudicelli, Differential effects of nitrovasodilators, K+channel openers and nicorandil on large and small coronary arteries in conscious dogs, *J. Cardiovasc. Pharmacol.* 20:S18 (1992).
5. P. Macho and S.F. Vatner, Effects of nitroglycerin and nitroprusside on large and small coronary vessels in conscious dogs, *Circulation* 64:1101 (1981).
6. H. Kanatsuka, C.L. Eastham, M.L. Marcus and K.G. Lamping, Effects of nitroglycerin on the coronary microcirculation in normal and ischaemic myocardium, *J. Cardiovasc. Pharmacol.* 19:755 (1992).
7. M.A. Kurz, K.G. Lamping, J.N. Bates, C.L. Eastham and M.L. Marcus, Mechanism responsible for the heterogeneous coronary microvascular response to nitroglycerin, *Circ. Res.* 23(suppl III):S99 (1991).
8. Y. Hayashi, H. Tomoike, K. Nagasawa, A. Yamada, H. Nishijima, H. Adachi and M. Nakamura., Functional and anatomical recovery of endothelium after denudation of coronary artery, *Am. J. Physiol.* 254:H1081 (1988).
9. D.A. Cox, J.A. Vita and C.B. Treasure, Atherosclerosis impairs flow-mediated dilatation of coronary arteries in humans, *Circulation* 77:43 (1989).
10. E.G. Nabel, A.P. Selwyn and P. Gonzale, Large coronary arteries in humans are responsive to changing in blood flow: an endothelium dependent mechanism that fails in patients with atherosclerosis, *J. Am. Coll. Cardiol.* 16:346 (1990).
11. J.E. Gage, O.M. Hess, T. Murakami, M. Ritter, J. Grimm and H.P. Krayenbuehl, Vasoconstriction of stenotic coronary coronary arteries during dynamic exercise in patients with classic angina pectoris: reversibility by nitroglycerin, *Circulation* 73:865 (1986).
12. E.G. Nabel, P. Ganz, J.B. Gordon, R.W. Alexander and A.P. Selwyn, Dilatation of normal and constriction of atherosclerotic coronary arteries caused by cold pressure test, *Circulation* 77:43 (1988).
13. E. Bassenge and J. Zanzinger, Nitrates in different vascular beds, nitrate tolerance, and interactions with endothelial function, *Am. J. Cardiol.*70:23B (1992).
14. D.J. Stewart, D. Elsner, O. Sommer, J. Holtz and E. Bassenge, Altered spectrum of nitroglycerin action in long-term treatment: nitroglycerin-specific venous tolerance with maintenance of arterial vasodepressor potency, *Circulation* 74:573 (1986).
15. S. Levi, F. Benedini, G. Bertolini, R. Cereda, G.C. Donν. G. Gromo and A. Sala, Synthesis and cardiovascular activity of 3-nitrooxyalkyl-2,3-dihydro-4H-1,3-benzoxazin-4-ones, a novel class of nitrate esters, XII Int. Symposium on Med. Chem. P-152,C-356 (1992).
16. C.M. Boulanger and P. Vanhoutte, Vascular effect of ITF 296 in dog arteries and veins, *in:* "ITF296 Internal Report" (1993).
17. J. Mizrahi, M. Bergamaschi and G. Gromo, Pharmacological profile of ITF 296, a new nitroester derivative with potent anti-anginal and selective coronary dilatation properties, *Proc. Brit. Pharmacol. Soc.* S16 (1993).
18. J.F. Giudicelli and A. Berdeaux, Compared effects of ITF 296, nitroglycerin and isosorbide dinitrate on coronary large conductance arteries and small resistance arterioles in the conscious dog. Effects of deendothelization, *in:* " ITF296 Internal Report" (1993).
19. A. Ueno and K. Nonaka, Differential effect of the novel nitrate derivative ITF 296 on large and small coronary arteries in the conscious dog: a comparative study with nitroglycerin and nicorandil, *in:* " ITF296 Internal Report" (1993).
20. E. Bassenge, Investigators report of coronary dilator response after acute and chronic administration of ITF 296, *in:* " ITF296 Internal Report" (1993).
21. P.W. Armstrong and J.A. Moffat, Tolerance to organic nitrates: clinical and experimental perspective, *Am. J. Med.* 74:73 (1983).
22. A. Berdeaux, B. Ghaleh, J.L. Dubois-Randɔ, B. Vignɔ, C. Drieu-la-Rochelle, L. Hittinger and J.F. Giudicelli, The role of vascular endothelium in exercise-induced dilation of large epicardial coronary arteries in conscious dogs, *Circulation* 89: in press (1994).

23. J. Duncker, P. Lindstrom and R.J. Bache, The novel nitrate ITF 296 preferentially increases subendocardial blood flow during exercise in the presence of a coronary artery stenosis, *in:* " ITF296 Internal Report" (1994).

24. R.J. Bache, P.A. McHale and J.C. Greenfield Jr., Transmural myocardial perfusion during restricted coronary inflow in the awake dog, *Am. J. Physiol,* 232:H645 (1977).

25. J. Rouleau, L.E. Boerboom, A. Surjadhana and J.I.E. Hoffman, The role of autoregulation and tissue diastolic pressure in the transmural distribution of left ventricular blood flow in anaesthetized dog, *Circ. Res.* 45: 804 (1979).

26. B.F.Robinson, Mode of action of nitroglycerin in angina pectoris: Correlation between haemodynamic effects during exercise and prevention of pain, *Br. Heart J.* 30:295 (1968).

27. J.H. Atterhog, L. Gekelund and A.L. Melin, Effect of nifedipine on exercise tolerance in patients with angina pectoris, *Eur.J. Clin. Pharmacol.* 8:125 (1975).

28. R.J. Bache and B.A. Tockman, Effect of Nitroglycerin and Nifedipine on subendocardial perfusion in the presence of a flow-limiting coronary stenosis in the awake dog, *Circ. Res.* 50: 678 (1982).

NITRIC OXIDE IN AMPHIBIAN PHOTORECEPTORS

Karl-F. Schmidt and Gottfried N. Nöll

Physiologisches Institut
Justus-Liebig-Universität
Aulweg 129
35392 Giessen, Germany

INTRODUCTION

The purpose of photoreceptors is the conversion of light into an electrical signal that controls the release of transmitter (glutamate) and thereby initiates a chain of physiological responses in other retinal neurons. The first step in the transduction cascade is the absorption of a photon by rhodopsin. Rhodopsin is mainly located in the plasma membrane of disks in the outer segment and consists of the chromophore 11-*cis*-retinal linked to the heptahelical protein opsin via a Schiff base to a lysin. Absorption of a photon isomerises retinal to the all-*trans*-conformation and converts rhodopsin to metarhodopsin II. Metarhodopsin II activates a cGMP-cleaving phosphodiesterase (PDE) via a specific G-protein (transducin). As a result of these enzymatic reactions the intracellular cGMP concentration is lowered and cGMP dissociates from the binding sites of the cGMP-dependent channels in the plasma membrane of the outer segment. The cGMP-dependent kation channels are open when the cGMP concentration in the photoreceptor is high in darkness. The channels close when the cGMP-level is lowered upon illumination and the inward current driven by a sodium-potassium pump in the inner segment is stopped. Interruption of this inward current, which is carried by sodium and calcium ions hyperpolarizes the membrane.

After a light flash the membrane potential and the cGMP-concentration of the photoreceptor cell is restored to preillumination levels. This flash response recovery is the result of several biochemical reactions. The activated rhodopsin is phosphorylated by a kinase and subsequently blocked by binding of arrestin[1,2]. Transducin autoregulates its activity by cleaving of GTP. The lifetime of the active PDE and the activity of the guanylate cyclase is presumed to be regulated via a calcium dependent negative feedback loop[3,4,5]. The closure of the cGMP-gated channels prevents calcium entry into the photoreceptor cell, while the sodium-calcium-potassium exchanger situated in the outer segment membrane continuously extrudes calcium. The light-dependent changes in the cGMP-metabolism are accompanied by a decreasing intracellular calcium concentration. Several models for the flash response recovery and the restoration of intracellular cGMP levels are based on this decrease of the cytosolic calcium level. The guanylate cyclase activity in vitro is enhanced by lowering of the calcium concentration. The required calcium levels are in a physiological range, but the regulatory pathway is not known[6,7,8,9].

Biochemical, Pharmacological, and Clinical Aspects of Nitric Oxide
Edited by B. A. Weissman *et al.*, Plenum Press, New York, 1995

103

The conductance of the cGMP-gated channel is affected by the extra- and intracellular calcium concentration[10,11], and the binding of cGMP to the channel protein is modulated by the intracellular calcium level[12]. The phosphodiesterase may be also subject to a calcium dependent regulation via a regulatory protein that interacts with rhodopsin kinase[13]. Other possible pathways for a calcium dependent negative feedback reaction have also been proposed[5,14], but some contradictory results make the role of calcium in the photoreceptor transduction process questionable and lead to the conclusion that calcium has multiple and complex effects on the recovery of photoresponses[15]. It is therefore reasonable to examine the role of other substances that may be linked to flash response recovery processes. It was demonstrated that two different types of guanylate cyclases exist in vertebrate photoreceptors. A particulate guanylate cyclase is controlled by the calcium level and a soluble guanylate cyclase is regulated by nitric oxide[16]. It was also shown that nitric oxide in photoreceptors is synthesized by nitric oxide synthase from L-arginine, as in other tissues[17].

The whole-cell patch clamp technique allows to apply intracellularly substances that interact with the NO-dependent pathway and to study their effects within the framework of the complete cell metabolism. Vertebrate photoreceptors are especially suitable for studies of a nitric oxide dependent regulation of the cGMP concentration because in these cells the cGMP-metabolism is directly reflected by the membrane voltage[18], and because both the nitric oxide synthase and the target enzyme of nitric oxide, the soluble guanylate cyclase were found in photoreceptors. Here we studied effects of sodium nitroprusside, NADPH, L-arginine and of nitric oxide synthase blockers on the membrane potential and light response recovery of isolated retinal rods from the frog (*Rana temporaria*).

METHODS

Rod outer segments with attached ellipsoids were isolated as described before[19] and incubated in: NaCl, 100 mM; KCl, 2.7 mM; $MgCl_2$, 0.5 mM; $CaCl_2$, 1 mM; glucose, 5 mM; HEPES, 10 mM; pH 7.8. Patch electrodes were filled with the following standard medium: KCl, 100 mM; $MgCl_2$, 0.5 mM; EGTA, 0.03 mM; GTP 1 mM; pCa 7.3; HEPES, 10 mM; pH 7.2. Other substances were added to this medium. The whole-cell access was obtained at the middle of the outer segment. The signals were amplified and processed by an EPC-7 system of List (Darmstadt, Germany). Diffuse light stimuli of saturating irradiance (2000 photons $s^{-1}\mu m^{-2}$, = 550 nm, duration = 30 ms) were provided by a light emitting diode.

The speed of flash response recovery [S_r] was defined as the ratio between response amplitude and response duration [mV/s]. This is reasonable, because the onset of the flash responses is very fast, in comparison to the offset. The initial underswing of the responses was not considered because this phenomenon is usually ascribed to voltage activated channels but not to the metabolism of nucleotides. The plateau phase of flash responses is determined by these channels and amounts to about -52 mV[20].

In the whole-cell configuration, an exchange of substances by diffusion between cytosol and pipette medium can affect the cell's function. The exchange of substances follows an exponential time course determined by both the molecular weight of the substance under study and the access resistance between pipette and cell[21]. When the membrane voltage of photoreceptor cells is recorded in the whole-cell configuration the loss of intracellular components is reflected by a membrane hyperpolarization and by a retardation of the flash response recovery. The alterations are following an exponential course with a time constant that varies with the size of the opening between cell and pipette. For a quantitative analysis a normalization procedure based on the measurement of the access resistance is required[19,22]. Therefore all quantitative data were corrected for an access resistance of 25 M.

RESULTS

When the whole-cell access to retinal rods is gained with pipettes containing the standard medium (including 1 mM GTP) an initial dark voltage [V_d] of about -10 mV is measured and the speed of the flash response recovery [S_r] is between 2 and 3 mV/s at the beginning. During the course of an experiment a spontaneous hyperpolarization accompanied by a reduction of flash response amplitudes is recorded and, in addition, a retardation of the flash response recovery occures (Fig. 1A, Table 1). The alterations of V_d and S_r follow an exponential time course according to the laws of diffusion and it is therefore likely that a diffusional loss of cytosolic components causes these alterations. Without GTP in the pipette medium the initial voltage is about -25 mV, the spontaneous hyperpolarization of the dark voltage is enhanced and proceeds more than 3 times faster. This result may indicate that a loss of intracellular nucleotides by diffusion into the pipette may be one reason for the spontaneous hyperpolarization[19], but it was not possible to achieve stable recording conditions simply by application of GTP.

Addition of sodium nitroprusside (0.01 - 0.3 mM) to the pipette mhas significant effects on the dark voltage and on the speed of the flash response recovery. The spontaneous hyperpolarization of V_d, observed under control conditions, is replaced by an initial depolarization followed by a relatively stable dark voltage and instead of a retardation, the response recovery S_r is accelerated during the course of an experiment. In the experiments with sodium nitroprusside the flash responses retained a needle like shape for more than 10 min and values of S_r exceeded 6 mV/s after 10 min recording (Fig. 1B, Table 1). When the membrane voltage in photoreceptors reflects the actual intracellular level of cGMP, it can be assumed that the modification of both, V_d and S_r, reflect different aspects of the cGMP-metabolism. The dark voltage may serve as an indicator of the intracellular cGMP level and the speed of flash response recovery may be representative for the turnover of cGMP. Under these assumptions the observed effects suggest that the concentration and the turnover of cGMP in retinal rods is enhanced by application of sodium nitroprusside[23].

Significant effects on the function of retinal rods were also observed upon application of NADPH. NADPH (0.1 mM) added to the pipette medium gives rise to marked depolarizations of the dark voltage. The speed of recovery is accelerated during the course of an experiment. The effects were similar to sodium nitroprusside, although the emerging picture was different in detail. The alterations of V_d and S_r did not follow an exponential course but showed a more complex behaviour. As it is shown in the example of Fig. 1C the cells kept the dark voltage relatively stable for the first recording period. The duration of this period differed in various experiments and ranged from 30 s to 200 s. This first period was followed by a relatively fast depolarization. The cells depolarized within less than 30 s from about -15 mV to about 0 mV and kept this dark voltage stable for more than 10 min while flash responses were still elicitable. In experiments with NADPH in the pipette medium the speed of repolarization was about 2.5 mV/s for the first flash responses. During the course of these experiments the speed of the repolarization increased and values of S_r exceeded 8 mV/s after 10 min. Other cofactors (NADH and FAD) were also tested, but no significant effects on the function of retinal rods were found.

When the pipette medium was complemented with the substrate of the NO-synthase L-arginine a slight stabilization of V_d was observed in some experiments, but this effect was not significant (Table 1). As shown in Fig. 1D, L-arginine (0.3 mM) added to the pipette medium prevented the prolongation of the flash responses and values of S_r remained constant between 2.2 and 2.5 mV/s during the course of the experiments.

Effects of intracellularly applied nitric oxide synthase inhibitors on dark voltage and flash responses of retinal rods where opposite to those described above upon application of sodium nitroprusside or NADPH.

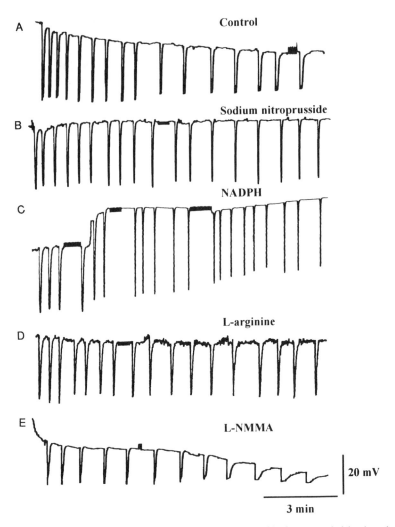

Figure 1. Alterations of the dark voltage and of photoresponses with time recorded in the whole-cell mode under control conditions (A), with 0.1 mM sodium nitroprusside (B), with 0.1 mM NADPH (C), 0.3 mM L-arginine (D), and with 0.1 mM L-NMMA (E) in the pipette filling solution. The steep downward deflections are responses to flashes of 30 ms duration and of saturating irradiance (ca. 2000 photons s^{-1}μm^{-2}, λ = 550 nm) provided by a light emitting diode. Access resistances were 25 M± 5 Ω in all experiments. Horizontal bars represent intervals of voltage clamp recordings. (This figure contains parts from Schmidt et al.[23] and Tsuyama et al.[24])

When nitric oxide synthase inhibitors were present in the recording pipette the spontaneous hyperpolarization of the dark voltage was accelerated and the speed of flash response recovery was reduced during the course of an experiment. Recordings from an experiment with the competitive inhibitor of nitric oxide synthase L-NMMA are shown in Fig. 1E. Two different arginine analogs L-NNA (L- -nitro-L-arginine, 100μM) and L-NMMA (Lω-monomethyl-arginine,100μM) were tested.

When L-NNA was used the time course of the hyperpolarization was less affected, but the retardation of the flash response recovery was similar to L-NMMA (Table 1). The results indicate that the concentration, as well as the turnover of cGMP is reduced by inhibition of nitric oxide synthase in retinal rods.

medium (experiments)	time constant [s]	difference [mV]	recovery [mV/s]
control (6)	412 ± 114	- 14.1 ± 5.7	0.61 ± 0.22
without GTP (11)	112 ± 32	- 25.4 ± 5.2	0.12 ± 0.06
nitroprusside 0.3 mM (5)	444 ± 132	+ 7.2 ± 6.2	7.20 ± 2.50
NADPH 0.1 mM (6)	------------*	+13.4 ± 5.2	8.30 ± 3.10
L-arginine 0.3 mM (5)	348 ± 64	- 16.1 ± 7.3	2.40 ± 0.40
L-NMMA 0.1 mM (4)	50 ± 21	- 37.3 ± 9.3	0.14 ± 0.05
L-NNA 0.1 mM (3)	317 ± 101	- 12.3 ± 4.3	0.16 ± 0.07

Table 1. *1st column*: time constant of the exponential alteration of the dark voltage, corrected for an access resistance of 25 Ω. Higher values indicate a more stable membrane potential. * time course of experiments with NADPH could not be fitted by exponentials. *2nd column*: amplitude of the time dependent hyper- (-) or depolarization (+) (difference between initial and final membrane potential). *3rd column*: speed of flash response recovery [S_r] after more than 10 min recording. At the beginning of an experiment the speed of recovery was between 2 and 3 mV/s. (Data partly from Schmidt et al.[23] and Tsuyama et al.[24])

The effects on the dark voltage of the two inhibitors were different. This may indicate that the dark activity of nitric oxide 8synthase of retinal rods is differentially inhibited by L-NMMA and L-NNA. The effects on the flash response recovery of both arginine analogs were similar and therefore it is likely that the activity of the enzyme during flash responses is equally affected by both inhibitors.

DISCUSSION

Cyclic GMP in photoreceptors is presumably synthesized by two enzymes: a particulate and a soluble guanylate cyclase. Cleavage of cGMP is due to a phosphodiesterase whose activity is controlled by a light dependent enzyme cascade. The activities of these three enzymes determine the cytoplasmic level of cGMP which, in turn, regulates the membrane current and the membrane voltage of vertebrate photoreceptors (see Fig. 2). In the present study two modifications in the behaviour of the membrane voltage were employed as indicators of the functional state of the photoreceptor cell: the slow spontaneous hyperpolarization in the dark and the speed of the recovery of flash responses.

If it is true that the membrane voltage at any given time reflects the intracellular level of cGMP, then one can assume that these two modifications may reflect different aspects of the photoreceptor's cGMP-metabolism. While the actual dark voltage can be used as an indicator of the intracellular cGMP level, the speed of the recovery phase of the flash responses may have a relation to the cGMP turnover.

The depolarization of the dark voltage and the acceleration of the flash response recovery caused by sodium nitroprusside on one hand, and the accelerated hyperpolarization and the prolongation of the recovery observed upon intracellular application of NO-synthase inhibitors on the other hand, suggest that these effects are linked to a nitric oxide dependent pathway.

The effects of sodium nitroprusside on the function of photoreceptors can be compared to the effects of light on the cGMP-metabolism. When photoreceptors are exposed to light the concentration of free cGMP is reduced while the turnover of cGMP is considerably increased[25,26].

Intracellular application of L-arginine did not significantly affect the course of the dark voltage but prevented the retardation of the flash response recovery. This could indicate that loss of L-arginine by diffusion is at least one of the reasons for the retardation of flash response recovery during whole-cell recording. While a minimum level of L-arginine seems to be essential for the normal flash responserecovery, it does not seem to be of great importance for the normal regulation of the dark voltage.

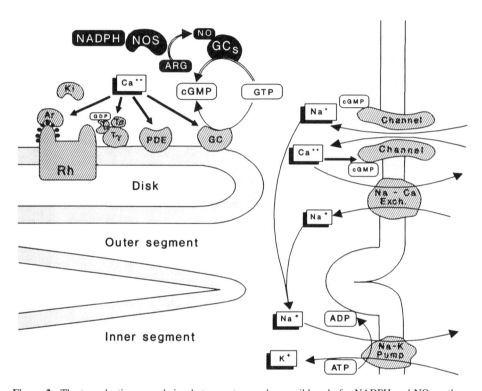

Figure 2. The transduction cascade in photoreceptors and a possible role for NADPH and NO-synthase. The connecting part between outer and inner segment and the first disk of a retinal rod is drawn. The scheme represents the situation during the flash response reco. Rhodopsin (Rh) is phosphorylated by rhodopsin kinase (Ki) and blocked by arrestin (Ar). Transducin (T) and the phosphodiesterase (PDE) are inactivated. The ligth-dependent kation channels gated by cGMP regulate the membrane potential and the intracellular calcium concentration, which has multiple effects on the transduction cascade (see introduction). Sodium is extruded by the sodium-potassium pumps in the plasma membrane of the inner segment. Calcium is extruded by sodium-calcium exchangers in the outer segment membrane. After a light flash the membrane potential and the cGMP-concentration of the photoreceptor cell is restored to preillumination levels by activating two types of guanylate cyclases: a particulate guanylate cyclase (GC) which is presumably regulated by a calcium dependent negative feedback loop and a soluble guanylate cyclase (GC_s) which is probably regulated via NADPH and a NO-synthase (NOS) producing nitric oxide (NO) from L-arginine (ARG).

The co-factor NADPH has surprisingly distinct effects: i. e. NADPH significantly depolarizes the membrane voltage and accelerates the recovery phase of the flash responses. One likely explanation of the NADPH effect is that it activates the photoreceptor NO-synthase in vivo, as it was found in vitro (Venturini et al. 1991). The complex time course of the NADPH action with its delay and the sudden drop of the voltage would then indicate, that a distinct level of NADPH in the cell! is required before the level of cGMP is raised. An enhanced level of NADPH in a light adapted photoreceptor cell could activate the guanylate cyclase indirectly via the NO-synthase, and in this way counterbalance an increased phosphodiesterase activity brought about by light dependent reactions. While the postulated role of NADPH requires further testing, it is clear that NADPH is a potent stimulus for the opening of cGMP-dependent channels in retinal rods. It is very likely that the activity of NO-synthase in photoreceptor cells has an influence on concentration and metabolic flux of cGMP in photoreceptors, which may be of relevance for flash response recovery and adaptation processes.

Acknowledgements: The authors are indebted to Prof. C. Baumann for continuous support. We wish to thank O. Becker and G. Schmandt for excellent technical assistance and B. Volkmann for preparation of the figures. The work was supported by the Deutsche Forschungsgemeinschaft (Schm 723/6-1).

REFERENCES

1. H. Kühn, Light-regulated binding of rhodopsin kinase and other proteins to cattle bovine photoreceptor membranes, *Biochem.* 17: 4389-4395 (1978).
2. H. Kühn, Light- and GTP-regulated interaction of GTP-ase and other proteins with bovine photoreceptor membranes, *Nature* 283: 587-589 (1980).
3. L. Lagnado and D. Baylor, Signal flow in visual transduction, *Neuron* 8: 995-1002 (1992).
4. E.N.Jr. Pugh and T.D. Lamb, Amplification and kinetics of the activation steps in phototransduction, *Biochim. Biophys. Acta* 1141: 111-149 (1993).
5. Y. Koutalos and K.W. Yau, A rich complexity emerges in phototransduction, *Curr. Opin. Neurobiol.* 3: 513-519 (1993)
6. K.-W. Koch and L. Stryer, Highly cooperative feedback control of retinal rod guanylate cyclase by calcium ions, *Nature* 334: 64-66 (1988).
7. Y. Horio and F. Murad, Solubilization of guanylyl cyclase from bovine rod outer segments and effects of lowering Ca2+ and nitro compounds, *J. Biol. Chem.* 266: 3411-3415 (1991).
8. H.-G. Lambrecht and K.-W. Koch, Phosphorylation of recoverin, the calcium-sensitive activator of photoreceptor guanylyl cyclase, *FEBS Letters* 294: 207-209 (1991).
9. H.-G. Lambrecht and K.-W. Koch, A 26 kD calcium binding protein from bovine rod outer segments as modulator of photoreceptor guanylate cyclase. *EMBO J.* 10: 793-798 (1991).
10. L.W. Haynes, A.R. Kay, and K.W. Yau, Single cyclic GMP-activated channel activity in excised patches of rod outer segment membrane, *Nature* 321: 66-70 (1986).
11. A. Zimmerman and D.A. Baylor, Cyclic GMP-sensitive conductance of retinal rods consists of aqueous pores, *Nature* 321: 70-72 (1986).
12. Y.T. Hsu and R.S. Molday, Modulation of the cGMP-gated channel of rod photoreceptor cells by calmodulin, *Nature* 361: 76-79 (1993).
13. S. Kawamura, Rhodopsin phosphorylation as a mechanism of cyclic GMP phosphodiesterase regulation by S-modulin. *Nature* 362: 855-857 (1993).
14. U.B. Kaupp and K.-W. Koch, Role of cGMP and Ca^{2+} in vertebrate photoreceptor excitation and adaptation, *Ann. Rev. Physiol.* 54: 153-175 (1992).
15. V.J. Coccia and R.H. Cote, Regulation of intracellular cyclic GMP concentration by light and calcium in electropermeabilized rod photoreceptors, *J. Gen. Physiol.* 103: 67-86 (1994).
16. A. Margulis, R.K. Sharma, and A. Sitaramayya, Nitroprusside-sensitive and insensitive guanylate cyclases in retinal rod outer segments, *Biochem. Biophys. Res. Comm.* 185: 909-914 (1992).
17. C.M. Venturini, R.G. Knowles, R.M.J. Palmer, and S. Moncada, Synthesis of nitric oxide in the bovine retina, *Biochem. Biophys. Res. Comm.* 180: 920-925 (1991).
18. E.E. Fesenko, S.S. Kolesnikov, and A.L. Lyubarski, Induction by cyclic GMP of cationic conductance in plasma membrane of retinal rod outer segment, *Nature* 313: 310-313 (1985).
19. K.-F. Schmidt, G.N. Nöll, and C. Baumann, Effect of guanine nucleotides on the dark voltage of single frog rods, *Visual Neurosci.* 2: 101-108 (1989).

20. C.R. Bader, D. Bertrand, and E.A. Schwartz, Voltage activated and calcium-activated currents studied in solitary rod inner segments from the salamander retina, *J. Physiol.* 331: 253-284 (1982).

21. M. Pusch and E. Neher, Rates of diffusional exchange between small cells and a measuring patch pipette, *Pflügers Arch.*, 411: 204-211 (1988).

22. K.-F. Schmidt, G.N. Nöll, P. Jacobi, and C. Baumann, Configuration of light responses in isolated retinal rods. A patch-clamp study, *Graefe's Arch. Clin. Exp. Ophthalmol.* 232: 153-161 (1994).

23. K.-F. Schmidt, G.N. Nöll, and Y. Yamamoto, Sodium Nitroprusside alters dark voltage and light responses on isolated retinal rods during whole-cell recording, *Visual Neurosci.* 9: 205-209 (1992).

24. Y. Tsuyama, G.N. Nöll, and K.-F. Schmidt, L-Arginine and nicotinamide adenine dinucleotide phosphate alter dark voltage and accelerate light response recovery in isolated retinal rods of the frog (*Rana temporaria*), *Neurosci. Letters* 149: 95-98 (1993).

25. A. Ames, T.F. Walseth, R.A. Heyman, M. Barad, R.M. Graeff, and N.D. Goldberg, Light-induced increases in cGMP metabolic flux correspondend with electrical responses of photoreceptors, *J. Biol. Chem.* 261: 13034-13042 (1986).

26. S.M. Dawis, R.M. Graeff, R.A. Heyman, T.F. Walseth, and N.D. Goldberg, Regulation of cyclic GMP metabolism in toad photoreceptors, *J. Biol. Chem.* 263: 8771-8785 (1988).

THE INVOLVEMENT OF L-ARGININE-NITRIC OXIDE PATHWAY IN THE ANTI-RICKETTSIAL ACTIVITY OF MACROPHAGELIKE CELLS

Avi Keysary[1], Chaya Oron[1], Miri Rosner[1] and Ben Avi Weissman[2]

[1]Department of Microbiology
[2]Department of Pharmacology
Israel Institute for Biological Research
P.O.B. 19, Ness Ziona,74100, Israel.

INTRODUCTION

Rickettsia conorii is an obligate, intracellular, gram-negative bacterium which causes Mediterranean spotted-fever. The encounter between rickettsia and macrophage can result either in the destruction of the cell due to rickettsial intracellular multiplication or in the destruction of the invading bacterium. The anti-rickettsial activity of the macrophage can be stimulated in two modes. The first, by treating the macrophages with cytokines such as γ-interferon (γ-IFN). The other, destruction of rickettsiae within the macrophage cell can be facilitated by treating the rickettsiae with specific-antibodies prior to their engulfment by the macrophage (Winkler and Turco, 1993).
Recombinant murine γ-IFN inhibited the growth of R. conorii in mouse macrophages. This activity was blocked by monoclonal antibodies to γ-IFN (Jerrells et al., 1986). R. conorii-infected mice which were γ-IFN-depleted became more susceptible to the bacterium (Li et al., 1987). It was demonstrated that mechanisms associated with NO synthase actions in macrophage are activated by γ-IFN. These mechanisms facilitate the elimination of various pathogens such as Leishmania major (Shawn et al., 1990), Francisella tularensis, (Fortier et al., 1992) Legionella pneumophila (Summersgill et al., 1992), Entamoeba histolytica (Jian and Cadee, 1992) and Ehrlichia risticii (Park and Rikihisa, 1992).
The mechanism(s) by which macrophages inhibit the growth of rickettsiae treated with anti-R. conorii antibodies is not clear yet. Nevertheless, it was demonstrated in macrophagelike cells which were infected with Rickettsia prowazekii that the rickettsiae destruction was respiratory-burst independent process (Keysary et al., 1988).
This work demonstrates that γ-IFN induces NO-synthase mechanisms which cause growth-inhibiton of R. conorii in a macrophagelike cell line. However, the growth-inhibition produced by the specific antibody-rickettsia binding is induced by a different mechanism.

Biochemical, Pharmacological, and Clinical Aspects of Nitric Oxide
Edited by B. A. Weissman *et al.*, Plenum Press, New York, 1995

111

MATERIALS AND METHODS

Rickettsia: R. conorii (Moroccan strain) stock was propageted in embryonated-egg yolk-sacs. Following trituration the rickettsiae were partially-purified by three differential centrifugations cycles. The rickettsiae were suspended in sucrose-phosphate-glutamate buffer (218 mM sucrose, 37.6 mM KH_2PO_4, 7.1 mM K_2HPO_4, 4.9 mM potassium glutamate, pH 7.0) and stored in -70°C.

Macropahgelike cell cultures: Mouse macrophagelike cell line J774A.1 was grown in Dulbecco modified Eagle medium supplemented with 10% fetal-calf serum, 2 mM glutamine and non-essential amino acids (Biological Industries, Beth-Haemek, Israel).

Infection of cells with rickettsiae: Ricketsiae were used to infect the macropahgelike cells in two paradigms:
1. Experiments in which cells were incubated with γ-IFN post-infection.
2. Experiments in which cells were infected with rickettsiae pretreated with antibodies.
In the first set of experiments, J774A.1 cells were seeded one day before infection into 96 well plates at a concentration of $1x10^5$ cells per well, in 0.1 ml medium. The cells were washed prior to infection with Hanks balanced salt solution supplemented with 0.1% gelatin and 5.0 mM L-glutamic acid (HBSSGG). Rickettsiae suspension (1:300 in HBSSGG, 0.1 ml) was added to each well. The plates were centrifuged at 500 x g for 15 min at 25°C and then incubated for 45 min at 34°C. The wells were washed three times with medium and then incubated with 0.25 ml medium containing test reagents: γ-IFN (Recombinant mouse γ-IFN, Genzyme, USA), N^G-monomethyl-L-arginine (MMLA) and L-arginine (Sigma). The infection rate achieved was 1.5-2.5 rickettsiae per cell. The cells were incubated at 34°C in humidified CO_2 incubator for 48 hours.

In experiments in which rickettsiae were pre-treated with antibodies, R. conorii suspensions in HBSSGG were incubated with anti-R. conorii IgG from hyper-immunized rabbit or with non-immune rabbit IgG for 15 minutes at 25°C. Cells were infected and maintained as described above.

Rickettsial count: The infected cells were scraped from duplicate wells, suspended in 0.02 ml medium, applied onto glass slides, dried and stained by a modification of Gimenez method (Wisseman et al., 1974). Fifty cells from each well were examined and the number of rickettsiae was determined. When there were more than 30 rickettsiae per cell, a value of 30 was assigned.

Nitrite determination: Supernatants from the wells were assayed for nitrite with the Griess reagent (Green et al., 1982). Sodium nitrite solutions were used for calibration.

RESULTS

Anti-rickettsial activity induced by γ-IFN
R. conorii multiply 18 fold in J774A.1 cells in 48 hours in medium containing 0.4 mM L-arginine. The presence of γ-IFN in the growing medium of the infected cell during the incubation time resulted in growth-inhibition of the rickettsia. γ-IFN at concentration of 5, 15, and 50 units per ml inhibited rickettsial growth by 53, 80 and 83%, respectively (Fig. 1). The anti-rickettsial effect of γ-IFN was associated with 6-fold increase of nitrite ion concentration in the mediun. Addition of MMLA (0.15-0.5 mM) abolished the interferon induced effect and reduced nitrite to control levels. High concentrations of L-arginine

112

(2.4 mM) restored the anti-rickettsial action of γ-IFN in the cells and in-addition, caused increase in nitrite formation (Fig 1).

Table 1: Effects of antibodies on rickettsial growth in macrophagelike cells.

Pre-treatment	Rickettsiae per cell on day 3 post-infection[1,2]
none	≥30
non-specific rabbit IgG (250 μg/ml)	≥30
anti-R. conorii rabbit IgG (1500 μg/ml)	0.6 ± 0.2
anti-R. conorii rabbit IgG (150 μg/ml)	0.7 ± 0.6
anti-R. conorii rabbit IgG (15 μg/ml)	≥30

[1]Results are expressed as mean ± S.D. of 3 - 5 determinations.
[2]Initial infection rate was 2.3 ±1.0 rickettsiae per cell.

Anti-rickettsial activity induced by antibodies

Rickettsiae treated with specific-IgG failed to multiply in J774A.1 cells, while untreated rickettsiae or rickettsiae treated with rabbit-IgG, which are not anti-R. conorii, multiplyed successfully in the macrophage cells (Table 1). No changes in nitrite ion levels in the different treatments groups were observed (≤1 μM). The presence of MMLA (0.25 mM) in the medium had no effect on the cellular anti-rickettsial activity.

DISCUSSION

results achieved in this study suggest the involvement of the NO-synthase pathway in the γ-IFN induced anti-rickettsial activity in macrophagelike cells. Both rickettsial growth-inhibition and nitrite production are significantly reduced in the presence of MMLA - a competitive inhibitor of NOS. Furthermore, excess of L-arginine restore the anti-rickettsial effect of γ-IFN and the nitrite production. It is assumed that the nitrogen intermediates produced by the NOS cause intracellular iron loss and inhibit the action of several critical iron containing enzyme such as aconitase of citric acid cycle (Drapier and Hibbs, 1986), mitochondrial electron transport chain oxidoreductase (Drapier and Hibbs, 1988) and ribonucleotide reductase of DNA synthesis (Krohenbuhl, 1980). Also γ-IFN was found to limit iron availibilty by down-regulation of transferrin receptors on macrophages surface (Lane et al., 1991).

Antibodies-treated rickettsiae killling by macrophagelike cells does not involve the NO synthase pathway since it was not inhibited by synthase inhibitor (MMLA) and nitirite synthesis was not observed during this process.

This study demonstrates that anti-rickettsial activity in macrophagelike cells may be the consequence of more then one mechanism or induced by different mechanisms.

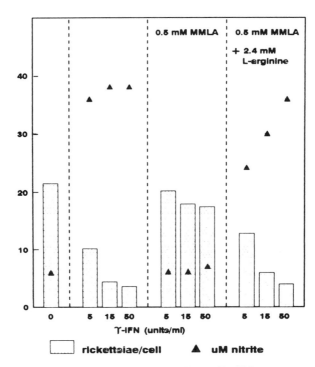

Figure 1: Effect of γ-IFN on R. conorii growth in J774A.1 cells. Values represent the means of 3 independent experiments.

REFERENCES

Drapier, J.-C., and Hibbs, J.B, Jr. 1986. Murine cytotoxic activated macrophages inhibit aconitase in tumor cells. J. Clin. Invest. 78:790-797.

Drapier, J.-C., and Hibbs, J.B., Jr. 1988. Differentiation of murine macrophages to express nonspecific cytotoxicity for tumor cells results in L-arginine-dependent inhibition of mitochondrial iron-sulfur enzymes in the macrophage effector cells. J. Immunol. 140:2829-2838.

Fortier, A.H., Polsinelli, T., Green, S.J., and Nacy, C.A. 1992. Activation of macrophages for destruction of Francisella tularensis: Identification of cytokines, effector cells, and effector molecules. Infect. Immun. 60:817-825.

Green, L.C., Wagner, D.C., Glogowski, J., Skipper, P.L., Wishnok, J.S. and R. Tannenbaum, S.R. 1982. Analysis of nitrate, nitrite, and [15N] nitrate in biological fluids. Anal. Biochem. 126:131-138.

Jerrells, T.R., Turco, J., Winkler, H.H., and Spitalny, G.L. 1986. Neutraliztion of lymphokines-mediated antirickettsial activity of fibroblasts and macrophages with monoclonal antibody specific for murine interferon gamma. Infect. Immun. 51:355-359.

Jian, Y.L. and Cadee, K. 1992. Macrophage cytotoxicity against Entamoeba histolytica trophozoites is mediated by nitric oxide from L-arginine. J. Immunol. 148:3999-4005.

Keysary A., McCaul T.F., and Winkler H.H. 1988. Roles of the Fc receptor and respiratory burst in killing of Rickettsia prowazekii by macrophagelike cell lines. Infect. Immun. 57:2390-2396.

Krohenbuhl, J.E. 1980. Effects of activated macrophages on tumor target cells in discrete phases of the cell cycle. Cancer Res. 40:4622-4627.

Lane, T.E., Wu-Hsieh, B.A., and Howard, D.H. 1991. Iron limitation and the gamma interferon-mediated antihistoplasma state of murine macrophages. Infect. Immun. 59:2274-2278.

Li, H., Jerrells, T.R., Spitalny, G.L. and Dieffenbach, C.W. 1987. Gamma interferon as a crucial host defense against Rickettsia conorii in vivo. Infect. Immunol. 55:1252-1255.

Park, J. and Rikihisa, Y. 1992. L-Arginine-dependent killing of intracellular Ehrlichia risticii by macrophages treated with gamma interferon. Infect. Immun. 60:3504-3508.

Shawn, J.G., Meltzer, M.S., Hibbs, J.B Jr. and Nacy, C.A. 1990. Activated macrophages destroy intracellular Leishmania major amastigotes by an L-arginine-dependent killing mechanism. J. Immunol. 144:278-283.

Summersgill, J.T., Powell, L.A., Buster, B.L., Miller, R.D. and Ramirez, J.A.. 1992. Killing of Legionella pneumophila by nitric oxide in interferon-activated macrophages. J. Leukoc. Biol. 52:625-629.

Winkler, H.H., and Turco, J. 1993. Rickettsiae and Macrophages, in: "Macrophage-Pathogen Interactions," B.S. Zwilling, and T.K. Einstein, eds., Marcel Dekker, Inc. New-York. pp:401-414.

Wisseman, C.L., Jr., Waddel, A.D., and Walsh, W.T. 1974. Mechanisms of Immunity in typhus infections. IV. Failure of chicken embryo cells in culture to restrict growth of antibody- sensityzed Rickettsia prowazekii. Infect. Immun. 9:571-575.

MODULATION OF LDL AND oxy-LDL CATABOLISM BY NO-DONORS AND PGE$_2$ IN HUMAN PERIPHERAL BLOOD LYMPHOCYTES AND RAT MACROPHAGES

Aldona Dembinska-Kiec, Iwona Wybranska, Barbara
Miszczuk-Jamska, Ewa Baczynska, Jadwiga Hartwich,
and Pawel Goldsztajn.

Department of Clinical Biochemistry of the Collegium Medicum
Jagiellonian University Cracow
Grzegorzecka 16
31501 Cracow
Poland

INTRODUCTION

One of the substances important for homeostasis, released by vascular endothelial cells, is the Endothelium Derived Relaxing Factor (EDRF/NO) (1). It resembles the biological activity of PGI$_2$, such as vasodilation, inhibition of platelet aggregation and adhesion, but the cellular "second messenger" for this mediator is c-GMP. Both PGI$_2$ and EDRF/NO activity were found to be decreased in atherosclerosis (1). The EDRF/NO activity can be substituted by nitrovasodilators (so called "NO-donors"), such as SIN-I or sodium nitroprusside (NaNP).

In contrast to the well-recognized influence of prostaglandins such as PGI$_2$ on low density lipoprotein (LDL) catabolism (2,3), there are only a few reports describing the influence of EDRF2/NO or NO-donors on LDL metabolism (4,5). PGE$_1$, PGE$_2$ or the stable PGI$_2$ analogue - Iloprost (2,3) have been reported to inhibit the binding of LDL to its receptor, inhibit LDL-receptor activity, inhibit the accumulation and degradation of LDL as well as biosynthesis of cholesterol by increasing c-AMP levels in different cells including the vascular smooth muscle, lymphocytes and macrophages.

In the present study we investigated the effect of NO-donors on the native LDL (n-LDL) catabolism in lymphocytes which bind and accumulate LDL only by the n-LDL receptor (similar to endothelial and smooth muscle cells of vessel wall) (6,7) and on the metabolism of oxidised LDL (oxy-LDL) which is removed from circulation by the scavenger receptor of macrophages (6-8).

Biochemical, Pharmacological, and Clinical Aspects of Nitric Oxide
Edited by B. A. Weissman *et al.*, Plenum Press, New York, 1995

MATERIALS AND METHODS

[125]I (5mCi) was purchased from NEN, Boston, MA. RPMI-1640 and Dulbecco's modified Eagle's medium (DMEM) was purchased from Gibco (Grand Island, NY, USA). All other chemicals were from Sigma (St Louis, MO, USA).

Venous, citrated (1:9) blood of healthy volunteers was used for the separation of lymphocytes (LT) by the Ficoll-Pague procedure. LT were suspended (2-4x10[6] cells/ml) in RPMI 1640 medium containing penicillin (100 U/ml), streptomycin (100 μg/ml) and transfered (1 ml) to 35 mm dishes (NUNC). Cells were incubated in the presence of 10% fetal calf serum (FCS)-LT with the low LDL receptor activity (LRA), or in the presence of 10% of lipoprotein deficient serum (LPDS)-LT with the high LDL receptor activity (HRA) for 22 hrs at 37°C in 5% CO_2 atmosphere.

Monocyte-derived, abdominal residual macrophages, were obtained from Wistar rats by peritoneal lavage and suspended (5x10[6] cells/ml) in RPMI 1640 medium containing 10% FCS, glutamine (4 mM), penicillin (100 U/ml), streptomycin (100 μg/ml) and amphotericin B (0.25 μg/ml). One ml of cell suspension was transfered to tissue culture (35 mm) dishes. Following 16 hrs incubation at 37°C in CO_2 atmosphere the non-adherent cells were removed by several washing steps with RPMI medium.

Human n-LDL samples (density 1,019-1.063 g/ml) were obtained from pooled plasma of normolipidemic subjects and prepared by differential ultracentrifugation. Oxydation of LDL (oxy-LDL) was performed by coincubation with 5 μM $CuSO_4$ at 37°C for 10 hrs. n-LDL and oxy-LDL were labelled with ^{125}I by the Iodogen method. The final specific activity was in the range of 50 to 100 cpm/ng of LDL protein.

Catabolism of n-LDL by LT with LRA or with HLA activity was performed by measurement of the receptor activity and cellular accumulation of LDL. The LDL receptor activity was monitored according to Goldstein and Brown (7,8). Briefly, 20 μg of [125]I n-LDL were added to each dish containing LT with LRA or HRA activity, with or without a 25-fold excess of unlabelled LDL. Then, cells were incubated for 6 hrs at 37°C and the LDL receptor activity was measured by differences in radioactivity of cellular fractions coincubated with or without an excess of unlabelled LDL. The amount of radioactivity measured in LT incubated without unlabelled LDL were taken as the total cellular accumulation of n-LDL by LT. Similarily, the estimation of cellular accumulation of oxy-LDL by macrophages was performed by coincubation of 100 μg/ml of ^{125}I oxy-LDL with monolayer macrophages for 6 hrs at 37°C in CO_2 atmosphre.

For the measurement of the radioactivity in cells, cells were washed three times with a ten fould excess of PBS and centrifuged (800 x g for 15 min at 4°C). The final cell pellet was suspended in 1 N NaOH and radioactivity was measured in a LKB β-counter.

The effect of NO-donors (NaNP: 0-300 μM, SIN-1: 0-300 μM or PGE_2: 0-300 μM), or N[G]monomethyl-L-Arginine (L-MMA), aa potent and specific inhibitor of NO-synthase (3 μM in macrophages only) on LDL catabolism, was carried out by performing the above mentioned the incubations in the presence of these agents.

The results are presented as a percentage of values obtained for cells incubated in the medium containing 10% LPDS (100%).

All results are presented as mean ± SD. Statistical analysis was calrried oue by Student's t-test and considered as significant at p< 0.05.

RESULTS

Preincubation of LT with LRA in the presence of NaNP resulted in a dose-dependent decrease of n-LDL receptor activity and cellular accumulation of n-LDL (Fig. 1). This effect was also observed when PGE_2 was used instead of the NO-donor (results not shown).

Preincubation of LT with LPDS increased the LDL receptor activity by 40% (from 609± 61 ng of LDL/mg of cell protein to 1040±105 ng of LDL/mg of cell protein). NaNP dosedependently prevented the up-regulation of LDL receptor activity. The preincubation with LPDS also increased the ability of "starving" cells to accumulate n-LDL (from 3745± 376 ng of LDL/mg of cell protein to 78011±7800 ng of LDL/mg of cell protein). In these experimental conditions (LT with HRA), the effect of NaNP was biphasic. Up to 100 µM inhibition was observed, while at 300 µM activation of n-LDL receptor activity was obtained (Fig. 2). Under identical experimental conditions PGE_2 inhibited both the n-LDL receptor activity and cellular n-LDL accumulation by LT with HRA (results not presented).

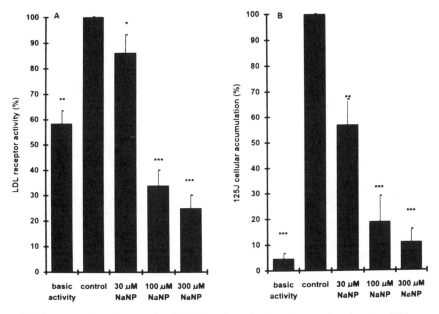

Figure 1: Effects of sodium nitroprusside (NaNP) on the induction of human lymphocyte n-LDL receptor activity (A) and ^{125}I n-LDL cellular accumulation (B). Lymphocytes used are with low n-LDL receptor activity. Mean ± SD from n=3-5 experiments carried out in triplicates. Statistical significance: *p<0.05; **p<0.02; ***p<0.001

In the absence of L-MMA, SIN-I up to 100 µM concentration did not affect the oxy-LDL accumulation by macrophages (Fig. 3), while SIN-l at a concentration of 300 µM as well as NaNP at all concentrations used, significantly increased the oxy-LDL accumulation by cells (Fig. 3).

Preincubation of cells with L-MMA significantly decreased NO biosynthesis (results not presented) and in addition, caused a significant increase in the accumulation of oxy-LDL by macrophages (Fig. 3B)

In the presence of L-MMA, SIN-I dose-dependently inhibited the accumulation of oxy-LDL by macrophages and prevented the NaNP-induced potentiation of oxy-LDL accumulation by these cells (Fig. 3B)

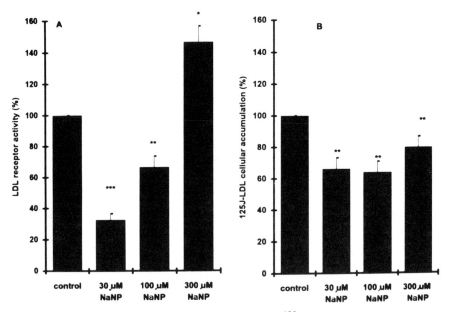

Figure 2: Effect of NaNP on n-LDL receptor activity (A) and ^{125}I-LDL cellular accumulation (B) in lymphocytes with high LDL-receptor activity. Mean ± SD, n=3-5 experiments carried out in triplicates. Statistical significance: *p <0.05; **p< 0.02; ***p<0.001.

DISCUSSION

In this study we have denonstrated that NO-donors can supress the n-LDL receptor activity as well as n-LDL intracellular accumulation in peripheral blood lymphocytes. Similar inhibitory effect was observed when the cellular activity of n-LDL receptor was low. However, at high B/E receptor activity states, a biphasic ieffect of NaNP was observed, which may suggest that high concentrations of NO (or NO-donors) can accelerate the cellular accumulation of n-LDL by cells with HRA.

In aedition, we found that the decrease in NO biosynthesis following preincubation of macrophages with L-MMA due to an augmented intracellular accumulation of oxy-LDL, suggesting that endogenously formed NO protects macrophages (the precursors of foam cells) against lipid accumulation. Under these experimental conditions (a decreased amount of endogenous NO), SIN-1 dose-dependently inhibited the increased accumulation of oxy-LDL by macrophages, probabley by substituting endogenous NO. However, in the preserved production of endogenous NO, both SIN-I and NaNP augmented the accumulation of oxy-LDL by macrophages, suggesting that a high NO/NO-donor concentration may potentiate the intracellular accumulation of lipids.

The mechanism(s) of NO/NO-donors effect on LDL catabolism is yet unknown and this study did not answer the open questions. The accumulation of c-AMP in fibroblasts arterial smooth musce cells, macrophages and lymphocytes elicited by prostanoids, cholera toxin, forscolin or direct application of dibutyryl-cAMP, was reported to be associated with a decrease in n-LDL-receptor binding activity, and the accumulation of oxy-LDL by macrophages (2,3).

Cytokines, such as Interferon-γ or TNF-α and endotoxin which were found to stimulate biosynthesis of EDRF/NO (1), bring about an accumulation of lipids in plasma (9), a process which may underly the mechanism(s), and could also explain the decreased uptake of LDL b8y the peripheral cells. Interferon-γ was also found to inhibit the development of atherosclerosis in rabbits. VanLenten et al.., (5) demonstrated that LPS, a potent inducer of NO synthase in macrophages, at concentration as low as 1 ng/ml, selectively prevents the expression of the scavenger receptor activity, and inhibits oxy-LDL binding and accumulation in human monocyte/macrophages. High concentration of L6PS (e.g.100 ng/ml) completely prevented the uptake of oxy-LDL, but had no effect on n-LDL binding, secretion of apoE and phagocytic activity of macrophages (5).

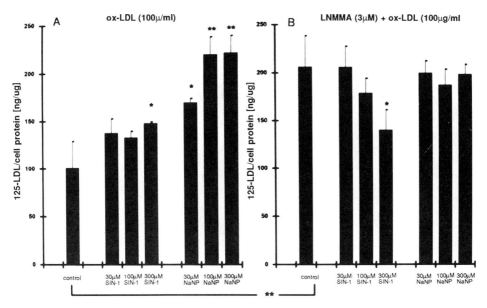

Figure 3: Effects of SIN-1 or NaNP on the cellular accumulation of ^{125}I-oxy-LDL by macrophages without (A) or in the presence of 3 μM of L-MMA (B). Mean ± SD n=3-5 experiments carried out in triplicates. Statistical significance: *p<0.05; **p<0.001

The increased LDL-binding at high NO concentrations may be relate4d to the toxic deformation of either the receptor on cell membrane. Another change might occur on the LDL molecule by NO itself (binding to serine -SH groups) (11) or by the ONOO- , generated from NO and OH- ions (1). Ut should be noted that the biphasic effect of NO was described in several experimental models. The cytoprotective effect of the different NO-donors at low (up to 100 μM) concentrations and the toxic effect at higher (below 300 μM) concentrations were observed in the granular cells of the cerebellum and retina (12).

We conclude that similarily to prostacyclin, EDRF/NO and NO-donors may inhibit the development of atherosclerosis not only by the inhibition of platelet activity, but also by the protection of peripheral cells against the excessive accumulation of lipids. However, it is important to note that high concentrations of NO may be toxic for cells.

REFERENCES

1. S. Moncada, R.M.J. Palmer, and E.A. Higgs, Nitric oxide: Physiology, pathophysiology, and pharmacology. *Pharmacol. Rev.* 43:109 (1991).
2. D.P. Hajjar, and B.B. Wexler, Metabolic activity of cholesterol esters in aortic smooth muscle cells is altered by prostaglandins I2 and E2, *J. lip. Res.* 24:1176 (1983).
3. D. P. Hajjar, and K.B. Pomerantz, Signal transduction in atherosclerosis: integration of cytokines and the eicosanoid network, *FASEB* J. 6:2933 (1992).

4. A. Dembinska-Kiec, A. Zmuda, J. Marcinkiewicz, H. Sinzinger, and R.J. Gryglewski, Influence of NO-donor (SIN-1) on functions of inflammatory cells, *Agents Acions* 1/2:32 (1991).

5. B.J. vanLenten, A.M. Fogelman, J. Seager, E. Ribi, M. Haberland, and P. Edwards, Bacterial endotoxin selectively prevents the expression of scavenger-receptor activity on human monocyte macrophages, *J. ImmunoL* 6:3718 (1985).

6. J.L. Goldstein, and M.S. Brown, The low-densoty lipoprotein pathway and its relation to atherosclerosis, *Ann Rev. Biochem.* 46:897 (1977).

7. J.L. Goldstein, M.S. Brown, R.G.W. Anderson, D.W. Russel, and W.J. Schneider, Receptor-mediated endocytosis: concepts emerging from the LDL receptor system, *Annu. Rev.Cell.BioL* 1:1 (1985).

8. M.S. Brown, and J.L. Goldstein, A receptor-mediated pathway for cholesterol homeostasis, *Science* 232:34 (1986).

9. I. Gouni, K. Oka, J. Etienne, and L. Chan, Endotoxin-induced hypertriglyceridemia is mediated by suppression of lipoprotein lipase at a post-transcriptional level, *J. Lip. Res.* 34:139 (1993).

10. A. Wilson, R. Schaub, R. Goldstein, and P. Kuo, Suppression of aortic atherosclerosis in cholesterol fed rabbits by purified rabbit interferon, *Arteriosclerosis* 10:208 (1990).

11. W. Jessup, D. Mohr, S.P. Gieseg, R.T. Dean, and R. Stocker, The participation of nitric oxide in cell freeand its restriction of macrophage-mediated oxidation of low-density lipoprotein, *Biochim. Biophys. Acta.* 1180:73 (1992).

12 M.F. Haberecht, D.A. Redburn, M. Nakane, and H.H.H.W. Schmidt, Immunocytochemical and histochemical localization of nitric oxide and soluble guanylyl cyclase in rabbit retina, *Endot.* 1:7 (1993).

THE ROLE OF NITRIC OXIDE IN NONADRENERGIC NONCHOLINGERGIC NEURAL RELAXATION OF MAMMALIAN AIRWAY SMOOTH MUSCLE

Louis Diamond, Ralph J. Altiere, Greg Lindsay, and David C. Thompson

University of Colorado Health Sciences Center
School of Pharmacy
4200 East Ninth Avenue
Denver, Colorado 80262-0238, USA

INTRODUCTION

Extensive evidence accumulated over the past two decades has documented the existence of an inhibitory nervous system in the airways of most mammalian species, including man, that is neither adrenergic nor cholinergic. Because the neurotransmitter of this system has not been identified with certainty, the system continues to be referred to as the nonadrenergic noncholinergic (NANC) inhibitory system. Most recently, attention has been focused on nitirc oxide (NO) as a possible transmitter of NANC inhibitory responses in the airways. This paper will succinctly review relevant background information regarding the airway NANC inhibitory system as well as current evidence advocating or disputing a role for NO in NANC inhibitory nerve-mediated relaxation of airway smooth muscle. Results from our own laboratory will be integrated with data reported by other investigators in an effort to present the reader with a balanced perspective on this intriguing, yet controversial topic.

THE AIRWAY NANC INHIBITORY SYSTEM

Stimulation of the autonomic innervation of smooth muscle typically results in either contraction or relaxation. Historically, these effects were considered to result from the release of norepinephrine from postganglionic sympathetic nerves or acetylcholine from postganglionic parasympathetic nerves. The discovery that certain smooth muscle effector tissues continue to respond to autonomic nerve stimulation following complete blockade of both adrenergic and cholinergic pathways led to the present concept of the existence of NANC nerves. Two types of NANC nerves have been identified in airway smooth muscle from several different species. One type is associated with relaxation (bronchodilation) and the other with contraction (bronchoconstriction). The nature of the neurotransmitters utilized by these nerves has been the subject of intense investigation, as has been the

Biochemical, Pharmacological, and Clinical Aspects of Nitric Oxide
Edited by B. A. Weissman *et al.*, Plenum Press, New York, 1995

queshon of whether or not the nerves serve important physiological or pathophysiological functlons.

NANC nerves which when activated cause bronchoconstriction were initially called NANC excitatory nerves. Subsequently, these nerves were demonstrated to be sensory in origin and to release tachykinins upon stimulation; hence they were given the name "tachykininergic". Tachykininergic nerves do not appear to be of major significance in the control of human airway smooth muscle tone in either health or disease. However in some animal species, such as the guinea pig, tachykininergic nerves may be involved in the regulation of bronchomotor tone.

NANC nerves which when stimulated produce bronchodilation are known as NANC inhibitory nerves. The extrinsic supply to these nerves appears to have parasympathetic origins within the central nervous system. Various transmitter substances have been proposed for NANC inhibitory nerves including purines (e.g., ATP), peptides (e.g., VIP) and, most recently, NO. Because human airway smooth muscle lacks sympathetic innervation, there has been much speculation that NANC inhibitory nerves may serve an important homeostatic role in man, controlling basal bronchomotor tone as well as moderating responses to environmental or patho-physiological spasmogenic stimuli.

NEUROTRANSMISSION IN THE AIRWAY NANC INHIBITORY SYSTEM

Methods of Study

Insight into the nature of the airway NANC inhibitory system neurotransmitter has been gleaned from a variety of *in vivo* and *in vilro* studies. Experiments conducted *in vivo* rely on indirect estimations of the contractile state of airway smooth muscle (e.g., by measuring airflow resistance during spontaneous or artificial ventilation) and are difficult to control because of the large number of known and unknown endogenous substances that can impinge upon smooth muscle tissue and alter its responsiveness. Further, patterns of extrinisic innervation of airway smooth muscle vary within and across species, making it difficult to isolate and stimulate nerves that subserve specific regions of the tracheobronchial tree. Consequently, most studies of the airway NANC inhibitory system have been conducted *in vitro* using segments of freshly removed airway tissues suspended in constant temperature organ baths.

To initiate neurotransmitter release from autonomic nerves in an isolated airway preparation, plate electrodes are placed on either side of the tissue and a voltage is applied. This technique is known as transmural or electrical field stimulation (EFS). By adjusting the amplitude, duration and frequency of EFS, it is possible to selectively depolarize and stimulate nerves without similarly affecting muscle. However, it is not possible to selectively stimulate different types of autonomic nerves and thus EFS results in the release of multiple neurotransmitters. Changes in the contractile state of airway smooth muscle tissue brought about by release of autonomic neurotransmitters can be monitored using appropriate physiological instruments such as force-displacement transducers and polygraphic recorders. Confirmation that observed responses are neurogenic (as opposed to myogenic) in origin can be obtained by demonstrating their disappearance after treatment with tetrodotoxin, an agent that selectively prevents depolarization of neuronal cell membranes.

Transmitter Candidates

Using combinations of the in vivo and in vitro techniques described above, various workers have attempted to characterize the neurotransmitter released by NANC inhibitory nerves in airway smooth muscle. Because of widespread interest in ATP as an inhibitory transmitter in the gastrointestinal tract, early experiments in airway tissues focused on this purine. However, little evidence was found in support of ATP and attention quickly turned to peptides, and particularly to VIP which had been localized in airway nerves and shown to be an effective airway smooth muscle relaxant. After more than a decade of research, the precise role of VIP in airway NANC inhibitory nerve neurotransmission remains unclear. At present, the preponderance of opinion favors a role for VIP in guinea pig airways and possibly in airways of other animal species, but not in human airways. With the advent of the general concept of gaseous neurotransmission, many laboratories undertook studies to evaluate NO as a possible transmitter of airway NANC inhibitory responses. What follows is a summary of the evidence reported to date either supporting or refuting such a role for NO.

NITRIC OXIDE AS THE AIRWAY NANC INHIBITORY NEUROTRANSMITTER

Evidence in Support

Two major requirements for establishing a substance as a neurotransmitter are: 1) demonstration of its presence and/or the presence of its biosynthetic enzymes within nerve terminals associated with the effector tissue and 2) demonstration that exogenous adminstration of the substance produces a physiological response that closely mimics the response that occurs when the transmitter is released endogenously as a result of nerve stimulation. In the case of NO and the NANC inhibitory system in airway smooth muscle, both of these requirements appear to have been fulfilled.

The enzyme responsible for the synthesis of NO from L-arginine is nitric oxide synthase (NOS). Using both NADPH- diaphorase histochemistry and immunocyto-chemistry, Fischer et al. (1993) demonstrated NOS-containing nerve fibers in the smooth muscle layer of the guinea pig trachea, a tissue known to have a functional NANC inhibitory system. Likewise, Hassall and colleagues (1993) found a major population of paratracheal neurons in the guinea pig trachea that were capable of generating NO. Kobzik et al. (1993) examined samples of human lung tissue using techniques similar to those used by Fischer et al. and were able to demonstrathe presence of NOS in nerve fibers associated with smooth muscle cells in large, cartilaginous airways. These airways also are known to possess functional NANC inhibitory innervation.

The results of *in vitro* and *in vivo* studies in a variety of species, including man, have shown that exogenous administration of authentic NO produces effects on airway smooth muscle that mimic those produced by electrical stimulation of NANC inhibitory nerves. However, the potency of NO as an airway smooth muscle relaxant varies between species and between airway tissues within a given species (see succeeding section). In isolated segments of cat trachea, our laboratory has shown that NO is capable of reversing bethanechol-induced contractions in a concentration-dependent manner (figure 1). The relaxant action of NO is unaffected by prior administration of NOS inhibitors indicating that these compounds, which block the relaxation response to NANC inhibitory nerve stimulation in cat trachea (as shown below), do not act via a post-synaptic mechanism unrelated to inhibition of NO synthesis. In anesthetized and mechanically ventilated guinea pigs, Dupuy and colleagues (1992) found that breathing 300 ppm NO for six minutes decreased baseline pulmonary resistance by only about 10 percent; but when an intravenous infusion of methacholine was used to induce bronchoconstriction, inhalation of NO for 10 minutes at concentrations ranging from 5 to 300 ppm produced rapid, potent and dose-dependent bronchodilation.

A third criterion for establishing a substance as a neurotransmitter requires documentation to show that interference with its biosynthesis leads to a decrease in physiologic response following stiumulation of nerves from which the substance is believed to be released. Several groups of investigators have reported a diminution or elimination of

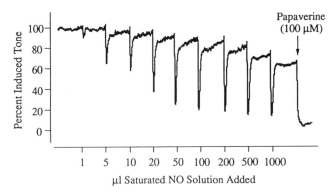

Figure 1. Nitric oxide-induced relaxant responses in isolated cat trachea contracted half-maximally with bethanechol. This level of tone is defined as 100% induced tone. At 10 min intervals, a saturated aqueous solution of NO was added to 14 ml tissue baths in the auantities indicated.

NANC inhibitory nerve-induced airway smooth muscle relaxation responses following administration of NOS inhibitors. The first such report was by Tucker et al. (1990) who showed that the NOS inhibitor, L-N^G-nitroarginine, attenuated alpha-chymotrypsin-resistant (i.e., non-VIP mediated) NANC relaxations of isolated guinea pig tracheal smooth muscle by as much as 89 percent at the highest concentration employed. The effect of L-N^G-nitroarginine was stereoselective and partially reversed by L-arginine. Subsequently, Li and Rand (1991) performed similar experiments and obtained essentially the same results. In our laboratory, the effects of NOS inhibition on NANC nerve-induced relaxation of isolated cat trachea were studied over a range of stimulation frequencies. Inhibition of NOS resulted in a leftward and upward shift in the NANC inhibitory nerve stimulation frequency response curve (Fig. 2). Fisher and associates (1993) also demonstrated a suppression of NANC relaxation responses in isolated cat trachea following NOS inhibition. Likewise, experiments in airways isolated from pigs and horses have demonstated a diminution of NANC nerve-mediated relaxation responses following inhibition of the NOS enzyme (Kannan and Johnson, 1992; Yu et al., 1994). Most importantly, studies in human trachea (Belvisi et al., 1992) and in central and peripheral human bronchi (Bai and Bramley, 1993; Ellis and Undem, 1992) have all confirmed a role for NO in the mediation of NANC inhibitory responses, albeit the question of whether NO is the sole mediator of NANC relaxations in human airways remains unanswered.

NITRIC OXIDE AS THE AIRWAY NANC INHIBITORY NEUROTRANSMITTER:

Evidence in Opposition

Although in many respects the data supporting a role for NO as the NANC inhibitory neurotransmitter in airway smooth muscle are quite compelling, other data cast substantial doubt on the neurotransmitter role of NO in this tissue. For example, Fischer et al. (1993) reported finding relatively greater numbers of nerves containing NOS in guinea

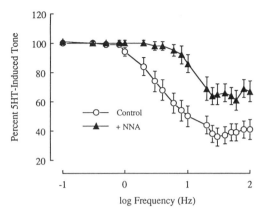

Figure 2. Partial inhibition of the NANC inhibitory response in cat trachea by the NOS inhibitor, L-N^G-nitroarginine (NNA). The tissue was treated with atropine, propranolol and guanethidine to abolish cholinergic and adrenergic nerve mediated responses and was half-maximally contracted with 5-HT (defined as 100% induced tone). NANC inhibitory responses were evoked by electrical field stimulation (10V, 0.3 msec for 5 sec at increasing frequencies as indicated).

pig bronchi than in trachea. This distribution pattern is in sharp contrast to the pattern revealed by functional studies which show the presence of NANC inhibitory nerves in guinea pig trachea but a virtual absence of such nerves in bronchi (Diamond and Altiere, 1988). Fischer and colleagues also observed that NOS was localized to the jugular and nodose ganglia of sensory nerves in the guinea pig, a finding inconsistent with the motor identity of NANC inhibitory nerves (as evinced by the fact that responses to their stimulation can be prevented by ganglionic blocking agents) (Diamond and O'Donnell, 1980).

Two other recent structural studies raise additional doubt regarding the role of NO as the NANC inhibitory transmitter in airway smooth muscle. Kobzik and colleagues (1993) reported finding NOS-containing nerves associated with airway smooth muscle in the rat lung and Dey et al. (1993) reported finding NOS-like immunoreactivity in a subpopulation of neurons within the nerve plexus of the ferret trachea. Taken together these findings suggest a role for NO in the regulation of airway smooth muscle in rat lung and ferret trachea. However, neither rat airways (Satchell, 1982) nor ferret trachea (McWilliam and Gray, 1990) possess a functional NANC inhibitory system. Responses evoked by activation of NANC inhibitory nerves in ferret trachea and bronchus are shown in figure 3. It is thus clear that the presence of NOS-containing nerve fibers is, in and of itself, insufficient to establish a functional role for NO in mediating airway smooth muscle responses to NANC nerve stimulation. It is possible, of course, that NO subserves a function other than, or in addition to, airway smooth muscle relaxation, not only in airway tissues that lack a NANC inhibitory system but in those that possess one as well.

The results of several functional studies also call into question the contention that NO serves as the neurotransmitter of airway NANC inhibitory nerves. For instance, cat experiments conducted in our laboratory have failed to show an effect of NOS inhibitors either on NANC relaxation responses in isolated segments of bronchi or on NANC bronchodilator responses in intact lungs (Diamond et al., 1992). To reconcile these results with those obtained in the isolated cat trachea, one must hypothesize that the cat tracheobronchial tree utilizes two different NANC inhibitory neurotransmitters (which intuitively seems unlikely) or that NO serves to modulate, rather than to mediate, NANC neurotransmission in cat airways. The possibility that NO does play a neuromodulatory role in the airways is supported by results from experiments in which the effects of NOS inhibition were evaluated on neurally-mediated tachykininergic excitatory responses in guinea pig bronchi. In these experiments, NOS inhibition attenuated and L-arginine restored excitatory responses to nerve stimulation, suggestinthat NO indeed might serve to

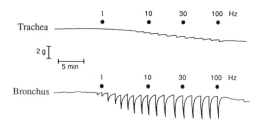

Figure 3. Representative tracings of NANC inhibitory responses in isolated segments of ferret trachea and mainstem bronchus. Tissues were treated with atropine, propranolol and guanethidine to abolish cholinergic and adrenergic nerve-mediated responses and were half-maximally contracted with 5-HT. NANC inhibitory responses were evoked by electrical field stimulation (10V, 0.3 msec for 5 sec at increasing frequencies as indicated). In contrast to the bronchus in which powerful NANC inhibitory responses were evoked, the trachea exhibited extremely weak responses.

modulate neural responses in the airways (Thompson et al., 1992). Additional functional evidence disputing a role for NO as the NANC inhibitory neurotransmitter derives from the studies of Hobbs et al. (1991). These workers examined the effects of hydroquinone, a free radical scavenger, on relaxation responses to NO and to NANC nerve stimulation in isolated guinea pig trachea. Hydroquinone nearly abolished responses to NO but had no discernible effects on responses to NANC nerve stimulation.

If NO serves as the airway NANC inhibitory neurotransmitter, it would be reasonable to expect airway tissues innervated by NANC nerves to exhibit comparable patterns of sensitivity to exogenously administered and endogenously released NO. However, this does not appear to be the case (Altiere et al., 1994). As shown in figure 4, compared to the cat trachea the guinea pig trachea is approximately 100 times less sensitive to exogenously administered NO. But when the sensitivity of these two tissues to endogenously released NANC transmitter is compared, only a two- to three-fold difference is seen with the cat trachea again being the more sensitive of the two. Results such as these, while by no means conclusive, add to the growing skepticism over claims that NO is the neurotransmitter of the airway NANC inhibitory system.

As a final note, it should be pointed out that no one to date has demonstrated release of NO from NANC airway nerves following stimulation. Such demonstration is fundamental to the establishment of NO as the NANC inhibitory neurotransmitter and, unless and until it is accomplished, the precise role of NO in the airways is likely to remain controversial.

SUMMARY

Mammalian airway smooth muscle is innervated by inhibitory nerves that release a NANC transmitter whose identity is unknown. Recent studies suggest the airway NANC transmitter may be NO. Three lines of evidence have been advanced in support of this notion including: 1) histological demonstration of the presence of NOS in nerves associated with airway smooth muscle; 2) an ability of exogenously administered NO to mimic the effects of NANC nerve stimulation; and 3) attenuation of NANC nerve-mediated airway smooth muscle relaxations following NOS inhibition and restoration of the relaxations following L-arginine administration. Evidence refuting a role for NO as the airway NANC neurotransmitter also has been advanced. This evidence includes: 1) histological demonstration of the presence of NOS in airway nerves that do not possess a functional NANC inhibitory system; 2) failure of NOS inhibitors to attenuate NANC

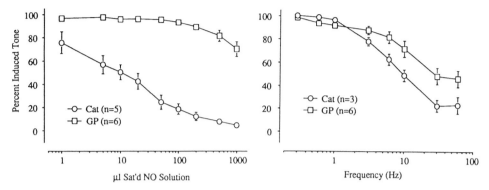

Figure 4. Species variations is response to NO and NANC inhibitory nerve activation. Tracheal segments from cat and guinea pig were treated with propranolol and guanethidine to inhibit adrenergic nerve-mediated responses and were half-maximally contracted with bethanechol (defined as 100% induced tone). Left panel: responses to NO were elicited by addition of increasing volumes of a saturated aqueous solution of NO to the 14 ml tissue baths. Right panel: NANC inhibitory responses were evoked by electrical field stimulation (10V, 0.3 msec for 5 sec at increasing frequencies as indicated).

nerve-mediated relaxations in airway tissues that do possess a functional NANC inhibitory system; 3) failure of pharmacological agents to modify NANC nerve-mediated and NO-mediated relaxations in a qualitatively similar manner; and 4) different relative sensitivities of airway tissues to NANC neurotransmitter and exogenous NO. Some of these discrepant findings may be accounted for if NO serves as a modulator (Gnder et al., 1992; Schuman and Madison, 1991), as opposed to a mediator, of NANC responses in the airways or if an NO complex (Gaston et al., 1994a and 1994b; Jansen et al., 1992), rather than NO itself, serves as the airway NANC neurotransmitter. Further study clearly is needed to determine the precise role of NO in the regulation of airway smooth muscle.

REFERENCES

Altiere, R.J., Diamond, L. and Thompson, D.C., 1994, Species variation in airway sensitivity to nitric oxide and nonadrenergic noncholinergic inhibitory nerve activation, *Am. J. Resp. Crit. Care Med.* 149:A594.

Bai, T.R. and Bramley, A.M., 1993, Effect of an inhibitor of nitric oxide synthase on neural relaxation of human bronchi. *Am. J. Physiol.* 264 *(Lung Cell. Mol. Physiol.* 8):L425.

Belvisi, M.G., Stretton, C.D., Miura, M., Verleden, G.M., Tadjkarimi, S., Yacoub, M.H. and Barnes, PJ., 1992, Inhibitory NANC nerves in human tracheal smooth muscle: a quest for the neurotransmitter. *J. Appl. Physiol.* 73:2505.

Dey, R.D., Mayer, B. and Said, S.I., 1993, Colocalization of vasoactive intestinal peptide and nitric oxide synthase in neurons of the ferret trachea. *Neurosci.* 54:839.

Diamond, L. and Altiere, R. J., 1988, Airway nonadrenergic noncholinergic inhibitory nervous system, *in:* "The Airways. Neural Control in Health and Disease,"M.A. Kaliner and P.J. Barnes, eds., Marcell Dekker, New York.

Diamond, L. and O'Donnell, M., 1980, A nonadrenergic vagal inhibitory pathway to feline airways. *Science* 208: 185.

Diamond, L., Lantta, J., Thompson, D.C. and Altiere, R.J., 1992, Nitric oxide synlhase inhibitors fail to affect cat airway nonadrenergic noncholinergic inhibitory (NANCI) responses. *Am. Rev. Resp. Dis.* 145:A382.

Dupuy, P.M., Shore, S.A., Drazen, J.M., Frostell, C., Hill, W.A. and Zapol, W.M., 1992, Bronchodilator action of inhaled nitric oxide in guinea pigs. *J. Clin. Invest.* 90:421.

Ellis, J.L. and Undem, BJ., 1992, Inhibition by L-N^G-nitro-L-arginine of nonadrenergic-noncholinergic-mediated relaxations of human isolated central and peripheral airways. *Am. Rev. Respir. Dis.* 146:1543.

Fischer, A. Mundel, P., Mayer, B., Preissler, U., Philippin, B. and Kummer, W., 1993, Nitric oxide synthase in guinea pig lower airway innervation. *Neurosci. Lett.* 149:157.

Fisher, J.T., Anderson, J.W. and Waldron, M.A., 1993, Nonadrenergic noncholinergic neurotransmitter of feline trachealis: VIP or nitric oxide? *J. Appl. Physiol.* 74:31.

Gaston, B., Drazen, J.M., Jansen, A., Sugarbaker, D.A., Loscalzo, J., Richards, W. and Stamler, J.S., 1994a, Relaxation of human bronchial smoolh muscle by S-nitrosothiols in vitro. *J. Pharmacol. Exp. Ther.* 268:978.

Gaston, B., Drazen, J., Loscalzo, J. and Stamler, J.S., 1994b, The biology of nitrogen oxides in the airways. *Am. J. Respir. Crit. Care Med.* 149:538.

Grider, J.R., Murthy, K.S., Jin, J.-G. and Maklouf, G.M., 1992, Stimulation of nitric oxide from muscle cells by VIP: prejunctional enhancement of VIP release. *Am. J. Physiol.* 262:G774.

Hassall, C.J.S., Saffrey, M.J. and Burnstock, G., 1993, Expression of NADPH-diaphorase activity by guinea-pig paratracheal neurones. *NeuroReport* 4:49.

Hobbs, AJ., Tucker, J.F. and Gibson, A., 1991, Differentiation by hydroquinone of relaxations induced by exogenous and endogenous nitrates in non-vascular smooth muscle: role of superoxide anions. *Br. J. Pharmacol.* 104:645.

Jansen, A., Drazen, J., Osborne, J.A., Brown, R., Loscalzo, J. and Stamler, J.S., 1992, The relaxant properties in guinea pig airways of S-nitrosothiols. *J. Pharmacol. Exp. Ther.* 261:154.

Kannan, M.S. and Johnson, D.E., 1992, Nitric oxide mediates the neural nonadrenergic, noncholinergic relaxation of pig tracheal smooh muscle. *Am. J. Physiol.* 262 (*Lung Cell. Mol. Physiol.* 2):L511.

Kobzik, L., Bredt, D.S., Lowenstein, CJ., Drazen, J., Gaston, B., Sugerbaker, D. and Stamler, J.S., 1993, Nitric oxide synthse in human and rat lung: immunocytochemical and histochemical localization. *Am. J. Respir. Cell Mol. Biol.* 9:371.

Li, C.G. and Rand, M.J., 1991, Evidence that part of the NANC relaxant response of guinea-pig trachea to electrical field stimulation is mediated by nitric oxide. *Br. J. Pharmacol.* 102:91.

McWilliam, P.N. and Gray, S.J., 1990, The innervation of tracheal smooth muscle in the ferret. *J. Auton. Nerv. Syst.* 30:233.

Satchell, D., 1982, Non-adrenergic, non-cholinergic nerves in mammalian airways: their function and the role of purines. *Comp. Biochem. Physiol.* 72C: 189.

Schuman, E.M. and Madison, D.V., 1991, A requirement for the intercellular messenger nitric oxide in long-term potentiation. *Science* 254:1503.

Thompson, D.C., Lantta, J., Diamond, L. and Altiere, R.J., 1992, A nitric oxide synthase inhibitor modulates neural responses in guinea pig airways. *Am. Rev. Resp. Dis.* 145:A382.

Tucker, J.F., Brave, S.R., Charalambous, L., Hobbs, A.J. and Gibson, A., 1990, L-N^G-nitro-arginine inhibits non-adrenergic, non-cholinergic relaxations of guinea pig isolated tracheal smooth muscle. *Br. J. Pharmacol.*

Yu, M., Wang, Z., Robinson, N.E. and LeBlanc, P.H., 1994, Inhibitory nerve distribution and mediation of NANC relaxation by nitric oxide in horse airways. *J. Appl. Physiol.* 76:339.

NITRIC OXIDE: A PUTATIVE MODULATOR OF MUSCARINIC RECEPTOR IN THE AIRWAYS SMOOTH MUSCLES

Nahum Allon and Yaakov Meshulam

Israel Inst. Biol. Res.
Department of Pharmacology
Ness-Ziona 70450, ISRAEL

INTRODUCTION

In 1987 nitric oxide (NO) was identified as an important endothelium-derived muscle relaxant (Ignarro et al., 1987; Palmer et al., 1987). NO, produced by the endothelium from arginine, act as a local vasodilator by diffusing into vascular smooth muscle and incorporating intracellularly with the heme present in guanylyl cyclase (Ignarro, 1989). This activates the guanylyl cyclase and results in an increased synthesis of cyclic GMP (cGMP) and consequent relaxation of smooth muscle cells.

In recent years, a growing number of evidence suggests an additional function of NO in down regulating smooth muscle hyperreponsiveness to acetylcholine (ACh). Inhibition of NO synthesis by the specific inhibitor L-NMMA, potentiate the tracheal smooth muscle's contraction, induced by cholinergic nerve stimulation (Palmer et al., 1988; Moncada et al., 1989; Johns et al., 1990). Inhibition or reduction of this contraction was mediated by NO like factor or by exogenous administration of NO or sodium nitroprusside (SNP), an agent releasing NO (Moncada, 1992). Moreover, inhibition of NO activated guanylyl cyclase by methylene blue, potentiated cholinergic induced contraction (Martin et al., 1985; Ignarro et al., 1989), whereas reduction of cholinergic-induced contraction was observed when a stable analogue of cGMP was added. These observations suggest that endogenous NO modulate cholinergic contraction through a cGMP-dependent mechanism.

NO may exert its inhibitory effects presynaptically on the nerve terminals or postsynaptically on the ACh receptors. In order to distinguish between these two sites, two experimental methods of muscle stimulation were employed; electrical stimulation (field or nerve stimulation) and ACh induced contraction. The results seemed to be species specific and preparation dependent. Administration of NO synthase or guanylyl cyclase inhibitors to isolated trachea enhanced ACh release from cholinergic nerve terminals in response to electrical stimulation (Brave, 1991; Sekizawa, 1993) but had no effect on ACh induced smooth muscle contraction. Administration of external NO, reduced the contraction response to both ACh and electrical stimulation in a dose

Biochemical, Pharmacological, and Clinical Aspects of Nitric Oxide
Edited by B. A. Weissman *et al.*, Plenum Press, New York, 1995

131

dependent manner, but with higher sensitivity to electrical stimulation (Sekizawa, 1993). Gao and Vanhoutte (1993), had demonstrated an increase in ACh induced trachea contraction following treatment with L-N^G-nitro arginine (NOArg) in isolated third order bronchial segment of a dog. Thus, the nature of the NO effect on the postjunctional receptors that modulate cholinergic stimulation is not clear and its role in-vivo is yet unknown. The present study was aimed to characterize the extant of modulation of cholinergic response by NO in anesthetized and artificially ventilated guinea pig and to evaluate its possible role in controlling trachea smooth muscle tone and hypersensitivity.

METHODS

Male, Dunkin-Hartley guinea-pigs (400-700 g) were anesthetized intraperitoneally with sodium pentobarbital (35 mg/kg) and mechanically ventilated (respirator model 683, Harvard Apparatus) through a tracheal cannula to 60 breaths/min and a tidal volume of 8 ml/kg. Polyethylene catheters were inserted into the left Jugular vain for the intravenous administration of drugs and the right femoral artery for the measurements of blood pressure.

Insufflation pressure was measured with differential transducer (Gould) connected to the sidearm of the tracheal cannula. Tidal air flow was measured by connecting a Fleish no. 000 pneumotachygraph to the tracheal cannula and monitoring the pressure loss across the device with a Statham differential transducer. Tidal volume was determined by electrical integration of the air-flow signal.

Following the surgical procedure, the animal was allowed to stabilize (while ventilated) for about 1 h. Deep anesthesia was maintained by frequent injection of 0.5 ml of diluted sodium pentobarbital (1:3 in saline) sufficient to eliminate spontaneous breathing. Drugs were administered by rapid bolus injections through the jugular vain cannula.

RESULTS

Intravenous injection of ACh resulted in a transient increase in the insufflation pressure. Following the intravenous administration of ACh, a dose dependent increase in insufflation pressure was obtained (fig. 1).

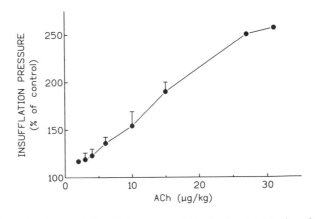

Figure 1. Dose dependent increase in insufflation pressure following iv administration of ACh (2-30μg/kg).

In order to block all uncontrolled electrical stimulation and concentrate on the effect of ACh induced contraction in the postjunctional receptors, tetrodotoxin (TTX 10 µg/kg) was injected iv, sufficient to eliminate most sodium dependent electrical conductance. Following TTX injection blood pressure dropped to 50% of the normal value and the occasional spontaneous breathings were eliminated. However, no change in the dose response curve of insufflation pressure was observed in response to iv injected ACh (Fig. 2).

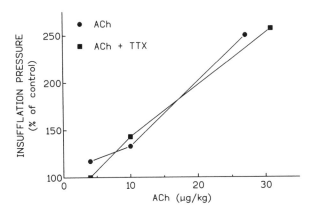

Figure 2. Pretreatment with TTX (10 µg/kg): No effect on the ACh dose dependent increase in insufflation pressure.

A single intravenous injection of 15 mg/kg NOArg resulted in a gradual increase (up to 30%) of airways basal tonus. Intravenous injection of ACh, 5-10 minutes later, resulted in a profound increase in insufflation pressure relative to the response induced by a similar dose of ACh, prior to the injection of NOArg (Fig. 3).

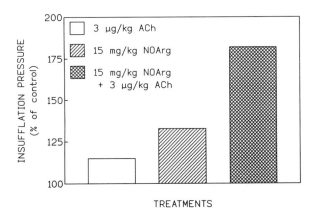

Figure 3. Modulation of trachea tone and responsiveness to ACh by NOArg. Response to single injection of ACh (3 µg/kg) before and 10 min after injection of NOArg (15 mg/kg).

The increase in responsiveness to ACh may be attributed (according to Starling low) to the elevated muscle tonus that increase the efficacy of the muscle contraction. In order to distinguish between direct increase in responsiveness and the increase attributed to elevated muscle tone, successive intravenous injection of small doses of NOArg (5 mg/kg every 10 min) were used. No change in basal airways insufflation pressure could be seen up to an accumulated dose of 20 mg/kg NOArg. However, testing the responsiveness of the airways smooth muscle to low dose of ACh, 5 min after each NOArg injection revealed a dose dependent (accumulated) increase in airways sensitivity (Fig. 4). TTX (10 µg/kg) previously shown to have no effect on muscle contraction induced by ACh alone, was also ineffective in altering the increase in sensitivity induced by NOArg.

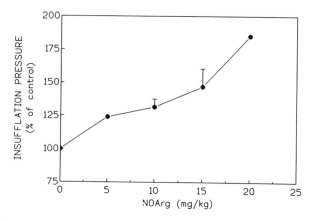

Figure 4. Dose dependent increase in trachea excitability to ACh by NOArg. The animals received 4 successive injections of NOArg (5 mg/kg), 10 min apart. The level of muscle contraction was tested 5 min. following each NOArg treatment, by an iv injection of ACh (6 µg/kg).

DISCUSSION

Cholinergic nerve stimulation resulted in contraction of tracheal smooth muscles and increase in lung resistance (Barnes, 1991). These smooth muscle contractions were potentiated by L-NMMA, a specific inhibitor of NO synthesis (Palmer et al., 1988; Moncada et al., 1989; Johns et al., 1990; Sekizawa et al., 1993). Smooth muscle contraction was reduced by the exogenous administration of NO or SNP (Moncada, 1992; Sekizawa et al., 1993). Moreover, methylene blue, an inhibitor of NO-activated guanylyl cyclase (Martin et al., 1985; Ignarro et al., 1989), potentiate cholinergic contraction. Thus, the data indicates that endogenous NO or NO-like factor modulate cholinergic contraction through a cyclic GMP dependent mechanism. In the present study we have shown that inhibition of NO syntase by NOArg, increased, independently, bronchial tone anpotentiated ACh induced bronchconstriction in anesthetized and ventilated guinea pigs. The smooth muscles contraction response to ACh and its modulation by NOArg, were not affected by pretreatment with 10 mg/kg TTX. Since this dose of TTX is known to block electrical conductance, this, may suggest that the modulation of smooth muscle excitability, in the guinea pigs, is restricted to the post synaptic region.

Sekizawa et al., (1993) demonstrated an increase in ACh release in isolated rat trachea treated with L-NMMA concomitant with a potentiation of the contraction induced by electrical field stimulation. ACh induced contraction was not affected by this treatment. Brave et al. (1991) showed that NOArg potentiated contraction induced by electrical field stimulation but had no effect on ACh release in guinea pigs trachea. Our results, confine the ACh effect to the post synaptic target by the TTX treatment, suggest that two independent processes are triggered by the NOArg: a) A gradual increase in airways tone in response to high doses of NOArg, administered in bolus injection and b) A potentiation of ACh induced contraction. The potentiation of ACh induced contraction was found to be sensitive to low doses of NOArg. Since the levels of airways smooth muscle tone is controlled by the balance between the bronchoconstriction and the bronchdilation mechanisms (Barnes, 1991), the increase in airways tone may be due to either or both the augmented release of excitatory ACh, and the modified muscarinic receptor. However, since the increase in airways tone was not affected by evident even after treatment with TTX, modification of the muscarinic receptor is more likely to be the major cause for the changes in ACh excitability.

Potentiation of ACh induced contraction was detected in our in-vivo guinea pigs' preparation but not in the isolated trachea of guinea pigs (Brave, 1991) or rats (Sekizawa, 1993). Since in the these in-vitro preparation only the upper air ways were tested this differences may localize the modulation of ACh response to the lower branches of the tracheal tree. This suggestion was supported by the finding that the potentiation of ACh induced contraction in response to NOArg treatment was seen in isolated third order bronchial segment of a dog (Gao and Vanhoutte, 1993).

The results indicate that regulation of ACh induced contraction may be attributed to postjunctional changes. Brave et al. (1991) and Sekizawa et al. (1993) have suggested that potentiation of cholinergic nerve endings by NO, is mediated via cGMP dependent mechanism (see also Martin et al., 1985; Ignarro et al., 1989). Since elevated levels of cGMP may act in the cell via multiple mediators (Schmidt et al., 1993), we tried to sort out those that may be relevant explanation for our model. A schematic representation of the combined effects of NO and cGMP that may down regulate the ACh intracellular changes is depicted in Fig. 5. In this model, three possible pathways for the modulation of ACh activity are presented: 1. A decrease in intracellular free Ca^{2+} that results in muscle relaxation (Clapp and Gurney, 1991); 2. An activation of protein kinase that results in the elevated protein phosphorylation (Yoshida et al., 1991) that in turn, may alter muscarinic receptor; and 3. Inhibition of cAMP phosphodiesterase that may result in elevation of cAMP levels (Ono and Trautwein, 1991), blocking Ca^{2+} influx. Indeed, the commonly used bronchodilators, the beta agonists relaxes smooth muscles through increased levels of cAMP in the cells. Each of these three pathways that is associated with elevated cGMP levels, may decrease the Ca^{2+} influx during cholinergic activation and may thus serve as candidates for the down regulation of the response to ACh.

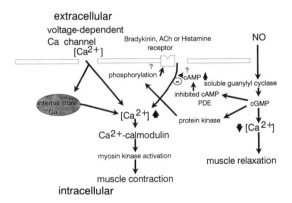

Figure 5. A schematic model demonstrating three putative pathways by which, elevated cGMP levels induced by NO may down regulate cholinergic induced smooth muscles contraction.

REFERENCES

Barnes, P.J., 1991, Pharmacology of airways smooth muscle, in The Lung scientific foundation, R.G. Crystal, J.B. West et al. (eds.), Raven press Ltd. New York.

Brave, S.R., Hobbs, A.J., Gibson, A. and Tucker, J.F., 1991, The influence of L-N^G- nitro-arginine on field stimulation induced contractions and acetylcholine release in guinea pig isolated tracheal smooth muscle, Biochem. Biophys. Res. Commun., 179:1017-1022.

Clapp, L.H. and Gurney, A.M., 1991, Modulation of calcium movements by nitroprusside in isolated vascular smooth muscle cells, Pflugers Arch., 418:462-470.

Gao, Y. and Vanhoutte, M., 1993, Attenuation of contractions to acetylcholine in canine bronchi by an endogenous nitric oxide-like substance, Br. J. Pharmacol., 109:887-891.

Ignarro, L.J., Byrns, R.E., Buga, G.M. and Wood, K.S., 1987, Endothelum-derived relaxing factor from pulmonary artery and vein possesses pharmacologic and chemical properties identical to those of nitric oxide radical. Circ. Res., 61: 866-879.

Ignarro, L.J., 1989, Heme-dependent activation of soluble guanylate cyclase by nitric oxide: regulation of enzyme activity by porphyrins and metalloporphyrins, Semi. Hematol., 26:63-76.

Johns, R.A., Peach, M.J., Linden, J. and Tichotsky, A., 1990, N^G-monomethyl L-arginine inhibits endothelium-derived relaxing factor-stimulated cyclic GMP accumulation on cocultures of endothelial and vascular smooth muscle cells by an action specific to endothelial cell, Circ. Res. 67:979-985.

Martin, W., Villani, G.M., Jothianandan, D. and Furchgott, R.F.,1985, Selective blockade of endothelium-dependent and glyceryl trinitrate-induced relaxation by hemoglobin and methylen blue in rabbit aorta, J. Pharmacol. Exp. Ther., 232:708-716.

Moncada, S., Palmer, R.M.J. and Higgs, E.A., 1989, Biosynthesis of nitric oxide from L-arginine, pathway for the regulation of cell function and communication, Biochem. Pharmacol., 38:1709-1715.

Moncada, S., 1992, The L-arginine; nitric oxide pathway, Acta Physiol. Scand., 145:201-227.

Ono, K. and Trautwein, W., 1991, Potentiation by cyclic GMP of beta-adrenergic effect on Ca^{2+} current in guinea pig ventricular cells, J. Physiol. 443:387-404.

Palmer, R.M.J., Ferrige, A.G. and Moncada, S.,1987, Nitric oxide release account for biological activity of endothelial-derived relaxing factor, Nature, 327:524-526.

Palmer, R.M.J., Rees, D.D., Ashton, D.S. and Moncada, S., 1988, L-arginine is the physiological precursor for the formation of nitric oxide in endothelium-dependent relaxation, Biochem. Biophys. Res. Commun. 153:1251-1256.

Schmidt, H.H.H.W., Lohmann, S.M. and Walter, U., 1993, The nitric oxide and cGMP signal transduction system: regulation and mechanism of action, Biochemica et Biophysica Acta, 1178:153-175.

Sekizawa, K., Fukushima, T, Ikarashi, Y., Maruyama, Y. and Sasaki, H., 1993, The role of nitric oxide in cholinergic neurotransmission in the rat trachea, Br. J. Pharmacol. 110:816-820.

Yoshida, Y., Sun, H.T., Cai, J.Q. and Imai, S., 1991, Cyclic GMP-dependent protein kinase stimulates the plasma membrane Ca^{2+} pump ATase of vascular smooth muscle via phosphorylation of a 240-kDa protein, J. Biol. Chem. 266:19819-19825.

COMPARATIVE EFFECTS OF N$^\omega$-NITRO-L-ARGININE, N$^\omega$-NITRO-L-ARGININE METHYL ESTER, AND N$^\omega$-NITRO-L-ARGININE BENZYL ESTER ON VASODILATOR RESPONSES TO ACETYLCHOLINE AND SUBSTANCE P

David Y. Cheng, Bracken J. DeWitt, Timothy J. McMahon,
Jose A. Santiago, Dennis B. McNamara and Philip J. Kadowitz

Department of Pharmacology
Tulane University Schoolof Medicine
New Orleans, LA 70112, U.S.A.

INTRODUCTION

Recent evidence suggests that the endothelium-derived relaxing factor first described by Furchgott and Zawadski (1980) is nitric oxide or a labile nitroso derivative. Nitric oxide is formed from L-arginine in cultured endothelial cells, and N^G-monomethyl-L-arginine (L-NMMA) was the first L-arginine analog shown to inhibit nitric oxide formation (Moncada et al., 1989). Since the discovery that L-NMMA inhibits nitric oxide synthase, a number of L-arginine analogs that block nitric oxide release have been developed (Ishii et al., 1990; Moore et al., 1990). The use of these compounds has provided important information on the role of nitric oxide in the regulation of cardiovascular function in *in vivo* experiments (Bellan et al., 1991;1993; McMahon et al, 1991; McMahon and Kadowitz, 1992;1993). Experiments with nitric oxide synthase inhibitors, including N$^\omega$-nitro-L-arginine (L-NA) and N$^\omega$-nitro-L-arginine methyl ester (L-NAME), have provided evidence that nitric oxide is involved in maintaining the pulmonary and peripheral vascular bed in a dilated state and in mediating vasodilator responses to acetylcholine, bradykinin, substance P, and other nitric oxide releasing agents (Bellan et al., 1991;1993; McMahon et al., 1991; McMahon and Kadowitz, 1993). However, recent studies have shown that L-NAME and other alkyl esters of L-NA are muscarinic receptor antagonists and suggest that these compounds are poor choices as nitric oxide synthase inhibitors in studies in which muscarinic receptors are not blocked (Buxton et al., 1992). Although L-NAME has been reported to inhibit responses to acetylcholine, bradykinin, and substance P in the pulmonary vascular bed of the cat, other studies show that L-NAME does not inhibit responses to endothelium-dependent vasodilator agents (Lippton et al., 1992). The present study was, therefore, undertaken to investigate and compare the effects of L-NA, which does not bind to muscarinic receptors (Buxton et al., 1992), with

Biochemical, Pharmacological, and Clinical Aspects of Nitric Oxide
Edited by B. A. Weissman *et al.*, Plenum Press, New York, 1995

those of L-NAME and N^{ω}-nitro-L-arginine benzyl ester (L-NABE), which are reported to bind to muscarinic receptors, in the pulmonary vascular bed of the intact-chest cat.

METHODS

Adult mongrel cats of either sex weighing 2.5-4.1 kg were sedated with ketamine hydrochloride (10-15 mg/kg i.m.) and were anesthetized with pentobarbital sodium (30 mg/kg i.v.). The animals were restrained in the supine position on a fluoroscopic table, and supplemental doses of anesthetic were administered as needed to maintain a uniform level of anesthesia. The trachea was intubated with a cuffed pediatric endotracheal tube, and the animals spontaneously breathed room air enriched with 95% O_2/5% CO_2. Systemic arterial (aortic) pressure was measured from a catheter inserted into the aorta from the femoral artery, and intravenous injections were made into a catheter positioned in the inferior vena cava from a femoral vein. For perfusion of the left lower lung lobe, a triple-lumen, 28 cm, 6F balloon perfusion catheter was passed under fluoroscopic guidance from an external jugular vein into the artery to the left lower lung lobe. After the animals had been heparinized (1,000 U/kg i.v.), the lobar artery was vascularly isolated by distension of the balloon cuff on the perfusion catheter. The lobe was perfused with a perfusion pump (model 1210, Harvard Instruments) by way of the catheter lumen beyond the cuff with blood withdrawn from a femoral artery. Lobar arterial pressure was measured from a second catheter port 5 mm beyond the cuff on the perfusion catheter. The perfusion rate was adjusted so that lobar arterial perfusion pressure approximated mean pressure in the main pulmonary artery and was not changed thereafter. The flow rate ranged from 28-45 ml/min, and left atrial pressure was measured with a radiopaque 6F double-lumen catheter passed transseptally into the left atrium. Mean vascular pressures, measured with Spectromed DTX Plus transducers zeroed at right atrial level, were recorded on a Grass model recorder after characteristic waveforms had been confirmed. These procedures have been described previously (McMahon and Kadowitz, 1993).

L-NA (Sigma Chemical Co., St. Louis, MO) was dissolved in acidified normal saline with sonication immediately before i.v. administration. L-NAME, L-NABE, acetylcholine chloride, and substance P (Sigma) were dissolved in normal saline. The thromboxane A_2 mimic, U46619 (Upjohn, Kalamazoo, MI) was dissolved in 100% ethanol at a concentration of 10 mg/ml and was diluted in 0.9% saline. The TXA_2 mimic was infused into the perfused lobar artery with a Harvard infusion pump at rates (50-360 ng/min) required to raise lobar arterial pressure to values of 35-42 mm Hg. S-nitroso-N-acetylpenicillamine (SNAP) was synthesized by Dr. Louis J. Ignarro (UCLA School of Medicine, Los Angeles, CA). Nitric oxide solutions in methanol were prepared by first bubbling 10 ml of reagent-grade methanol (EM Industries, Cherry Hill, NJ) for 20 min with nitrogen in a gas-tight reaction vial to remove dissolved oxygen. The methanol was then bubbled with nitric oxide gas (Hydrocarbon Technologies, Sulphur, LA) for 20 min and stored in a freezer in a gas-tight vial. The doses of nitric oxide administered are expressed only as volume (microliters) of nitric oxide solution injected. Felodipine (Astra-Merck, West Point, PA) was dissolved in 0.1 cremophore, 0.2 ml propylene glycol, and 0.7 ml Tris buffer, pH 7.4, to make a final concentration of 1 mg/ml.

Arterial blood gases and pH were measured with a Corning model 178 analyzer and were in the normal range. All hemodynamic data are expressed in absolute units and are presented as mean ± S.E. Responses represent peak changes, and data were analyzed using a one-way analysis of variance and Scheffe's F test or paired t-test. A P value of less than 0.05 was used as the criterion for statistical significance.

RESULTS

The inhibitory effects of L-NA, the methyl ester L-NAME, and benzyl ester L-NABE, on vasodilator responses to acetylcholine (0.1 μg) and substance P (1.0 μg) were compared in the pulmonary vascular bed of the cat. When lobar arterial pressure had been raised to a high steady value (35-42 mm Hg) with U46619, intralobar injections of acetylcholine and substance P caused significant decreases in lobar arterial pressure (Fig. 1). Following the administration of L-NA, L-NAME, and L-NABE at a dose of 100 mg/kg i.v., decreases in lobar arterial pressure in response to acetylcholine were reduced significantly by 51%, 58%, and 52%, respectively (Fig. 1). The decreases in lobar arterial pressure in response to intralobar injections of substance P were also reduced significantly by 44%, 49%, and 52% following administration of L-NA, L-NAME, and L-NABE, respectively, in a dose of 100 mg/kg i.v. (Fig. 1). The reductions in the vasodilator response to acetylcholine, when compared with the reduction in the response to substance P following administration of L-NA, L-NAME, and L-NABE, did not differ significantly.

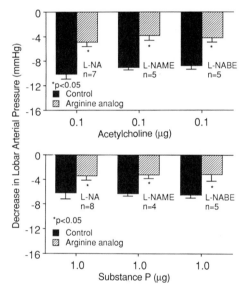

Figure 1. Influence of N$^{\omega}$-nitro-L-arginine (L-NA), N$^{\omega}$-nitro-L-arginine methyl ester (L-NAME), and N$^{\omega}$-nitro-L-arginine benzyl ester (L-NABE) on decreases in lobar arterial pressure in response to acetylcholine (A) and substance P (B) under elevated tone conditions. Responses were compared before and after administration of the nitric oxide (NO) synthase inhibitors(100 mg/kg i.v.). *P <0.05, significantly different from control; n indicates number of animals.

The decreases in lobar arterial pressure in response to acetylcholine were reduced significantly following administration of atropine (1 mg/kg i.v.), whereas the muscarinic receptor blocking agent had no significant difference on the pulmonary vasodilator response to substance P (Fig. 2).

The specificity of the inhibitory effects of L-NA, L-NAME, and L-NABE was assessed by investigating the actions of the three nitric oxide synthase inhibitors on vasodilator responses to various agents that act by endothelium-independent mechanisms, and these data are summarized in Fig. 3. Following administration of the nitric oxide synthase inhibitors in a dose of 100 mg/kg i.v., decreases in lobar arterial pressure in response to SNAP,adenosine, and felodipine were not significantly different from control responses, but the decrease in response to nitric oxide was potentiated when tone in the pulmonary vascular bed had been increased to similar levels with U46619 (Fig. 4). In addition to decreasing vasodilator responses to acetylcholine and to substance P, L-NA, L-NAME, and L-NABE, when administered in a dose of 100 mg/kg i.v., caused significant increases in lobar arterial and systemic arterial pressure without altering left atrial pressure. The peak increases in lobar arterial and systemic arterial pressures that occurred over a 20-46 min period following the administration of L-NA, L-NAME, and L-NABE, did not differ significantly from one another (Fig. 4).

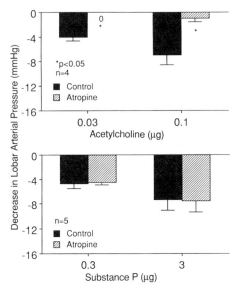

Figure 2. Influence of atropine on decreases in lobar arterial pressure in response to acetylcholine (A) and substance P (B). Responses were compared before and after administration of the muscarinic antagonist (1 mg/kg i.v.). *P <0.05, significantly different from control; n indicates number of animals.

In addition to studies in the pulmonary vascular bed, the effects of L-NA and L-NAME were investigated in the peripheral vascular bed of the cat (Santiago et al., 1994). In these experiments, injections of acetylcholine, bradykinin, and substance P into the mesenteric arterial perfusion circuit caused dose-related decreases in mesenteric arterial perfusion pressure. Following administration of L-NA or L-NAME doses in doses of 100 mg/kg i.v., vasodilator responses to acetylcholine, bradykinin, and substance P were decreased significantly. Vasodilator responses to acetylcholine (10 ng), bradykinin (30 ng), and substance P (10 ng) were reduced 52 ± 7, 66 ± 6, and 39 ± 7%, respectively, following administration of L-NA and 54 ± 8, 55 ± 10, and 26 ± 6%, respectively, following administration of L-NAME. The reductions in response to acetylcholine (10 ng), bradykinin (30 ng), and substance P (10 ng) were not significantly different following administration of either nitric oxide synthase inhibitors. The administration of L-NA or L-NAME resulted in a significant increase in mesenteric arterial and in systemic arterial pressures. Systemic and mesenteric arterial pressures rose in a progressive manner with time, and peak increases in mesenteric arterial perfusion pressure following administration of L-NA and L-NAME were observed to occur in 15-31 min.

The peak increases in mesenteric arterial and systemic arterial pressures in response to L-NA and L-NAME did not differ significantly after administration of the nitric oxide synthase inhibitors.

Following administration of the nitric oxide synthase inhibitors, vasodilator responses to SNAP, sodium nitroprusside, adenosine, and prostaglandin E₁ were not decreased. Vasodilator responses to SNAP were increased significantly at doses of 10 and 30 μg and responses to sodium nitroprusside were increased significantly at all doses studied following administration of the nitric oxide synthase inhibitors. The effects of the

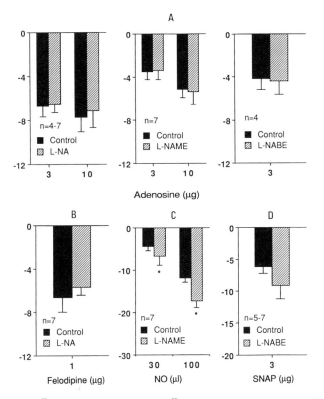

Figure 3. Influence of N$^{\omega}$-nitro-L-arginine (L-NA), N$^{\omega}$-nitro-arginine methyl ester (L-NAME), and N$^{\omega}$-nitro-L-arginine benzyl ester (L-NABE) on decreases in lobar arterial pressure in response to adenosine (A), felodipine (B), nitric oxide (NO; C), and S-nitroso-N-acetylpenicillamine (SNAP; D) under elevated tone conditions. Responses were compared before and after administration of NO synthase inhibitors (100 mg/kg i.v.). *P <0.05, significantly different from control; n indicates number of animals.

muscarinic receptor antagonist, atropine, on vasodilator responses to acetylcholine, bradykinin, and substance P were compared; and following administration of atropine in a dose of 1 mg/kg i.v., vasodilator responses to acetylcholine were reduced significantly whereas vasodilator responses to bradykinin and substance P were not changed following administration of the muscarinic receptor antagonist.

DISCUSSION

Results of the present study show that L-NA, L-NAME, and L-NABE increase lobar arterial pressure and attenuate decreases in lobar arterial pressure in response to acetylcholine and substance P but do not reduce responses to vasodilator agents that act by various endothelium-independent mechanisms.

Inasmuch as pulmonary blood flow and left atrial pressure were maintained constant, the changes in lobar arterial pressure reflect changes in pulmonary lobar vascular resistance. The results of the present study demonstrate that the three nitric oxide synthase inhibitors increase pulmonary vascular resistance, decrease pulmonary vasodilator

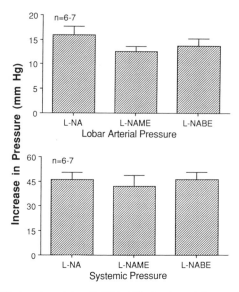

Figure 4. Influence of N^{ω}-nitro-L-arginine (L-NA), N^{ω}-nitro-L-arginine methyl ester (L-NAME), and N^{ω}-nitro-L-arginine benzyl ester (L-NABE) on lobar arterial pressure (A) and systemic pressure (B) in the absence of U46619 infusion. Peak responses were measured over 20-46 min and compared before and after administration of NO synthase inhibitors (100 mg/kg i.v.). *P <0.05, significantly different from control; n indicates number of animals.

responses to acetylcholine and substance P, and do not decrease vasodilator responses to agents that induce vasodilation by diverse endothelium-independent mechanisms.

The present data show that the three nitric oxide synthase inhibitors, L-NA, L-NAME, and L-NABE, do not markedly differ in their ability to inhibit vasodilator responses to the endothelium-dependent agents and to increase baseline tone in the pulmonary vascular bed of the cat. These results are of interest in view of the recent finding that L-NAME and other alkyl esters of L-NA possess muscarinic receptor blocking activity (Buxton et al., 1992). Many studies have employed L-NAME, and the observation that alkyl esters of L-NA are muscarinic receptor antagonists suggests that the interpretation of the results of studies with L-NAME may be difficult because of its muscarinic receptor blocking properties (Broten et al., 1992; Gardiner and Bennett, 1992; Buxton et al., 1992; Smith et al., 1992; White et al., 1993). The results of the present study showing a similar pattern of inhibitory activity of L-NA, which does not possess muscarinic receptor blocking activity, with that of L-NAME and L-NABE, which bind to muscarinic receptors, may suggest that the muscarinic receptor blocking properties of the alkyl esters is small when compared with the inhibitory effects on nitric oxide synthase in resistance vessel elements in the feline pulmonary vascular bed (Buxton et al., 1992). These data may suggest that the relative effects of alkyl esters of L-NA on muscarinic receptor function and on nitric oxide synthase activity may depend on the tissue or vascular bed studied. The hypothesis that the relative effects of alkyl esters of L-NA on muscarinic receptor function and on nitric oxide synthetase activity were dependent on

142

specific vascular bed studied was explored in the mesenteric vascular bed of the cat (Santiago et al., 1994). The results of these studies show that L-NAME and L-NA had a similar inhibitory effect on vasodilator responses to acetylcholine inthe mesenteric vascular bed (Santiago et al., 1994). In addition, L-NAME and L-NA had a similar inhibitory effect on mesenteric vasodilator responses to bradykinin and substance P and increased mesenteric arterial perfusion pressure to a similar extent (Santiago et al., 1994). The results of studies in the mesenteric vascular bed are similar to results in the pulmonary vascular bed and indicate that the relative effects of L-NA and L-NAME on muscarinically mediated vasodilator responses are not dependent on the specific vascular bed studied in the cat. It has been reported that L-NAME is rapidly converted to L-NA in several species (Huber et al., 1992; Krejcy et al., 1993). It is, therefore, not surprising that L-NA and L-NAME have similar patterns of effect on responses to acetylcholine, substance P, and on increases in systemic and lobar arterial pressures in the cat. The observation that only about 50% of the vasodilator response to acetylcholine can be blocked by L-NA or L-NAME in the hindquarters mesenteric and pulmonary vascular beds of the cat, whereas the response can be abolished by atropine, suggests that a muscarinic receptor-mediated mechanism in addition to nitric oxide release may play a role in mediating vasodilator responses to acetylcholine in these systems (Bellan et al., 1991;1993). However, the nature of these additional mechanisms that may involve release of a hyperpolarizing factor or other mechanisms is uncertain at the present time. It has been reported recently that L-NAME does not inhibit vasodilator responses to acetylcholine or bradykinin in the pulmonary vascular bed of the cat. The reason for the difference in results in the studies of Lippton et al. (1992) and the present study is uncertain but is not due to difference in species or experimental preparation used, although a different anesthetic agent was employed in the two studies. The increases in lobar arterial and systemic arterial pressure in response to L-NA, L-NAME, and L-NABE in the present study were similar and provide support for the hypothesis that "tonic release of nitric oxide" serves to maintain both the pulmonary and peripheral vascular beds of the cat in a dilated state. However, the magnitude of the change in systemic vascular resistance cannot be determined since cardiac output was not measured and systemic vascular resistance could not be calculated.

In conclusion, the results of the present investigation show that L-NA, L-NAME, and L-NABE possess a similar pattern of inhibitory activity on pulmonary vasodilator responses to acetylcholine, suggesting that all three agents can be used to study muscarinic receptor-mediated nitric oxide release in the pulmonary vascular bed of the intact-chest cat. Results of studies with L-NA and L-NAME in the mesenteric vascular bed are similar to results in the pulmonary vascular bed and provide support for the hypothesis that alkyl esters of L-NA do not block muscarinic receptors in the cat.

Acknowledgments

The authors wish to thank Ms. Janice Ignarro for editorial assistance. The studies were supported by National Institutes of Health grants HL15580 and HL46737 and a grant from the American Heart Association.

REFERENCES

Bellan, J.A., McNamara, D.B., and Kadowitz, P.J., 1993, Differential effects of nitric oxide synthesis inhibitor on vascular resistance and responses to acetylcholine in the cat, *Am. J. Physiol. 264(Heart Circ. Physiol. 33)*:H45.

Bellan, J.A., Minkes, R.K. McNamara, D.B., and Kadowitz, P.J., 1991, N^{ω}-nitro-L-arginine selectively inhibits vasodilator responses to acetylcholine and bradykinin in cats, *Am. J. Physiol. 260(Heart Circ. Physiol. 29)*:H1025.

Broten, T.P., Miyashiro, J.K., Moncada, S., and Feigl, E.O., 1992, Role of endothelium-derived relaxing factor in parasympathetic coronary vasodilation, *Am. J. Physiol. 262(Heart Circ. Physiol. 31)*:H1579.

Buxton, I.L.O., Cheek, D.J., Eckman, D., Westfall, D.P., Sanders, K.M., and Keef, K.D., 1992, N^G-nitro-L-arginine ester and other alkyl esters of arginine are muscarinic receptor antagonists, *Circ. Res.* 72:387.

Furchgott, R.F., and Zawadski, J.V., 1980, The obligatory role of endothelial cells in the relaxation of arterial smooth muscle by endothelial cells in the relaxation of arterial smooth muscle by acetylcholine, *Nature (Lond.)* 288:373.

Gardiner, S.M., and Bennett, T., 1992, Involvement of nitric oxide in the regional haemodynamic effects of perindoprilat and captopril in hypovolaemic brattleboro rats, *Br. J. Pharmacol.* 107:1181.

Huber, S., Grohs, J.G., Schwarzacher, S., and Raberger, G., 1992, Oral N^G-nitro-L-arginine in conscious dogs: 24 hour hypertensive response in relation to plasma levels, *Amino Acids* 2:225.

Ishii, K., Chang, B., Kerwin, J.F., Huang, Z.J., and Murad, F., 1990, N^{ω}-nitro-L-arginine: a potent inhibitor of endothelium-derived relaxing factor formation, *Eur. J. Pharmacol.* 179:219.

Krejcy, K., Schwarzacher, S., and Raberger, G., 1993, Distribution and metabolism of N^G-nitro-L-arginine and N^G-nitro-L-arginine methyl ester in canine blood *in vitro*, *Naunyn-Schmiedeberg's Arch. Pharmacol.* 347:342.

Lippton, H.L., Hao, Q., and Hyman, A., 1992, L-NAME enhances pulmonary vasoconstriction without inhibiting EDRF-dependent vasodilation, *J. Appl. Physiol.* 73:2432.

McMahon, T.J., Hood, J.S., Bellan, J.A., and Kadowitz, P.J., 1991, N^{ω}-nitro-L-arginine methyl ester selectively inhibits pulmonary vasodilator responses to acetylcholine and bradykinin, *J. Appl. Physiol.* 71:2026.

McMahon, T.J., and Kadowitz, P.J., 1992, Pulmonary vasodilator responses to vagal stimulation is blocked by N^{ω}-nitro-L-arginine methyl ester in the cat, *Circ. Res.* 70:364.

McMahon, T.J., and Kadowitz, P.J., 1993, Analysis of responses to substance P in the pulmonary vascular bed of the cat, *Am. J. Physiol. 264(Heart Circ. Physiol. 33)*:H394.

Moncada, S., Palmer, R.M.J., and Higgs, E.A., 1989, Biosynthesis of nitric oxide from arginine. A pathway for the regulation of cell function and communication, *Biochem. Pharmacol.* 38:1709.

Moore, P.K., Al-Swayeh, O.A., Chong, N.W.S., Egands, R.A., and Gibson, A., 1990, L-N^{ω}-nitroarginine (L-NOARG), a novel L-arginine-reversible inhibitor N^{ω} of endothelium-dependent vasodilation *in vitro*, *Br. J. Pharmacol.* 99:408.

Santiago, J.A., Garrison, E.A., and Kadowitz, P.J., 1994, Comparative effects of N-nitro-L-arginine and N^W-nitro-L-arginine methyl ester on vasodilator responses to acetylcholine, bradykinin, and substance P, *Eur. J. Pharmacol.* 254:207.

Smith, R.E., Palmer, R.M., Bucknall, C.A., and Moncada, S., 1992, Role of nitric oxide synthesis in the regulation of coronary vascular tone in the isolated perfused rabbit heart, *Heart Cardiovasc. Res.* 26:508.

White, D.G., Gurden, J.M., Penny, D.M., Roach, A.G., and Watts, I.S., 1993, The effect of N^G-nitro-L-arginine methyl ester upon basal blood flow and endothelium-dependent vasodilation in the dog hindlimb, *Br. J. Pharmacol.* 108:763.

VASCULAR RESPONSES TO ENDOTHELIN-1 IN CONSCIOUS RATS: MODULATION BY ENDOGENOUS NITRIC OXIDE

Janos G. Filep[1], Alain Fournier[2], and Eva Foldes-Filep[1]

[1]Research Center, Maisonneuve-Rosemont Hospital,
Department of Medicine, University of Montreal
Montreal, P.Q., Canada H1T 2M4 and
[2]Institut National de la Recherche Scientifique-Sante,
Montreal, P.Q., Canada H9R 1G6

INTRODUCTION

The vascular endothelium is an active site for the production of many active substances essential in the regulation of vascular tone and reactivity. For instance, endothelial cells release endothelium-derived relaxing factor (EDRF), now characterized as nitric oxide (NO) (Ignarro et al., 1987; Palmer et al., 1987) and endothelin-1 (ET-1) (Yanagisawa et al., 1988). The continuous release of NO from endothelium (Ignarro, 1989) appears to play an important role as an intrinsic modulator of vascular tone, blood flow (Ignarro, 1989) and microvascular permeability in the mesenteric (Kubes and Granger, 1992) and coronary circulation (Filep et al., 1993b).

ET-1 has been implicated in a wide variety of physiologic functions, particularly those involving the cardiovascular system. These actions include vasoconstriction, vasodilation, secretion of biologically active compounds and mitogenesis (see Simonson and Dunn, 1992). Recently, we have shown that ET-1 is capable of enhancing protein extravasation in the coronary, pulmonary, gastrointestinal and renal circulation (Filep et al., 1991). The observation that ET-1 releases NO from guinea pig or rat isolated perfused lungs (de Nucci et al., 1988) led to the hypothesis that NO may mediate the vasodilator and vasodepressor responses to ET-1. However, *in vivo* studies using the NO synthase inhibitors, N^G-monomethyl-L-arginine (L-NMMA) (Palmer et al., 1988) and N^G-nitro-L-arginine methyl ester (L-NAME) (Moore et al., 1990) resulted in conflicting results since both significant inhibition of the depressor and vasodilator actions of ET-1 (Whittle et al., 1989; Gardiner et al., 1990) and failure of L-NMMA to attenuate the depressor response to ET-1 (Gardiner et al., 1989) have been described. The objectives of this study were to determine (1) whether NO mediates the depressor and attenuates the pressor action of ET-1 and (2) whether inhibon of NO synthesis compromises ET-1-induced increases in microvascular albumin permeation in the conscious rats.

Biochemical, Pharmacological, and Clinical Aspects of Nitric Oxide
Edited by B. A. Weissman *et al.*, Plenum Press, New York, 1995

MATERIALS AND METHODS

Experimental protocols

The experiments were performed on conscious, chronically catheterized male Wistar rats weighing 220-310 g. The preparation of animals has been described in detail elsewhere (Filep and Filep-Th, 1986).

Previous experiments showed that L-NMMA and L-NAME at a dose of 25 and 2 mg/kg, respectively, evoked near maximal (93-97 %) increase in mean arterial blood pressure (MABP) in conscious rats (Filep et al., 1993a). Therefore, these doses of L-arginine analogues were used in the present experiments. In the first series of studies, the ability of L-NMMA and L-NAME to modify ET-1 (1 nmol/kg)-induced changes in MABP was determined. In order to directly compare the ET-1 responses before and after NO synthesis blockade, in some animals MABP was either elevated by an infusion of noradrenaline (620-820 µg/kg/min) to levels observed following treatment with L-arginine analogues or L-NAME-induced elevation of MABP was titrated to normotensive levels with diazoxide (90 µmol/kg) or hydralazine (1.2-1.5 µmol/kg) before injection of ET-1.

In subsequent experiments, albumin extravasation was quantitated by measuring the extravasation of Evans blue dye which binds to plasma albumin. In this series of experiments, Evans blue dye (20 mg/kg) was injected i.v. together with ET-1 (1 nmol/kg) or its vehicle into animals pretreated with L-NAME (2 mg/kg) or during noradrenaline infusion. Ten min after injection of ET-1 the rats were anaesthetized and were perfused with 0.9 % NaCl to remove the excess of intravascular dye. Then portions of various organs were excised, and tissue Evans blue content was determined following extraction as described previously (Filep et al., 1991).

Drugs and chemicals

ET-1 was synthesized in our laboratories by solid-phase methodology. The purity of the preparation was greater than 97 % as determined by high performance liquid chromatography. All other chemicals were purchased from Sigma Chemical Co. (St. Louis, MO, USA) with the exception of L-NMMA which was obtained from Research Biochemicals International (Natick, MA, USA).

Statistical analysis

Results are expressed as means ±S.E.M. Statistical evaluation of the data were performed by one-way analysis of variance using ranks (Kruskal-Wallis test) followed by Dunn's multiple contrast hypothesis test to compare various treatments to the same control. A $p<0.05$ level was considered significant for all tests.

RESULTS

Effects of L-NMMA and L-NAME on the depressor and pressor responses to ET-1

As well established, ET-1 (1 nmol/kg) produced an initial transient decrease in MABP followed by a sustained pressor action. Neither L-NAME nor L-NMMA affected the depressor action of ET-1, whereas L-NAME, but not L-NMMA significantly decreased the magnitude of the pressor response to ET-1 compared to the effects of ET-1 in control rats (fig. 1a). Elevation of MABP by an infusion of noradrenaline to levels comparable to those seen after L-NAME or L-NMMA, significantly enhanced the depressor effect and decreased the pressor action of ET-1 compared to ET-1-induced changes in control animals (fig. 1a). L-NMMA and L-NAME caused about 40-50% inhibiton of the depressor response to ET-1 and a significant increase in the pressor action of ET-1 compared to the effects of ET-1 in rats receiving noradrenaline infusion (fig. 1a). Similarly, a statistically significant inhibition of the depressor and a significant potentiation of the pressor effect of ET-1 were detected in animals treated with L-NAME plus hydralazine or L-NAME plus diazoxide compared to the effects of ET-1 in control (untreated) animals (fig. 1b).

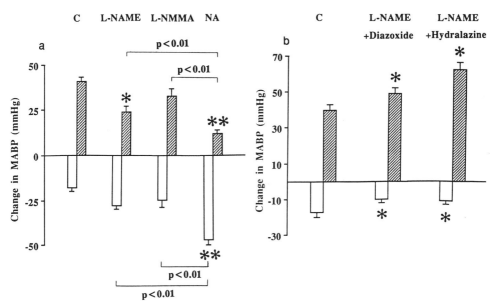

Figure 1. Endothelin-1-induced maximum decrease (open columns) and peak increase (hatched columns) in mean arterial blood pressure (MABP) in conscious rats. (a) The animals were pretreated with L-NAME (2 mg/kg) for 10 min, L-NMMA (25 mg/kg) for 2 min, noradrenaline (NA, 620-820 ng/kg/min) for 10 min or 0.9 % NaCl (control, C) before bolus i.v. injection of ET-1 (1 nmol/kg). MABP were 110±3 mmHg (n=8), 152±5 mmHg (n=8), 149±4 mmHg (n=6) in control, L-NAME, L-NMMA and noradrenaline-treated animals, respectively, before injection of ET-1. (b) Following injection of L-NAME (2 mg/kg), the elevated MABP was restored to normotensive levels with diazoxide (90 μmol/kg) or hydralazine (1.2-1.5 μmol/kg) before injection of ET-1 (1 nmol/kg). MABP were 110±3 mmHg (n=6), 107±2 mmHg (n=6) and 109±5 mmHg (n=5) in control animals receiving vehicle of L-NAME (C) and in rats treated with L-NAME plus diazoxide or L-NAME plus hydralazine, respectively. Values are means with S.E.M. * p<0.05, ** p<0.01 (compared to control by Dunn's multiple contrast hypothesis test) (Reprinted from Filep et al., Br. J. Pharmacol. 110:1213-1221, 1993 with the permission of the Publisher).

Effects of L-NAME on albumin extravasation

Injection of L-NAME (2 mg/kg) evoked increases (up to 280 %) in albumin extravasation in the large airways, heart, kidney and gastrointestinal tract, whereas no significant changes were detected in the pulmonary parenchyma, skeletal muscle and dorsal skin (table 1).

Maintenance of MABP at the level observed following L-NAME administration by infusion of noradrenaline did not enhance albumin extravasation, except in the pulmonary circulation, where noradrenaline induced similar increases in tissue Evans blue content as L-NAME (table 1).

Effects of L-NAME on ET-1-induced albumin extravasation

In agreement with our previous studies, injection of ET-1 (1 nmol/kg) produced a significant increase in albumin extravasation in most vascular beds studied (table 1). When ET-1 was injected following L-NAME, albumin extravasation was markedly potentiated (up to 550 %) in the bronchial, coronary, gastric, duodenal and renal vascular beds (table 1). Unlike L-NAME, noradrenaline infusion enhanced ET-1-induced albumin extravasation only in the pulmonary circulation (table 1). However, albumin leakage elicited by noradrenaline plus ET-1 in the bronchi and parenchyma was somewhat lower than that seen following L-NAME plus ET-1 (table 1). In the trachea, pancreas and liver, the effects of ET-1 and L-NAME were additive (table 1). Combined administration of L-NAME and ET-1 evoked significant increases in albumin extravasation in the pulmonary parenchyma and skeletal muscle, where neither L-NAME nor ET-1 alone affected albumin permeation (table 1).

DISCUSSION

The present experiments were designed to study the role of endogenous NO in mediating and/or modulating the vascular responses to ET-1 by using NO synthase inhibitors. The evaluation of the degree of inhibition of NO production *in vivo* is hindered by the lack of reliable methods for quantitation of endogenous NO production in experimental animals. Large increases in mean arterial blood pressure elicited by L-arginine analogues (Aisaka et al., 1989; Rees et al., 1989; Whittle et al., 1990; Hecker et al., 1990) are considered to indicate that the resultant decrease in endothelial NO production is responsible for the elevation of blood pressure. L-NMMA and L-NAME are believed to inhibit NO biosynthesis via the competitive inhibiton of NO synthase. Accordingly, the effects of L-NAME and L-NMMA on blood pressure and albumin extravasation can be effectively reversed by L-arginine, but not by D-arginine (Moore et al., 1990; Vargas et al., 1991, Filep et al., 1993a). These observations coupled with the findings that the biologically inactive enantiomer, D-NAME did not affect blood pressure and permeability (Filep et al., 1993a) would indicate that the effects of L-NAME can be attributed to inhibition of endogenous release of NO from endothelial and other cells.

In order to rule out the confounding influence of varying blood pressure and vascular tone on the ET-1 responses between control and L-NMMA or L-NAME-treated subjects, mean arterial blood pressure was either elevated by a constant infusion of noradrenaline in control animals to comparable levels as seen after L-arginine analogues or the elevated blood pressure in L-NAME-treated animals was titrated to normotensive levels by using the endothelium-independent vasodilators, diazoxide or hydralazine. In these paradigms, blunting, but not complete inhibition of the depressor action and potentiation of the ET-1 pressor response could be demonstrated. These observations indicate that ET-1-induced NO release is responsible, at least partly, for the depressor action of the peptide and that endogenous NO blunts the pressor action of ET-1 in the conscious rat.

TABLE 1. Effects of L-NAME and noradrenaline (NA) on ET-1-induced albumin extravasation in selected vascular beds in conscious rats.

ORGAN	C (n=6)	ET-1 (n=6)	L-NAME (n=6)	L-NAME plus ET-1 (n=5)	NA (n=6)	NA plus ET-1 (n=6)
Trachea	62±6	64±9	108±12*	110±10*	118±21*	123±10*
Upper bronchi	47±6	125±11*	104±9*	227±38**	161±28*	183±23*
Lower bronchi	49±5	140±8*	112±10	238±25**##	168±19*	194±26*
Pulmonary parenchyma	81±7	101±7	110±8	261±30**	135±13	162±7**
Left ventricle	78±11	144±11*	163±15*	461±40**##	109±15	243±40**
Right atrium	99±5	221±27*	187±12*	468±25**##	105±7	274±16**
Liver	53±5	71±6	110±10**	114±13**#	58±4	83±6
Spleen	118±8	190±6*	195±23*	238±25*	113±8	186±7*
Pancreas	38±5	48±6	100±12	126±15**##	43±5	46±6
Kidney	57±9	112±22*	136±20*	315±24**##	70±6	146±23*
Stomach	71±5	130±9*	155±25*	307±33**##	77±6	136±27*
Duodenum	90±9	164±10*	252±21**	326±34**#	102±16	216±16*
Skeletal muscle	46±4	51±9	68±10	72±8*	61±6	71±8
Dorsal skin	32±5	34±7	43±4	45±6	41±4	44±7

Values are presented as Evans blue dye, μg/g tissue (dry weight) means ±S.E.M. The animals were given L-NAME (2mg/kg), noradrenaline (620-820 μg/kg/min) or 0.9 % NaCl (C, control) for 10 min before bolus i.v. injection of ET-1 (1 nmol/kg) plus Evans blue dye (20 mg/kg).
The rats were anaesthetized and were perfused with 0.9 % NaCl 10 min after injection of ET-1. The permeability measurement was made 15 min after injection of ET-1. * p<0.05, ** p<0.01 (compared to control by Dunn's multiple contrast hypothesis test); # p<0.05, ## p<0.01 (compared to NA plus ET-1).

The present study confirms and extends previous observations that L-NAME causes a rapid increase in albumin extravasation in the cat mesenterium (Kubes and Granger, 1992) and rat coronary circulation (Filep et al., 1993b). Our data show that L-NAME also enhances albumin extravasation in the large airways, liver, spleen, pancreas and kidney. These effects of L-NAME are not simply a consequence of elevations in systemic blood pressure and consequently an increase in perfusion pressure as noradrenaline infusion did not mimick the permeability effect of L-NAME with the exception of the lung. Acute generalized vasoconstriction elicited by noradrenaline or L-NAME would result in rapid increases in left atrial end diastolic pressure and consequently in pulmonary pressure.

Elevation of pulmonary pressure (over 40 cm H_2O) would lead to widening and disruption of the endothelial junctions, and thereby would promote protein leakage (Tsukimoto et al., 1990). However, one should keep in mind that capillary hydrostatic pressure is not the primary determinant of mediator-stimulated protein extravasation (Grega et al., 1986) provided that the endothelial layer is intact. Indeed, L-NAME-induced increases in transcapillary protein fluxes were associated with a slight decrease in capillary hydrostatic pressure in the cat ileum (Kubes and Granger, 1992). On the other hand, albumin extravasation could probably be masked by arterial vasoconstriction elicited by L-NAME. This might explain the failure of L-NAME to induce albumin extravasation in the skeletal muscle and dorsal skin.

Inhibition of NO synthesis by L-NAME resulted in enhanced albumin leakage in response to ET-1. Although high pressure-induced structural changes in the capillaries may explain the permeability enhancing effect of L-NAME in the pulmonary circulation, the mechanism by which inhibition of NO production increases protein extravasation ii other vascular beds remains unclear. Since interendothelial cell gap formation and consequently opening of the large-pore system appears to be the major determinant of protein extravasation in inflammation (Grega et al., 1986), it is plausible to assume that L-NAME treatment leads to gap formation. Although the mechanism by which NO could regulate vascular permeability is unknown at present, several possibilities warrant attention. Under physiological conditions, the continuous release of NO from endothelial cells maintains the vasculature in a state of "active vasodilation", prevents adhesion of platelets and neutrophil granulocytes to the endothelium and may also scavenge small amounts of superoxide released by endothelial cells (Zweier et al., 1988). Decreased NO production promotes adhesion of platelets and neutrophil granulocytes to the endothelium (Radomski et al., 1987; Kubes et al., 1991), an event that is known to induce endothelial dysfunction (Lefer et al., 1991). Another possibility is that inhibition of NO synthesis would allow for a local accumulation of superoxide, which is known to alter microvascular integrity (Del Maestro et al., 1981). In addition, activated neutrophil granulocytes may also contribute to accumulation of superoxide. It is not known at present whether inhibition of NO production in inflammatory cells could lead to their activation, which in turn release substances that can increase fluid and protein extravasation.

The present findings may have relevance to pathological conditions associated with endothelial dysfunction, e.g. reperfusion of ischemic tissues. Loss of endothelium-dependent vasorelaxation due to reduced release or action of NO is one of the early events during reperfusion (Lefer et al., 1991). This would lead to enhanced vasoconstriction, accumulation of neutrophil granulocytes and oedema formation, which are characteristic features of the inflammatory response associated with reperfusion of ischemic tissues.

In conclusion, these observations indicate that endogenous NO mediates, in part, the vasodepressor effect and attenuates the vasopressor action of ET-1. Inhibition of NO production leads to an increase in albumin extravasation and potentiation of the permeability effect of ET-1 in the coronary, gastrointestinal and renal vascular beds of conscious rats.

Acknowledgements

This study was supported by the Medical Research Council of Canada and the Foundation of the Maisonneuve-Rosemont Hospital. A.F. and J.G.F. are scholars of the Fonds de la Recherche en Sant' du Qu'bec.

REFERENCES

Aisaka, K., S.S. Gross, O.W. Griffith and R. Levi, 1989, L-arginine availability determines the duration of acetylcholine-induced systemic vasodilation in vivo, Biochem. Biophys. Res. Commun. 163, 710.

Del Maestro, R.F., J. Bjork and K.E. Arfors, 1981, Increase in microvascular permeability induced by enzymatically generated free radicals. 1. In vivo study, Microvasc. Res. 22, 239.

de Nucci, G., R. Thomas, P. D'Orleans-Juste, E. Antunes, C. Walder, T.D. Warner and J.R. Vane, 1988, Pressor effects of circulating endothelin are limited by its removal in the pulmonary circulation and by the release of prostacyclin and endothelium-derived relaxing factor, Proc. Natl. Acad. Sci. USA 85, 979E.

Filep, J. and Fejes-Toth, 1986, Does vasopressin sustain blood pressure in conscious spontaneously hypertensive rats? Hypertension 8, 514.

Filep, J.G., E. Foldes-Filep, A. Rousseau, P. Sirois and A. Fournier, 1993a, Vascular responses to endothelin-1 following inhibition of nitric oxide synthesis in the conscious rats, Br. J Pharmacol. 110, 1213.

Filep, J.G., E. Foldes-Filep and P. Sirois, 1993b, Nitric oxide modulates vascular permeability in the rat coronary circulation, Br. J. Pharmacol. 108, 323.

Filep, J.G., M.G. Sirois, A. Rousseau, A. Fournier and P. Sirois, 1991, Effects of endothelin-1 on vascular permeability in the conscious rats: interactions with platelet-activating factor, Br. J. Pharmacol. 104, 797.

Gardiner, S.M., A.M. Compton, T. Bennett, R.M.J. Palmer and S. Moncada, 1989, N^G- monomethyl-L-arginine does not inhibit the hindquarters vasodilator action of endothelin-1 in conscious rats, Eur. J. Pharmacol. 171, 237.

Gardiner, S.M., A.M. Compton, P.A. Kemp and T. Bennett, 1990, Regional and cardiac haemodynamic responses to glyceryl trinitrate, acetylcholine, bradykinin and endothelin-1 in conscious rats: effects of N^G-nitro-L-arginine methyl ester, Br. J. Pharmacol. 101, 632.

Grega, G.J., S.W. Adamski and D.E. Dobbins, 1986, Physiological and pharmacological evidence for the regulation of permeability, Fed. Proc. 45, 96.

Hecker, M., J.A. Mitchell, H.J. Harris, M. Katsuma, C. Thiemermann and J.R. Vane, 1990, Endothelial cells metabolize N^G-methyl-L-arginine to L-citrulline and subsequently to L-arginine, Biochem. Biophys. Res. Commun. 167, 1037.

Ignarro, L.J., 1989, Biological actions and properties of endothelium-derived nitric oxide formed and released from artery and vein, Circ. Res. 65, 1.

Ignarro, L.J., G.M. Buga, K.S. wood, R.E. Byrns and G. Chaudhuri, 1987, Endothelium-derived relaxing factor produced and released from artery and vein is nitric oxide, Proc. Natl. Acad. Sci. USA 84, 9265.

Kubes, P. and D.N. Granger, 1992, Nitric oxide modulates microvascular permeability, Am. J. Physiol. 262, H611.

Kubes, P., N. Suzuki and D.N. Granger, 1991, Nitric oxide: an endogenous modulator of leukocyte adhesion, Proc. Natl. Acad. Sci. USA 88, 4651.

Lefer, A.M., P.S. Tsao, D.J. Lefer and X.L. Ma, 1991, Role of endothelial dysfunction in the pathogenesis of reperfusion injury after myocardial ischemia, FASEB J. 5, 2029.

Moore, P.K., O.A. Al-Swayeh, N.W.S. Chong, R.A. Evans and A. Gibson, 1990, N^G-nitro-L-arginine: a novel, L-arginine reversible inhibitor of endothelium-dependent vasodilation in vitro, Br. J. Pharmacol. 99, 408.

Palmer, R.M.J., A.G. Ferrige and S. Moncada, 1987, Nitric oxide release acounts for the biological activity of endothelium-derived relaxing factor, Nature 327, 524.

151

Palmer, R.M.J., D.P. Rees, D.D. Ashton and S. Moncada, 1988, L-arginine is the physiologic precursor for the formation of nitric oxide in endothelium-dependent relaxation, Biochem. Biophys. Res. Commun. 153, 1251.

Radomski, M.W., R.M.J. Palmer and S. Moncada, 1987, Endogenous nitric oxide inhibits human platelet adhesion to vascular endothelium, Lancet ii, 1057.

Rees, D.D., R.M.J. Palmer and S. Moncada, 1989, Role of endothelium-derived nitric oxide in the regulation of blood pressure, Proc. Natl. Acad. Sci. USA 86, 3375.

Simonson, M.S. and M.J. Dunn, 1992, The molecular mechanisms of cardiovascular and renal regulation by endothelin peptides, J. Lab. Clin. Med. 119, 622.

Tsukimoto, K., D. Mathieu-Castello, R. Prediletto and J.B. West, 1990, Structural basis of increased permeability of pulmonary capillaries with high transmural pressures, Am. Rev. Respir. Dis. 141, A297.

Vargas, H.M., J.M. Cuevas, L.J. Ignarro and G. Chaudhuri, 1991, Comparison of the inhibitory potencies of N^G-methyl, N^G-nitro and N^G-amino-L-arginine on EDRF function in the rat: evidence for continuous basal EDRF release, J. Pharmacol Exp. Ther. 257, 1208.

Whittle, B.J.R., J. Lopez-Belmonte and D.D. Rees, 1989, Modulation of the vasodepressor action of acetylcholine, bradykinin, substance P and endothelin in the rat by specific inhibiton of nitric oxide formation, Br. J. Pharmacol. 98, 646.

Yanagisawa, M., H. Kurihara, S. Kimura, Y. Tomobe, M. Kobayashi, Y. Mitsui, Y. Yazaki, K. Goto and T.Masaki, 1998, A novel potent vasoconstrictor peptide produced by vascular endothelial cells, Nature 332, 411.

STIMULATION OF ENDOGENOUS NO-PRODUCTION INFLUENCES THE DILATION OF THE CAPILLARY MICROVASCULATURE IN VIVO

Wilhelm Bloch, Dirk Hoever, and Klaus Addicks

Department of Anatomy I
University of Cologne
Joseph-Stelzmann-Str.9
D-50123 Cologne, Germany

INTRODUCTION

In the last two decades it has been shown that endothelial cells, especially microvascular endothelial cells possess contractile filaments (Becker 1969; Drenckhan et al., 1986). Investigations revealed a varying amount of microtubules and microfilamentes within the cytoplasm of the endothelial cells (for review, Hammersen, 1980). The composition of such microfilaments has been identified by immunostaining with antibodies which are specific for actin, myosin, alpha-actinin and tropomyosin by Drenckhan (1983 and 1986) in mammilian endothelial cells. The discovery of such contractile elements in the endothelial cells supports the findings of many researchers, who demonstrated a regulation of capillaries by endothelial cell motility By means of vitalmicroscopical studies in mesenterial capillaries of different species (Zweifach et al., 1934; Joris et al., 1972; Addicks et al., 1979; Lübbers et al., 1979; Weigelt and Schwarzmann, 1981; Wolff and Dietrich, 1985) Results from DeClerk et al. (1981) and Morel et al. (1989) show that a lot of mediators relax and contract endothelial cells in culture.

At the moment, one of the important and interesting mediators of smooth muscle containing vessels which have an regulativ effect on endothelial cells is nitric oxide (Oliver, 1992). The effect of nitric oxide on the functional system of endothelial cells of the capillary is not known. Therefore the interest in studies on the effect of nitric oxide on capillaries is growing. Interestingly the distribution of the NO-producing enzyme NO-synthase displays a decreasing expression of the enzyme with a decrease of vessel diameter and an absence of NO-synthase in the endothelium of the capillaries of the heart (Addicks et al., in press) The model we used provides the possibility to study the regulation of capillaries by nitric oxide in relation to coronary flow. The studies comprised of an investigation of capillary diameter regulation by basal and stimulated NO-release. The use of NO-donors as sodiumnitroprussid (SNP) and glyceroltrinitrate

Biochemical, Pharmacological, and Clinical Aspects of Nitric Oxide
Edited by B. A. Weissman *et al.*, Plenum Press, New York, 1995

153

(GTN) with different release mechanisms and localisations (Feelisch and Noack, 1987; Sellke et al., 1990) provided the possibility to study the independence from the flow of the effect nitric oxide has on capillaries. In contrast to SNP, GTN cannot release NO in smaller arteries, arterioles and capillaries.

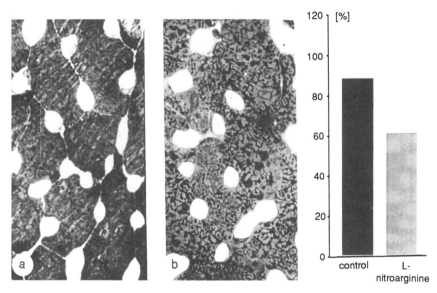

Figure 1. Semithin sections of papillary muscle which were cut transversally to the long axis of capillaries (C) show no differences of capillary diameter between the control group (1a) and the L-NA treated group (1b). The graph (1c) shows a decrease of coronary flow of more than 30% in contrast to the morphological findings of unchanged capillary diameters.

MATERIALS AND METHODS

Hearts from 12-16 week old male Wistar rats weighing 350-400g were isolatedly perfused. The rats were anaestetized with carbon dioxide (CO_2) and were then killed by cervical dislocation. Following the opening of the chest the heart was quickly excised after cannulation of the aorta and retrogradely perfused according to the Langendorff technique. The hearts were perfused at a constant pressure of 60cm H_2O with a modified Krebs Henseleit buffer: $CaCl_2$ 1,8mmol/l, $MgCl_2$ 1,05mmol/l, KCl 5.35mmol/l, NaCl 136.9mmol/l, NaH_2PO_4 0.42mmol/l, Glucose 10.1mmol/l, $NaHCO_3$ 23.8mmol/l prewarmed to 37°C and equilibrated with 95% O_2/5% CO_2. The hearts were allowed to beat spontaneously. To study the pharmacological effects of endogenously supplied nitric oxide (NO) on terminal exchange vessels, the hearts were perfused alone and in combination with bradykinin 10^{-7}M and L-nitroarginine 10^{-4}M. For the investigation of flow independent effect of nitric oxide on capillaries the NO-donors SNP 10^{-5}M, SNP 10^{-6}M and GTN 5×10^{-5}M were administered. Experimental groups with animals matched in age and weight were created and compared with corresponding controls receiving saline only. The experimental groups and the corresponding controls were equilibrated for 20 minutes. After the equilibration period coronary flow was monitored for 10min and 25min. The two groups under L-nitroarginine alone or in combination with bradykinin were perfused with L-nitroarginine since starting at the 10th minute. The switch-over time for substance was the 25th minute point. The coronary flow was registrated for 10min and the capillary diameters were measured after 5min or 20min respectively.

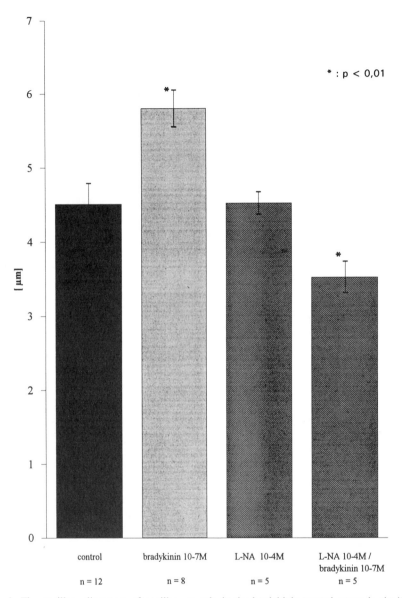

Figure 2. The capillary diameters of papillary muscle in the bradykinin treated group is significantly increased against the respective control after 30min isolated pressure constant heart perfusion with addition of bradykinin 10^{-7}M for the last 5minutes and following perfusion fixation at the same pressure. After pretreatment with L-nitroarginine 10^{-4}M from 10min and bradykinin 10^{-7}M treatment from 25 to 30min the dilation of capillaries is completly abolished. Furthermore bradykinin 10^{-7}M itself reduces the diameter of capillaries. The administration of L-nitroarginine 10^{-4}M alone from 10 to 30min shows no difference against control.

Following the perfusion at constant pressure with the modified Krebs-Henseleit solution, the hearts were perfused with a 0.1M cacodylate buffered 2%

glutaraldehyde/2% paraformaldehyde fixative via the cannula located within the aorta near the coronary ostia. The perfusion pressure was kept at 60cm H_2O. Left papillary muscle was removed and subsequently fixated in the same fixative followed by postfixation in 2% osmium tetroxide buffered at pH 7.3 with 0.1M sodium cacodylate for 2 hours at 4°C. The specimens were rinsed in cacodylate buffer three times, then block stained in 1% uranyl acetate in 70% ethanol for 8 hours, dehydrated in a series of graded ethanols and embedded in araldite. Semithin slices of plastic embedded papillary muscles were stained with methylene blue and examined by a computer aided morphometrical analysis-unit (Leica CBA8000). Ultrathin slices (30-60 nm) were obtained with a diamond knife on a Reichert ultramicrotome, placed on copper crids, and examined with a Zeiss EM 902A electron microscope.

MORPOMETRIC ANALYSIS

Morphometric data was collected on randomly sampled transverse sections which consisted exclusively of muscle fibres and terminal exchange vessels (diameter 1-26μm) from the left papillary muscles. The papillary muscles are particulary suitable for a stereological analysis (Mattfeldt and Mall, 1984), since an axis of anisotropy can be detected. Capillary diameter were measured on a Leitz Medilux microscope connected with a Leitz CBA8000 image analysing system. The capillary diameter [μm], was measured by recording the smallest profile diameter as the closest approximation of the true diameter. For each animal 400 profiles were examined.

RESULTS

The inhibition of basal NO-production with L-nitroarginine 10^{-4}M did not show a morphological change of capillary diameter. This stands in contrast to a decrease of coronary flow by 30% (Fig. 1). It also could be shown morphometrically that there was no basal NO-effect on the capillaries. There was no significant difference in capillary diameter between the control group (4.51±0.23μm, n=8) and the L-nitroarginine treated group (4.68±0.14μm, n=5). In contrast to the basal NO-release the stimulation of the endogenously applied NO with bradykinin (for 5minutes) not only leads to an increase of coronary flow by 50% but also leads to a remarkable increase of capillary diameter. The morphometric analysis showed an increase in diameter from control (4.5±0.28μm, n=12) to bradykinin treated hearts (5.80±0.25μm, n=8). Pretreatment with L-nitroarginine completly abolishes the bradykinin effect on the capillaries. After pretreatment with L-nitroarginine bradykinin itself reduces the diameter of capillaries (3.52±0.21μm, n=5) (Fig. 2). In combination with light microscopical and morphometrical examination the ultrastructural investigation shows structural alterations of the capillaries against the control groups. In the control group hearts the capillaries were embedded in the myocardium. There was only small interstitum and the luminal surface is nearly regular (Fig. 3a). The bradykinin treated papillary muscle displayed capillaries with a small endothelium that were surrounded by an interstitial celft (Fig. 3b). Like in the·bradykinin treated hearts the interstitium of L-NA/bradykinin treated group is extended too (Fig. 3c). The results of the modulation of endogenous NO-release gave neither evidence for flow dependent nor flow independent dilation of the capillaries. To investigate the direct effect of NO on the capillaries the flow parameter is adjusted to be equal in the SNP and GTN treated groups. The adjusted flow is 30-40% higher than the flow in the control group. Morphological studies show a dilation of capillaries in the SNP treated group

(SNP 10^{-5}M, $5.34\pm0.23\mu$m, n=5; SNP 10^{-6}M, $5.32\pm0.14\mu$m, n=5) in comparison with the control ($4.51\pm0.31\mu$m, n=10) in accordance with the increased coronary flow. Contrarily, the administration of GTN ($4.61\pm0.31\mu$m, n=7) leads to an equally increased coronary   flow but no dilation of capillaries. The findings were verified morphometrically. There is a significant increase of capillary diameter in both of the SNP treated groups and no dilation under the influence of GTN though there was an equipotent increase of coronary flow (Fig. 4). Upon electronmicroscopical examination the SNP treated papillary muscles displayed no extended interstitium (Fig. 3d).

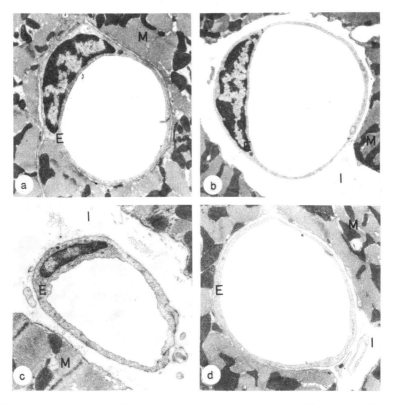

Figure 3. The ultrastructural investigation shows structural alterations of capillary endothelium (E) and surrounding interstitium (I). **3a** In control hearts the capillaries are embedded in the myocardium (M). There is only small interstitium and the luminal surface is nearly regular. **3b** The capillaries of bradykinin treated papillary muscle have a small endothelium (E) and are surrounded by an interstial cleft (I). **3c** In contrast in the L-NA pretreated and bradykinin treated group a wide endothelium (E) can be found and the luminal surface is irregular. As with the bradykinin treated hearts the interstitium (I) is extended. **3d** SNP treated muscle show no increase of interstitium (I), a small endothelium (E) and a nearly regular luminal surface.

DISCUSSION

This study is the first to report on the directly regulative effect of NO on intracardial capillaries. The results indicate that an NO-release exceeding the basal endogenous NO-release has a direct regulativ effect on the capillary microvasculature.

The model we used for demonstrating a functional change in capillary diameter is a combination of a functional experiment and a morphometrical study. It gives a unique chance to study capillary regulation in the heart. Two major methodical questions must be answered before the results can be evaluated:

1. Which influence does the fixation have on the vessel diameter? Comparative vitalmicroscopical and morphometrical studies after fixation and embedding conducted by Rhodin (1986) on mesenteric microvessels showed that intraarterial perfusion preserved the prefixative dimensions of the various segments and the ultrastructure of the cells.

2. Whether the fiber shorting in working myocardium has an influence of capillary diameter? In rat myocardium Poole (1992) demonstrated a lack of change in capillary diameter at different contraction states that is corresponding to our own findings which showed no correlation between ultrastructurally measured sarcomere length and light microscopically observed capillary diameter in rat hearts after isolated heart perfusion (data not shown). Therefore it is to accept that the measured capillary diameters reflect a functional state of capillaries independent from the contraction of the myocardium.

This study gives a functional correlate to earlier investigations of endothelial motility in culture by many groups (DeClerk et al., 1981; Morel et al., 1989; Boswell et al. 1992; Oliver, 1992). But there are differences between endothelial cells from large-vessels and from microvessels. Particulary endothelial cells from microvessels show motility which is responsible for the effect of the NO-donor SNP (Morel et al., 1989). But the endogenous endothelial production of NO also relaxes endothelial cells of bovine aorta in culture (Oliver, 1992). The present studies demonstrate that endogenously produced NO has not only an effect on endothelial cells in culture but also, has a regulative effect on the endothelial cells in the functional system of a capillary under stimulated conditions. The lacking effect of basally supplied NO on capillaries in contrast to the remarkable effect on coronary flow which is regulated by resistance vessels containing smooth muscle, is corresponding to the distribution of NOS in coronary vessels. It is suggested that there is a decreasing expression of endothelial NOS in the arterial vessels going along with the decrease in vessel diameter. The capillaries seem to be free of NOS (Addicks et al., in press). Furthermore it has been shown that the inhibition of basal endogenous NO-release causes a decrease in coronary flow which is not necessarily followed by a contraction of the capillaries. It is suggested that the stimulated NO-release upstream from the capillary system causes a luminal overflow high enough to directly regulate the following vessels. In the bradykinin treated group however a passive effect through increased flow cannot be excluded. This assumtion of a direct NO effect on capillaries is supported by the results of the experiments with the NO-donors SNP and GTN. There is a distinct effect of the spontaneously NO-releasing SNP (Feelisch and Noack, 1987) on coronary flow and capillary diameter. GTN however, being unable to convert nitroglycerin into NO in small microvessels (Sellke et al., 1990) has an equipotent increase of coronary flow but no relaxing effect on capillaries. These results show that an increase of coronary flow does not necessarily lead to a dilation of capillary microvasculature. Local differences in the release of the unstable NO by SNP and GTN are responsible for variations in the degree of relaxation of capillaries of the heart. The decrease of capillary diameter under L-NA and Bradykinin is suggested to be a NO-independent effect of bradykinin on capillary endothelium. This is in accordance with the observed contractile properies of bradykinin on microvascular endothelium in cell culture (Morel et al., 1989).

The bradykinin induced NO-release acts as a feedback mechanism in capillary contraction induced by this peptide (Oliver, 1992).

There are several suggestions for the meaning of capillary autoregulation. The contractility may influence local tissue perfusion (Ragan et al., 1988) and contribute to the autoregulation of blood flow in microvessels (Morel et al., 1989). Furthermore there is evidence for regulation of permeability by bradykinin and NO induced endothelial motility (Oliver et al., 1992).

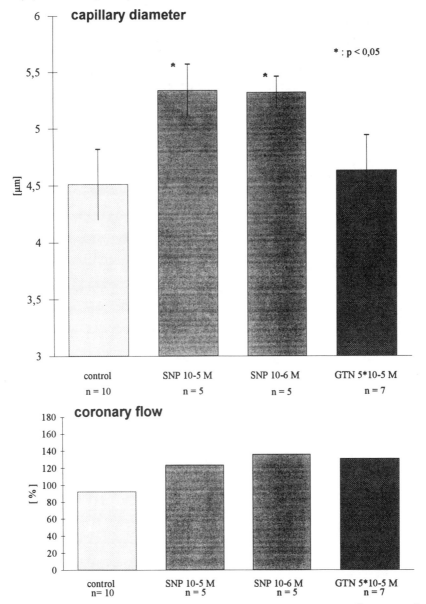

Figure 4. An equipotent increase of coronary flow 30-40% is achieved with SNP 10^{-5}M, SNP 10^{-6}M and GTN $5x10^{-5}$M. The increase of coronary flow is followed by a significant dilation of capillaries in the SNP treated groups, whereas in the equipotent increase of coronary flow in the GTN treated group is not followed by an extension of capillaries.

The electronmicroscopical observations of the capillary endothelium in the bradykinin treated groups also give hints for an increase of endothelial permeability by bradykinin. But there is no clear evidence for modulation of permeability by endogenously produced and exogenously administered NO.

In summary it is to indicate that an NO-release which is exceeding the basal endogenous NO-delivery has a regulativ effect on capillary microvasculature. The lack of modulation of capillary microvasculature by basal supplied NO is corresponding to the endothelial distribution of NOS. We suggest that in contrast to basal NO-release the bradykinin stimulated endothelial NO-release lead to a luminal overflow of NO in larger arterial vessels high enough upstream to regulate the following NO-synthase free capillaries. Bradykinin itself contracts the capillaries by a NO-independent mechanism. The presented results demonstrate a capillary autoregulation in the heart independent of coronary flow.

REFERENCES

Addicks, K., Weigelt, H., Hauck, G.G., and Lübbers D.W., 1979, Light- and electronmicroscopic studies with regard to the role of intraendothelial structures under normal and inflammatory conditions, Bibl. Anat. 17:32-35.

Addicks, K., Bloch, W., and Feelisch, M., Nitric oxide modulates sympathetic neurotransmission at the prejunctional level, J. Microsc. Res. Tech. in press

Becker, C.G., and Murphy, G.E., 1969, Demonstration of contractile protein in endothelium and cells of the heart valves, endocardium, intima, arteriosclerotic plaques, and Aschoff bodies of rheumatic heart disease, Am. J. Path. 55:1-37.

Boswell, C.A., Majano, G., J oris, I., and Ostrom, K.A., 1992, Acute endothelial cell contraction in vitro: a comparsion with vascular smooth muscle cells and fibroblasts, Microvasc. Res. 43:178-191..

De Clerck, F., De Brabander, M., Neels, H., and Van de Velde, V., 1981, Direct evidence for the contractile capacity of endothelial cells, Thromb. Res. 23:505-520.

Drenckhan, D., and Wagner, J., 1986, Stress fibers in the splenic sinus endothelium in situ: molecular structure, relationship to the extracellular matrix, and contractility, J. Cell Biol. 102:1738-1747.

Drenckhan, D., 1983, Cell motility and cytoplasmic filaments in vascular endothelium, Prog. Appl. Microcirc. 1:55-70.

Feelisch, M., and Noack, E., 1987, Correlation between nitric oxide formation during degradation of organic nitrates and activation of guanylate cyclase, Eur. J. Pharmacol. 139:19-30.

Joris, I., Majno, G., and Ryan, G.B., 1972, Endothelial contraction in vivo: a study of the rat mesentry, Virch. Arch. 12:73-83.

Hammersen, F., 1980, Endothelial contractility-does it exist?, Adv. Microcirc 9:95-134.

Lübbers, D.W., Hauck, G., Weigelt, H., and Addicks, K., 1979, Contractile properties of frog capillaries tested by electrical stimulation, Bibl. Anat. 17:3-10.

Mattfeldt, T., and Mall, G., 1984, Estimation of length and surface of anisotropic capillaries, J. Microsc. 135:181-190.

Morel, N.M.L., Dodge, A.B., Patton, W.F., Herman, I.M., Hechtman, H.B., and Shepro, D., 1989, Pulmonary microvascular endothelial cell contractility on silicone rubber substrate, J. Cell Physiol. 141:653-659.

Oliver, J.A., 1992, Endothelium-derived relaxing factor contributes to the regulation of endothelial permeability, J. Cell Physiol. 151:506-511.

Poole, D.C., Batra, S., Mathieu-Costello, O., and Rakusan, K., 1992, Capillary geometrical changes with fiber shortening in rat myocardium, Circ. Res. 70:697-706.

Sellke, F.W., Myers, P.R., Bates, J.N., and Harrison, D.G., 1990, Influence of vessel size on the sensitivity of porcine coronary microvessels to nitroglycerin, Heart Circ. Physiol. 27:H515-H520.

Ragan, D.M.S., Schmidt, E.E., MacDonald, I.C., and Groom, A.C., 1988, spontaneous cyclic contractions of the capillary wall in vivo, impending red cell flow: A quantitative analysis. Evidence for endothelial contractility, Microvasc. Res. 36:13-30.

Rhodin, J.A.G., 1986, Perfusion and superfusion fixation on rat mesentry microvascular beds. Intravital and electron microscope analyses, J. Submicrosc. Cytol. 45:453-470.

Weigelt, H., and Schwarzmann, V., 1981, A new method for the simultaneous presentation of low and high magnification of icroscopic specimens: application to in vivo studies of mesenterial capillaries, Microsc.Acta 85:161-173.

Wolff, E.K., and Dietrich, H.H., 1985, In vivo micro application to capillaries in frog mesentery, Microc., Endothelium, Lymphatics 2:607-615.

Zweifach, B.W., 1934, A micro-manipulative study of blood capillaries, Anat.Rec. 59:83-108.

INDUCTION OF NADPH - DIAPHORASE - ACTIVITY WITH ENDOTOXIN IN RAT HEART AND SPLEEN IN VIVO

W. Bloch, *G. Dickneite, A. Krahwinkel, F. Dobers and K. Addicks

Department of Anatomy I
University of Cologne
Joseph-Stelzmann-Str.9
D -50123 Cologne, Germany

*Research Laboratories of Behringwerke AG
P.O.Box 11 40
D-35001 Marburg, Germany

INTRODUCTION

There is evidence to assume a participation of an inducible NO-synthase (iNOS) in lipopolysaccharide (LPS)-induced shock (Thiemermann and Vane, 1990). Nitric oxide (NO) has been proposed as a mediator of hypotension in septic shock (Julou-Schaeffer et al., 1990; Kilbourn et al., 1990). The distribution of iNOS under LPS-treatment in vivo however has not been exactly localized. Nevertheless there is evidence for an expression of the inducible NO-synthase in a variety of cells including vascular smooth muscle cells (Fleming et al., 1991), macrophages (Green et al., 1990), neutrophils (McCall et al., 1989) and endothelial cells (Ohshima et al., 1992). To investigate the effect of iNOS in the vascular system and blood regulation we examined the expression of iNOS in the spleen and the heart of LPS-treated rats after the onset of the hypodynamic phase. The method used was NADPH-diaphorase-staining which selectively stained the different isoforms of NOS (Hope et al., 1991; Kobzik et al., 1993; Myatt et al., 1993). The differentation of iNOS endothelial and neuronal NOS was followed by comparison of the untreated control rats and the LPS-treated rats.

MATERIAL AND METHODS

Female CD rats (Charles River-Wiga, Sulzfeld, Germany) were anesthetized i.p. initially with a mixture of 80mg/kg Ketamin and 4mg/kg Xylazin and given a

Biochemical, Pharmacological, and Clinical Aspects of Nitric Oxide
Edited by B. A. Weissman *et al.*, Plenum Press, New York, 1995

161

maintenance dose of 20mg/kg/h Ketamin and 1.0 mg/kg/h Xylazin as an i.v. infusion. Body temperature was maintained at 37°C with a heated underblanket.

After a stabilization period of 30min, in the substance group rats were infused with LPS (500µg/kg/hr) via the tail vein. Blood pressure, heart rate and respiration rate were continously recorded. As soon as the shock phase changed from hyperdynamic to hypodynamic, which occured between the 3rd and 4th hour after LPS-infusion the hearts were perfused in situ with 500ml of ice-cold phosphate buffered saline (PBS, pH 7.4).

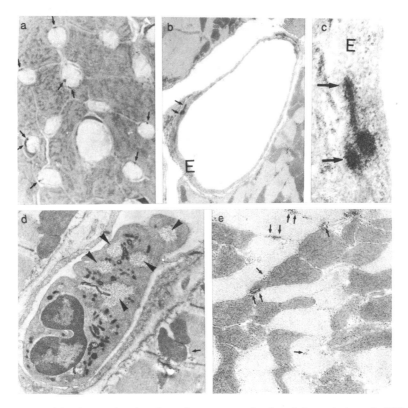

Figure 1a-d (a) Light micrographs of portions of transverse section from left ventriculare of a LPS-treated rat shows dark blue plaques (➜) in capillary wall which represents a positive NADPH-diaphorase staining. The light microscopic investigation shows no NADPH-diaphorase reaction products in myocytes. NADPH-diaphorase staining is a marker for different isoforms of nitric oxide synthase (NOS).
(b) Electronmicroscopic observation shows dark plaques (➜) in capillary endothelium (E). At higher magnification the NADPH-diaphorase reaction products impress as cloudy structures (➜) (c) and black granulars in the endothelium (E). (d) An intravascular located granulocyte contains NADPH-diaphorase reaction products (➜). (e) NADPH-diaphorase reaction products impress as black granulars (➜) in the sacroplasm of myocytes.

This was done after opening the chest via a cannula inserted directly into the left ventricle. Then 1000ml of a fixative containing 4% paraformaldehyde in 0.1 M phosphate buffer (pH 7.4) were administered. Hearts and spleens were excised, postfixed with 4% paraformaldehyde in 0.1 M phosphate buffer at 4°C overnight and then placed in PBS containing 18% sucrose. Free-floating 40-50µm vibratome sections were incubated in 100ml 0.1 M Tris/HCl buffer pH 8.0 containing 50mg reduced nicotinamide adenine dinucleotide phosphate (NADPH), 100mg nitroblue tetrazolium (NBT), 125mg monosodium maleate and 0.2% Triton X-100 at 37°C for 1hour, then washed briefly in

PBS. For the corresponding controls, NADPH was omitted from the incubation medium. For light microscopy, vibratome slices were directly examined or previously embedded in araldit for the production of semi-thin sections of 3-4 µm. For ultrastructural examination, the slices were postfixed with 2% osmium tetroxide in 0.1 M PBS for 20min at 4°C. This procedure led to the formation of poorly soluble osmium-coordinated complexes with the formazan, generated from NBT by the NADPH-d activity, appearing as black spots at the ultrastructural level. Following a thorough washing in 0.1 M phosphate buffer for 30 minutes, the slices were dehydrated conventionally in a graded ethanol series and finally infiltrated with and embedded in araldite. Ultrathin sections (30-60nm) were obtained with a diamond knife on a Reichert ultramicrotome, placed on copper crids, and examined with a Zeiss EM 902A electron microscope.

RESULTS

The examination of the spleens and hearts showed positive NADPH-diaphorase staining in untreated and treated organs, but the distribution of the NADPH-diaphorase activity was different. Hearts from untreated rats only showed positive staining in the endothelium of larger vessels and an absence of NADPH-diaphorase activity in endothelium of capillaries. In LPS treated rats not only larger vessel were NADPH-diaphorase positive but also a large number of capillaries (Fig. 1a,b,c). In myocytes NADPH-diaphorase reaction products was only found by electronmicroscopic observation (Fig. 1e). In smooth muscle there was no finding of NADPH-diaphorase activity at this point. In the spleen of untreated animals only a part of the vessel endothelium was weakly NADPH-diaphorase positive (Fig. 2a). Contrarily, in rats which received LPS, the positivly stained parts of vessels were more widespread. The smaller vessels in particular also showed extended NADPH-diaphorase activity in the endothelium. Furthermore the NADPH-diaphorase staining was positive in leucocytes of an extensive part of the lymphatic tissue (Fig. 2b) which were negativly stained in untreated rats. NADPH-diaphorase stained leucocytes were localized in the perilympathic zone adjacent to the white pulp within capillary structures and in the surrounding tissue in LPS-treated rats (Fig. 2b). Outside the spleen leucocytes also contain NADPH-diaphorase reaction products (Fig. 1d).

DISCUSSION

In septic shock hypotension is primarily caused by general dilation of the vessels and by impairment of the contractility of the heart (Artman et al., 1986). One of the factors thought to decrease the contractility of the heart (Balligand et al., 1993; Schulz et al., 1992) and to lead to a dilation of vessels (Palmer et al., 1987) is nitric oxide. Inducible NOS has been proposed as a mediator of hypotension in septic shock (Julou-Schaeffer et al., 1990). The results in the heart and spleen provides evidence for an increased and extended source of the endothial NO-release in septic shock especially in microvasculature which normally is free of endothelial NO-synthase in the rat heart (Addicks et al., in press). Endothelium may contribute as a source of increased NO-production which leads to the vasodilation in septic shock. In the early hypodynamic phase there is no evidence for a participation of smooth muscle in NO-release. In contrast to findings which has been shown that smooth muscle also displays an inducible production of NO (Fleming et al., 1991). Therefore a time delayed expression of iNOS in smooth muscles has to be considered. The electronmicroscopic observation elicits that myocytes are also concerned to the NO-production. The positive NADPH-diaphorase staining in spleen gives a hint that the lympathetic cells are also involved in the NO-production in this phase of septic shock. It is assumed that circulating und migrating leucocytes are involved in the development of hypotension in septic shock.

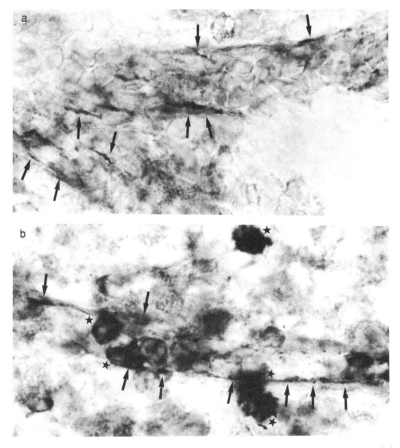

Figure 2a,b (a) The spleen of untreated rats shows only in a weak NADPH-diaphorase staining in the endothelium (➜) of a microvessel. The intravascular and extravascular lympathic cells are free of NADPH-diaphorase staining. (b) The spleen of a LPS-treated rat shows a distinct NADPH-diaphorase staining in the endothelium (➜) of an microvessel and there are positivly stained leucocytes (★) which are located intra- and extravasculary.

The morphologically investigated distribution of iNOS supported the assumption that direct vasodilation and also the extended expression of NOS in the heart especially in the capillaries and myocytes which causes an direct impairment of contractility, are involved in the origin of hypotension.

In summary, the positive NADPH-diaphorase activity at the onset of the hypodynamic state is a hint for the occurance of an inducible NO-synthase resulting in the depletion of vascular autoregulation in septic shock. Additionally there is evidence that the expression of iNOS is located in endothelium, myocytes and lymphatic tissue.

REFERENCES

Addicks, K., Bloch, W., and Feelisch, M., Nitric oxide modulates sympathetic neurotransmission at the prejunctional level, J. Microsc. Res. Tech. in press

Artman, M., Jackson, J.D., Boucek, R.J., Graham, T.P., and Boerth, R.C., 1986, Effects of endotoxin on coronary vascular in the isolated blood-perfused rabbit heart, Circ. Shock 19:13-22.

Balligand, J., Kelly, R.A., Mardsen, P.A., Smith, T.W., and Michel, T., 1993, Control of cardiac muscle cell function by an endogenous nitric oxide signaling system, Proc. Natl. Acad. Sci. 90:347-351.

Fleming, I., Gray, G.A., Schott, C., and Stoclet, J., 1991, Inducible but not constitutive production of nitric oxide by vascular smooth muscle cells, Eur. J. Pharmacol. 200:375-376.

Green, S.J., Mellouk, S., Hoffman, S.L., Meltzer, M.S., and Nacy, C.A., 1990, Cellular mechanisms of nonspecific immunity to intracellular infection: cytokine-induced synthesis of toxic nitrogen oxides from L-arginine by macrophages and hepatocytes, Imm. Lett. 25:15-20.

Hope, B.T., Michael, G.J., Knigge, K.M., and Vincent, S.R., 1991, Neuronal NADPH diaphorase is a nitric oxide synthase, Proc. Natl. Acad. Sci. 88:2811-2814.

Julou-Schaeffer, G., Gray, G.,A., Fleming, I., Schott, C., Parratt, J.R., and Stoclet J., 1990, Loss of vascular responsiveness induced by endotoxin involves L-arginine pathway, Am. J. Physiol. 259:H1038-H1043.

Kilbourn, R.G., Gross, S.S., Jubran, A., Adams, J., Griffith, O.W., Levi, R., and Lodato, R.F., 1990, N-methyl-L-arginine inhibits tumor necrosis factor-induced hypotension: implications for the involvement of nitric oxide, Proc. Natl. Acad. Sci. 87:3629-3662.

Kobzik, L., Bredt, D.S., Lowenstein, C.J., Drazen, J., Sugarbaker, D., and Stamler, J.S., Nitrix oxide synthase in human and rat lung: immunocytochemical and histochemical localization, Am. J. Respir. Cell Mol. Biol. 9:371-377.

McCall, T.B., Boughton-Smith, N.K., Palmer, R.M.J., Whittle, B.J.R., and Moncada, S., 1989, Synthesis of nitric oxide from L-arginine by neutrophils. release and interaction with superoxide anion. Biochem. J. 261:293-296.

1993, Immunohistochemical localization of nitrix oxide synthase in the human placenta, Placenta 14:487-495.

Ohshima, H., Brouet, I.M., Bandaletova, T., Adachi, H., Oguchi, S., Iida, S., Kurashima, Y., Morishita, Y., Sugimura, T., and Esumi, H., 1992, Polyclonal antibody against an inducible form of nitric oxide synthase purified from the liver of rats treated with propionibacterium acnes and lipopolysaccharide, Biochem. Biophys. Res. Commun. 187:1291-1297.

Palmer, R.M.J., Ferrige, A.G., and Moncada, S., 1987, Nitric oxide release accounts for the biological activity of endothelium-derived relaxing factor, Nature 327:524-526.

Schulz, R., Nava, E., and Moncada, S., 1992, Induction and potential biological relevance of a Ca2+-independent nitric oxide synthase in the myocardium, Br. J. Pharmacol. 105:575-580.

Thiemermann, C., and Vane, J.R., 1990, Inhibition of nitric oxide synthesis reduces the hypotension induced by bacterial lipopolysacharides in the rat in vivo, Eur. J. Pharmacol. 182:591-595.

VASCULOPROTECTIVE ACTIONS OF NITRIC OXIDE

Allan M. Lefer

Department of Physiology
Jefferson Medical College
Thomas Jefferson University
Philadelphia, PA 19107
U.S.A.

INTRODUCTION

Nitric oxide (NO) has been known to be an endogenously synthesized and released mediator of biological effects for only a short time. Since its original postulation as the active principle in endothelium-derived relaxing factor[1, 2] and its recent confirmation[3], NO has been shown to exert a wide variety of physiological effects. Table 1 lists the major known actions of NO in the cardiovascular system including the effects of NO on the heart, blood, and blood vessels. All of these effects occur in vivo and at concentrations in the low nanomolar range. Recently, NO has been measured in a perfused heart by Kelm and Schrader[4] who provided evidence that NO regulates coronary vascular tone at concentrations of 1-2 nM.

In assessing these cardiovascular effects of NO, one is impressed by the fact that all of these actions are pro-homeostatic and protect the circulatory system from perturbations in its normal function (i.e., oppose pathophysiological effects). The effects can be thought of as tending to maintain the patency of the microvasculature while autoregulating the macrovasculature and resisting clotting or obstructions of all blood vessels. There does not seem to be any major effect of NO on cardiac muscle except perhaps a modest effect on the beat-to-beat fine regulation of contractility by NO produced by the endocardial endothelium[5]. In this connection, authentic NO gas, at concentrations of 100 to 1000 nM, failed to exert a significant inotropic effect in isolated cardiac muscle (i.e., rat or cat papillary muscles)[6].

RESULTS AND DISCUSSION

Figure 1 illustrates a representative example of an experiment employing a rat isolated papillary muscle isolated from the left ventricle of a rat and an aortic ring isolated from the

Biochemical, Pharmacological, and Clinical Aspects of Nitric Oxide
Edited by B. A. Weissman *et al.*, Plenum Press, New York, 1995

167

same rat. These tissue preparations were suspended in Krebs-Henseleit solution in 5-ml muscle chambers at 37°C. Bubbling with 95% O_2+5% CO_2 was kept to a minimum. Both tissue preparations were stimulated with $2x10^{-6}$M norepinephrine, and NO gas was added to the chamber incrementally from 100 to 1000 nM NO.

The NO concentrations were determined with a specific NO electrode[7]. The aortic ring relaxed immediately to 52 nM NO and fully relaxed at 500 nM. However, the papillary muscle failed to relax to NO even at concentrations of 500 nM. Moreover, NO donors (i.e., organic nitrates that release NO physically in solution) including SPM-5185, CAS-735 and S-nitroso-acetylpenicillamine (SNAP) all provided essentially the same results.

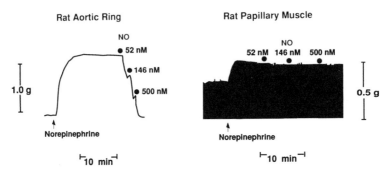

Figure 1. Representative recordings of responses of rat aortic ring and rat papillary muscle stimulated with $2x10^{-6}$M norepinephrine to nitric oxide (NO) gas. Concentrations of NO are indicated in nM. Force and time calibrations are shown. Note the full vasorelaxation of the aortic ring and only very small responses of the papillary muscle to 500 nM NO.

Thus, we are perplexed by the report of Finkel et al.[8] who reported a large negative inotropic effect in hamster papillary muscles to 50 mM L-arginine, the precursor of NO. We also obtained large negative inotropic effects in rat and cat papillary muscles experiments with 50 mM L-arginine, but also with D-arginine[6]. Thus, we think that the L-arginine effect is not due to nitric oxide but to some other action of arginine. In any event, NO does not exert a major negative inotropic effect under physiologic conditions[6].

Most of the other circulatory effects of NO can be considered to be useful in severe ischemia followed by reperfusion (i.e., so called "reperfusion injury"). This reperfusion injury is generally attributed to an early endothelial dysfunction, also known as the "endothelial trigger", followed later by infiltration of polymorphonuclear leukocytes, termed the "neutrophil amplification" step[9,10]. Recently, the link between endothelial dysfunction and the adherence of neutrophils to the endothelium was shown to be due to diminished basal nitric oxide release[11].

Several years ago, we speculated that the biological properties of NO suggested that NO acts to preserve the circulation, and following reperfusion of an ischemic vascular bed, there is an effective reduction in NO release (i.e., either a reduced synthesis of NO, or an enhanced destruction of NO by superoxide radicals)[12]. In order to test this hypothesis, we performed an experiment several years ahead of its time. We infused authentic NO gas, at low concentrations into the circulation near the ischemic-reperfused heart[13]. We calculated the concentration of NO in the coronary artery blood to be about 1-2 nM[13]. The results obtained were quite remarkable. We were able to markedly attenuated the post-reperfusion necrosis of the myocardium. Figure 2 illustrates these results.

Table 1: Cardiovascular Actions of Nitric Oxide

1.	Promotes vasodilation
2.	Quenches superoxide radicals
3.	Inhibits platelet aggregation
4.	Attenuates leukocyte adherence to the endothelium
5.	Prevents microvascular leakiness
6.	Attenuates vascular smooth muscle cell proliferation
7.	Enhances endothelial cell regeneration
8.	Exerts no significant cardiopressant effect

NO attenuated the area-of-necrosis indexed to the area-at-risk 70% in the NO treated group compared to the cats receiving the vehicle (p<0.01). This effect was at or just below the NO threshold for vasodilation, and thus the cardioprotective effect of NO could not be attributed to vasodilation. Subsequent experiments with NO donors[14, 15] and with the NO substrate, L-arginine[16] confirmed these findings and provided information on the mechanism of the cardioprotective effect. All indications are that the low concentrations of NO produced in all these experiments (i.e., sub-vasodilator concentrations) attenuate neutrophil adhesion to the endothelium and thus prevent neutrophil released mediators of cell injury. These mediators include, oxygen derived free radicals, elastase, and perhaps other substances as well[17]. Thus, the major protective effect of NO in all its forms, appears to be a vasculoprotective action. Further studies were then directed to a more detailed analysis of these vasculoprotective effects in ischemia-reperfusion states as well as other forms of vascular injury.

One of the earliest clues that endothelially derived nitric oxide played an important regulatory effect on leukocyte-endothelial interaction was provided by Kubes et al.[18]. These investigators investigated the cat mesenteric microvasculature using intravital microscopy. When the NO synthase inhibitor N[G]-mono-methyl arginine (L-NMMA) was given to cats, there was a striking increase in leukocyte adherence to the mesenteric venules. This increased adhesive effect could be blocked by the administration of a monoclonal antibody against CD18[18,] the common β-chain of the β$_2$ integrins, which are major adhesion molecules on the surface of the leukocyte. These findings opened the way for further studies on leukocyte-endothelium dynamics in ischemia-reperfusion.

Recently, our laboratory has studied the rat mesenteric microvasculature employing intravital microscopy[19]. This technique enables us to focus on small venules 30-50 µm in diameter, and to observe leukocyte flux (i.e., the number of leukocytes flowing past a certain point/minute), leukocyte rolling (i.e., the number of leukocytes slowing down and touching the endothelium), and leukocyte adherence (i.e., the number of leukocytes actually sticking to the venular endothelium. The venular endothelium is the major site of PMN adherence, although significant adherence also occurs in large coronary arteries[20]. N[G]-L-arginine-methyl ester (L-NAME) a nitric oxide synthase inhibitor was superfused over the mesenteric loop at a concentration of 100 µM. This resulted in a marked increase in leukocyte rolling at 30 minutes (Figure 3)[19]. This enhanced leukocyte rolling could be abolished by simultaneous intravenous addition of 100 µM L-arginine, the substrate for NO synthesis, but not by D-arginine a non-NO generating isomer of L-arginine Additionally, the L-NAME induced increase in leukocyte rolling was blocked by intravenous administration of a P-selectin neutralizing monoclonal antibody[21]. Additional studies also showed that increased leukocyte adherence and increased neutrophil accumulation (i.e., increased intestinal myeloperoxidase activity) also occurred with 100μM L-NAME superfusion of the rat mesentery[19]. All of these findings clearly signal a marked up-regulation of leukocyte-endothelial interaction in the absence of basal NO . production.

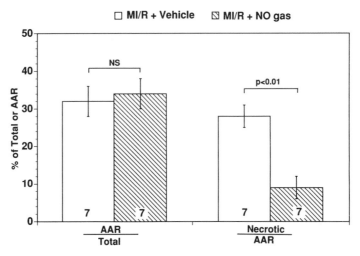

Figure 2. Cardioprotective effect of NO gas infused into cats subjected to 90 min of myocardial ischemia followed by 270 min of reperfusion. NO infusion started 30 min prior to reperfusion at a subvasodilator infusion rate. Note the significant attenuation of necrotic cardiac damage indexed to area-at-risk. Bar heights are means, brackets indicate ± SEM for six cats in each group.

These findings also suggest an up-regulation of leukocyte-endothelial adhesivity. In order to clarify the mechanism of this enhanced adhesive interaction, we found P-selectin expression was markedly up-regulated from 16 ± 5% of the venules to 54 ± 8% (p<0.01) of the mesenteric venules, 30 minutes after superfusion with L-NAME. Moreover, L-arginine attenuated the L-NAME induced up-regulation of P-selectin expression. Thus, P-selectin is a major player in the mediation of enhanced leukocyte-endothelial interaction when NO is suppressed. This is similar to the situation occurring in splanchnic ischemia-reperfusion in the rat[22] where a monoclonal antibody directed against P-selectin protects against reperfusion injury and increased leukocyte-endothelial interaction in mesenteric venules. Thus, NO exerts a microvasculoprotective effect in this setting.

We have also studied the role of nitric oxide in another model of vascular injury. This model involves producing a controlled vascular injury in the rat carotid artery by gently blowing a stream of N_2 gas into the lumen of the artery[23]. The stream of N_2 gas produces a rapid denudation of the endothelium with only a small amount of splaying of subendothelial connective tissue. The endothelium regenerates slowly, and neointimal proliferation occurs by increased migration of vascular smooth muscle cells into the intima. This pattern of vascular remodeling in response to injury has been termed "restenosis" since this type of injury occurs following coronary artery angioplasty. It can also be considered as an early manifestation of atherosclerosis. Seven days after this type of injury to the carotid artery, there is only modest regeneration of the endothelium and massive intimal proliferation, such that the intimal/medial ration, an index of proliferation, increased from 0.15 ± 0.03 to 0.84 ± 0.08 (p<0.01)[24]. Moreover, assessing the ability of the carotid artery endothelium to release nitric oxide, one finds that the vasorelaxant response of acetylcholine (ACh) an endothelium-dependent dilator decreased from 82±6% to 20±5% in injured arteries (p<0.01) with no change in the vasodilator response to sodium nitrite, a direct vasodilator. Thus, the injured artery has a massively dysfunctional endothelium, and cannot release adequate amounts of nitric oxide. This was confirmed for basal NO release by quantifying the constrictor responses of the isolated carotid artery rings to the NO synthase inhibitor, L-NAME.

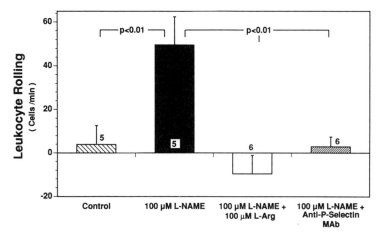

Figure 3. Numbers of leukocytes rolling (L-NAME induced) along rat mesenteric venules observed by intravital microscopy. All values were recorded 30 min following the treatments indicated. Bar heights are means, brackets indicate ±SEM, numbers in bars are of numbers of rats studied in each group.

We further studied this model of arterial injury by intravenously infusing injured rats with a nitric oxide donor (SPM-5185), cysteine containing compound which was previously shown to be effective in attenuating myocardial reperfusion injury in cats[14]. This NO donor, but not its non-NO donating control compound (i.e., SPM-5267), infused for the seven days following carotid artery intimal injury at doses below vasodilator doses (i.e., 10 µg/day) effectively prevented neointimal formation and promoted endothelial regeneration. Fig. 4 shows representative recordings taken from isolated rat carotid artery rings in response to ACh and NaNO$_2$. Arteries isolated from sham injured rats show full vasorelaxation to both ACh and NaNO$_2$. Arteries from injured rats given only 0.9% NaCl over the seven days show almost no vasorelaxation to ACh but a full vasorelaxation to NaNO$_2$ indicating an endothelial dysfunction rather than a vascular smooth muscle injury. The active NO donor SPM-5185 restored normal vasorelaxation responses to ACh, whereas the control non-NO donating compound SPM-5267 was ineffective, indicating that it is not the organic backbone of the molecule that exerts the vasculoprotective effect[24]. Additionally, SPM-5185 was found to exert an anti-proliferative effect on cultured rat vascular smooth muscle cells[24]. This anti-proliferative effect may be important in preventing restenosis of the injured carotid artery. These results are also consistent with the results of McNamara et al.[25] who showed that L-arginine can prevent restenosis in injured rabbit femoral arteries. Therefore, NO exerts yet another type of vasculoprotective effect.

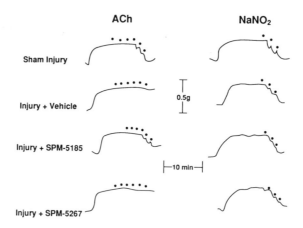

Figure 4. Representative recordings of isolated rat carotid artery rings from rats subjected to sham injury or intimal injury induced by blowing a stream of N_2 over the intimal surface. Arteries were isolated 7 days after sham injury or injury and treatment with vehicle (0.9% NaCl), SPM-5185 a cysteine NO donor or SPM-52367 a non-NO donating control. Time and force calibrations are shown. Vasorelaxation responses to U-46619 stimulated carotid rings are shown to 10 μM ACh and 100μM $NaNO_2$. Only SPM-5185 restored endothelium-dependent responses to ACh.

In summary, nitric oxide plays a multifaceted roll in vascular homeostasis including important protective effects on the microvasculature in its interaction with formed elements of the blood, in regulating microvascular permeability in preventing oxidant induced vascular injury, and in preventing pathological macrovascular remodeling in response to injury. Many applications of these important effects to disease states are evident including reperfusion injury, atherosclerosis, coronary artery disease, and circulatory shock. Future work is needed to clarify these situations and to examine the mechanisms of the disease states as they relate to nitric oxide. These endeavors should prove to be fruitful pursuits for biomedical researchers in the future.

Acknowledgement

Supported in part by Research Grant No. GM45434 from the National Institutes of Health

REFERENCES

1. Palmer, R.M.J., A.G. Ferrige and S. Moncada, Nitric oxide release accounts for the biological activity of endothelium-derived relaxing factor, Nature 327:524-526, 1987.
2. Ignarro, L.J., G.M. Buga, K.S. Wood, R.E. Byrns and G. Chaudhuri, Endothelium-derived relaxing factor produced and released from artery and vein is nitric oxide, Proc. Nat. Acad. Sci. U.S.A. 84:9265-9269, 1987.
3. Feelisch, M., M. te Poel, R. Zamora, A. Deussen and S. Moncada, Understanding the controversy over the identity of EDRF, Nature 368:62-65, 1994.

4. Kelm, M. and J. Schrader, Control of coronary vascular tone by nitric oxide, Circ. Res. 66:1561-1575, 1990.
5. Brutsaert, D.L. and L.J. Andries, The endocardial endothelium, Am. J. Physiol. 263:H985-H1002, 1992.
6. Weyrich, A.S., X-l. Ma, M. Buerke, T. Murohara, V.E. Armstead, J.N. Nicolas, A.P. Thomas, D.J. Lefer, J. Vinten-Johansen and A.M. Lefe, Physiologic concentrations of nitric oxide do not elicit an acute negative inotropic effect in unstimulated cardiac muscle, Circ. Res., 1994. (Submitted for Publication)
7. Tsukahara, H., D.V. Gordienko and M.S. Goligorsky, Continuous monitoring of nitric oxide release from human umbilical vein endothelial cells, Biochem. Biophys. Res. Commun. 193:722-729, 1993.
8. Finkel, M.S., C.V. Oddis, T.D. Jacob, S.C. Watkins, B.G. Hattler and R.L. Simmons, Negative inotropic effects of cytokines on the heart mediated by nitric oxide, Science 257:387-389, 1992.
9. Lefer, A.M., P.S. Tsao, D.J. Lefer and X-l. Ma, Role of endothelial dysfunction in the pathogenesis of reperfusion injury following myocardial ischemia, FASEB J. 5:2029-2034, 1991.
10. Bulkley, G.B, Mediators of splanchnic organ injury: Overview and perspective, In: "Splanchnic Ischemia and Multiple Organ Failure," Edward Arnold Publishers, London, 1989.
11. Ma, X-l., A.S. Weyrich, D.J. Lefer and A.M. Lefer, Diminished basal NO release after myocardial ischemia and reperfusion promotes neutrophil adherence to coronary endothelium, Circ. Res. 72:403-412, 1993.
12. Rubanyi, G. and P.M. Vanhoutte, Superoxide anions and hyperoxia in activate endothelium-derived relaxing factor, Am. J. Physiol. 250:H822-H827, 1986.
13. Johnson, G. III, P.S. Tsao and A.M. Lefer, Cardioprotective effects of authentic nitric oxide in myocardial ischemia with reperfusion, Crit. Care Med. 19:244-252, 1991.
14. Siegfried, M.R., C. Carey, X-l. Ma and A.M. Lefer, Beneficial effects of SPM-5185, a cysteine-containing NO donor in myocardial ischemia-reperfusion, Am. J. Physiol. 263:H771-H777, 1992.
15. Siegfried, M.R., J. Erhardt, T. Rider, X-l. Ma and A.M. Lefer, Cardioprotection and attenuation of endothelial dysfunction by organic nitric oxide donors in myocardial ischemia-reperfusion, J. Pharmacol. Exptl. Therap. 260:668-675, 1992.
16. Weyrich, A.S., X-l. Ma and A.M. Lefer, The role of L-arginine in ameliorating reperfusion injury after myocardial ischemia in the cat, Circulation 86:279-288, 1992.
17. Buerke, M., A.S. Weyrich and A.M. Lefer, Isolated cardiac rat myocytes are sensitized by hypoxia/reoxygenation to neutrophil released mediators of cell injury, Am. J. Physiol. 266:H128-H136, 1994.
18. Kubes, P., M. Suzuki and D.N. Granger, Nitric oxide: An endogenous mediator of leukocyte adhesion, Proc. Natl. Acad. Sci. U.S.A. 88:4651-4655, 1991.
19. Davenpeck, K., T. Gauthier and A.M. Lefer, Exogenous nitric oxide attenuates leukocyte-endothelial interaction via P-selectin in splanchnic ischemia-reperfusion, FASEB J. 8:A894, 1994.
20. Lefer, D.J., K. Nakanishi, J. Vinten-Johansen, X-l. Ma and A.M. Lefer, Cardiac venous endothelial dysfunction after myocardial ischemia and reperfusion in dogs, Am. J. Physiol. 263:H850-H856, 1992.
21. Weyrich, A.S., X-l. Ma, D.J. Lefer, K.H. Albertine and A.M. Lefer, In vivo neutralization of P-selectin protects feline heart and endothelium in myocardial ischemia and reperfusion injury, J. Clin. Invest. 91:2620-2629, 1993.
22. Davenpeck, K., T. Gauthier, K.H. Albertine and A.M. Lefer, Role of P-selectin in microvascular leukocyte-endothelial interaction in splanchnic ischemia-reperfusion, Am. J. Physiol., 1994. (In Press)
23. Dryski, M., E. Mikat and T.D. Bjornsson, Inhibition of intimal hyperplasia after arterial injury by heparins and heparinoid, J. Vasc. Surg. 5:623-633, 1988.
24. Guo, J-p., K. Milhoan, R.S. Tuan and A.M. Lefer, Beneficial effect of SPM-5185, a cysteine-containing NO donor in rat carotid artery intimal injury, Circ. Res., 1994. (In Press)
25. McNamara, D.B., B. Bedi, H. Aurora, L. Tena, L.J. Ignarro, P.J. Kadowitz and D.L. Akers, L-arginine inhibits balloon catheter-induced intimal hyperplasia, Biochem. Biophys. Res. Commun 193:291-296, 1993.

NITRIC OXIDE: AN ENDOGENOUS INHIBITOR OF BALLOON CATHETER-INDUCED INTIMAL HYPERPLASIA

Dennis B. McNamara, Harmeet Aurora, Brenda Bedi,
Thomas Osgood, Raphael Santiago, I-L. Chen,
Philip J. Kadowitz and Donald L. Akers

Departments of Pharmacology and Medicine
Tulane University School of Medicine
1430 Tulane Avenue
New Orleans, LA 70112, U.S.A.

INTRODUCTION

Regrowth of a neoendothelial vascular lining and intimal hyperplasia (IH) occur subsequent to balloon catheter injury to the vascular wall (Eldor et al., 1981; Barone et al., 1989; Weidinger et al., 1990; Saroyan et al., 1992). Prostacyclin (prostaglandin I_2, PGI_2) and nitric oxide (NO) are formed by the endothelium and have been reported to inhibit vascular smooth muscle proliferation (Garg and Hassid, 1989). However, the *in vivo* relationship between IH and PGI_2 or endothelium-derived relaxing factor (EDRF) [which is thought to be NO] formation by the neoendothelium has yet to be firmly established. Earlier studies have demonstrated that balloon catheter-induced injury to the vascular wall is associated with a decrease (Eldor et al., 1981), an increase (Mehta et al., 1982), or no change in PGI_2 formation (Hoover et al., 1989). Additionally, balloon catheter-induced injury has been reported to produce an initial decrease in EDRF generation with a return to control by 4 weeks, although the recovery of endothelium-dependent relaxation appears to depend on the severity of the initial injury (Weidinger et al., 1990). Others have shown a persistent defect in the response to various endothelium-dependent vasodilators (Shimokawa et al., 1987). Thus, although there is evidence that balloon injury and subsequent IH can alter both PGI_2 and EDRF generation, there is little information on the effect of balloon catheter-induced vascular injury on the generation of PGI_2 and EDRF in animals that received the same degree of injury. Therefore, the present study was undertaken to investigate the time course of recovery of vascular generation of PGI_2 and EDRF following catheter-induced injury. We also tested the hypothesis that administration of LARG, the precursor of NO, inhibits balloon catheter-induced IH.

Biochemical, Pharmacological, and Clinical Aspects of Nitric Oxide
Edited by B. A. Weissman *et al.*, Plenum Press, New York, 1995

METHODS

Operative Preparation and Harvesting of Aortae

Male New Zealand White rabbits weighing between 2 and 4 kg were randomly divided into 6 groups, as previously published (McNamara et al., 1993). One group was sham operated and received treatment with LARG (0.5 g/kg/day); another group underwent balloon catheter injury and received no treatment; another group underwent balloon catheter injury and received LARG (0.5 g/kg/day); two groups underwent balloon catheter injury and received LARG plus LNAME (0.5 g/kg/day or 0.1 g/kg/day); another group underwent balloon catheter injury and received LNAME (0.5 g/kg/day). Treatment with LARG was initiated 2 days prior to induction of catheter injury whereas treatment with LNAME was initiated the day of injury. Animals were sacrificed at the indicated times after induction of catheter injury. LARG and LNAME were administered in the drinking water or by gavage. The animals were anesthetized with ketamine HCl (20 mg/kg i.m.). Through an arteriotomy in the superficial femoral artery, a 4 French embolectomy catheter was passed until the tip was positioned in the ascending aorta. The balloon was inflated with water and withdrawn to the level of the abdominal aorta. This procedure was then repeated 3 additional times (Saroyan et al., 1992; Light et al., 1993a,b).

At the time of sacrifice, the animals were euthanized with a lethal dose of pentobarbital (150 mg i.v. push), and the thoracic aortae were removed. After removal, the aortae were fixed in glutaraldehyde.

Histological Studies

Arterial specimens were embedded in paraffin, sectioned at 5 micron intervals, and stained with the Verhoeff-Van Gieson stain for elastic tissue.

PGI_2 Formation Studies

Vascular segments were incubated with or without 20 μM [1-^{14}C] arachidonic acid for 1h. The products were assayed by radiometric thin layer chromatography or radioimmunoassay, as previously published (Saroyan et al., 1992; Light et al., 1993a,b). PGI_2 formation was assayed by 6-keto-$PGF_{1\alpha}$, the stable metabolite of PGI_2.

Organ Bath Studies

The 3-mm rings were suspended from Grass FT03C force-displacement trans-ducers in Krebs buffer at 37°C for isometric force measurements (Saroyan et al., 1992; Light et al., 1993a,b). Relaxation with 10^{-7} to 10^{-5} M ACh, followed by 10^{-5} M nitroglycerin (NTG), was tested in rings submaximally contracted with phenylephrine. Results for each are expressed as percent relaxation or contraction from the baseline contraction produced by phenylephrine. The relaxant response to ACh was utilized as a bioassay for NO formation. The response to NTG, which releases NO, was utilized as a bioassay for the ability of the vascular smooth muscle to relax in response to NO.

Measurement of IH

In order to obtain a semiquantitative measurement of IH, specimens prepared for light microscopy as described above were examined morphometrically using videomicroscopy and computerized digital image analysis system [Optimas, BioScan, Inc., Edmonds, WA] (Saroyan et al., 1992; Light et al., 1993a,b). The absolute area of the intima, as defined by the tissue between the lumen of the vessel and the internal elastic membrane, was divided by the absolute area of the media between the internal and external elastic membranes to obtain the intima to media (I/M) ratio for each specimen.

Data Analysis

Data obtained from within a group were averaged and reported as mean ± S.E. The data were analyzed using analysis of variance and the Scheffe F-test to determine if differences existed between groups. A P <0.05 with 95% confidence intervals was considered significant. The n refers to the number of animals in a group.

RESULTS

Catheter-Induced Injury Without In Vivo Treatment

Intimal Hyperplasia. No IH was noted in control thoracic aortae. However, following catheter injury, IH developed progressively with time (fig. 1). Initiation of reendothelialization with a layer of hyperplastic endothelial cells (identified by Factor VIII related antigen staining) overlaying subendothelial fibrosis and IH were present at 2-3 weeks after injury (data not shown; Saroyan et al., 1992).

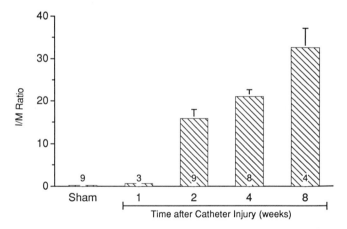

Figure 1. Time course of IH development in thoracic aorta after catheter injury.

PGI$_2$ Formation. Both basal (data not shown) and arachidonic acid stimulated 6-keto-PGF$_{1\alpha}$ formation by thoracic aortic rings (fig. 2) were attenuated initially; however, formation returned to control levels by 3 weeks after injury.

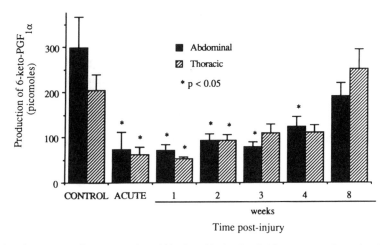

Figure 2. Time course of recovery of arachidonic acid-stimulated 6-keto-PGF$_{1\alpha}$ formation by thoracic aortic rings after catheter injury.

ACh-Induced Relaxation (Bioassay for NO Formation). The relaxant response to 10^{-6} M ACh was markedly attenuated in animals that were sacrificed up to 8 weeks following catheter-induced injury (fig. 3). The response to 10^{-5} M NTG was not altered by catheter-induced injury (data not shown; Light et al., 1993a,b).

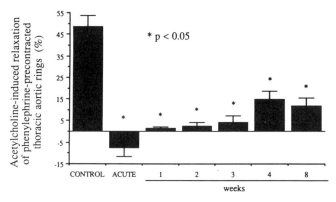

Figure 3. Time course of recovery of ACh-induced relaxation of thoracic aortic rings after catheter injury.

Catheter-Induced Injury With In Vivo LARG Treatment (0.5 g/kg/day)

Intimal Hyperplasia. The data in figure 4 indicate that *in vivo* LARG treatment for 2 weeks attenuates IH development. Moreover, this effect of LARG is reversed by treatment with LNAME (0.5 g/kg/day) concomitantly with LARG (fig. 4) but not by LNAME (0.1 g/kg/day; data not shown). Administration of LNAME (0.5 g/kg/day) for 2 weeks following injury significantly increased the intimal area as compared to the no treatment group (2.13 ± 0.26 cm^2 vs. 1.52 ± 0.12 cm^2, P = 0.0129).

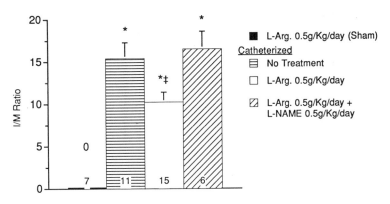

Figure 4. Attenuation of IH development in thoracic aortic rings by administration of LARG to rabbits prior to and following catheter injury. LNAME = 0.5 g/kg/day.

DISCUSSION

The present data indicate there is a different time course of recovery of PGI$_2$- and EDRF-generating capacity following balloon catheter-induced injury (Saroyan et al., 1992). Both basal and arachidonic acid-stimulated PGI$_2$ generation returned to control levels at 3 weeks; however, EDRF generation remained depressed by 75% and development of IH was progressive over the 8-week study. These data suggest that endogenously generated neoendothelial NO rather than PGI$_2$ may play a more important role in inhibiting IH.

Exogenously administered LARG attenuated the development of IH (McNamara et al., 1993). This effect was reversed by LNAME, suggesting the conversion of LARG to NO by NO synthase (NOS) is the mechanism by which LARG inhibited IH. The observation that administration of LNAME alone significantly increases intimal area in catheterized animals suggests that NO produced from endogenous LARG may play a role in attenuating IH. The inducible form of NOS has been reported to be formed in the blood vessel wall 24 h after catheter injury (Joly et al., 1993). It is interesting to speculate the induction of NOS (which is substrate- not agonist-driven) and conversion of LARG to NO by this isoform underlies the inhibition of IH by LARG. These data further suggest administration of LARG may be therapeutically beneficial in preventing restenosis following revascularization attempts employing balloon catheter.

Acknowledgments

The authors thank Ms. Janice Ignarro for editorial assistance.
This work was supported in part by NIH grants HL15580 and HL46737 and grants-in-aid from the American Heart Association and the American Heart Association-Louisiana, Inc.

REFERENCES

Barone, G.W., Conerly, J.M., Farley, P.C., Flanagan, T.L., and Kron I.L., 1989, Endothelial injury and vascular dysfunction associated with the Fogarty balloon catheter, *J. Vasc. Surg.* 9:422.

Eldor, A., D.J. Falcone, D.P. Hajjar, C.R. Minick, and B.B. Weksler, 1981, Recovery of prostacyclin production by de-endothelialized rabbit aorta, *J. Clin. Invest.* 67:735.

Weidinger, F.Z., J.M. McLenachan, M.I. Cybulsky, J.B. Gordon, H.G. Rennke, N.K. Hollenberg, J.T. Fallon, P. Ganz, and J.P. Cooke, 1990, Persistent dysfunction of regenerated endothelium after balloon angioplasty of rabbit iliac artery, *Circulation* 81:1667.

-L. Chen, M.Y. Vaccarella, D.J. Bang, P. Kvamme, S. Singh, S.V. Scalia, M.D. Kerstein, P.J. Kadowitz, and D.B. McNamara, 1992, Differential recovery of prostacyclin and endothelium-derived relaxing factor after vascular injury, *Am. J. Physiol. 262(Heart Circ. Physiol.* 31):H1449.

Garg, U.C., and A. Hassid, 1989, Nitric oxide-generating vasodilators and 8-bromo-cyclic GMP inhibit mitogenesis and proliferation of cultured rat vascular smooth muscle cells, *J. Clin. Invest.* 83:1774.

Mehta, P., J. Mehta, and D. Hay, 1982, Thromboxane and prostacyclin generation by intact human vessels in response to balloon catheter trauma, *Prostaglandins Leukotrienes Med.* 9:539.

Hoover, E.L., B. Kharma, M. Ross, H. Webb, K. Fain, I. DiMaio, A. Ketosugbo, and H-K. Hsu, 1989, Cyclooxygenase activity in the thoracoabdominal aorta after 24 hours of intraaortic balloon counterpulsation: an assessment of the effects of localized mechanical trauma, *Vasc. Surg.* 23:175.

Shimokawa, H., L.L. Aarhos, and P.M. Vanhoutte, 1987, Porcine coronary arteries with regenerated endothelium have a reduced endothelium-dependent responsiveness to aggregating platelets and serotonin, *Circ. Res.* 61:256.

McNamara, D.B., B. Bedi, H. Aurora, L. Tena, L.J. Ignarro, P.J. Kadowitz, and D.L. Akers, 1993, L-Arginine inhibits balloon catheter-induced intimal hyperplasia, *Biochem. Biophys. Res. Commun.* 193:291.

Light, J.T., Jr., J.A. Bellan, M.P. Roberts, S.D. Force, I-L. Chen, M.D. Kerstein, P.J. Kadowitz, D.B. McNamara, 1993a, Heparin treatment enhances the recovery of neoendothelial acetylcholine-induced vascular relaxation after balloon catheter injury in the rabbit aorta, 1993a, *Circulation* 88:413.

Light, J.T., J.A. Bellan, I-L. Chen, L.L. Longenecker, W.A. Murphy, D.H. Coy, P.J. Kadowitz, and D.B. McNamara, 1993b, Angiopeptin enhances acetylcholine-induced relaxation and inhibits intimal hyperplasia after vascular injury, *Am. J. Physiol.* 265 *(Heart Circ. Physiol.* 34):H1265.

Joly, G.A., V.B. Schini, and P.M. Vanhoutte, 1992, Balloon injury and interleukin 1ß induce nitric oxide synthase activity in rat carotid arteries, *Circ. Res.* 71:331.

GENERATION AND ROLES OF NITRIC OXIDE IN ANAPHYLAXIS

Yaakov Ashkenazy[2], Valentin Witzling[2], Yitchak Abend[3],
Sandra Moshonov[1], and Uriel Zor[1]

[1]Department of Hormone Research
 The Weizmann Institute of Science, Rehovot
 Departments of Internal Medicine
[2]Wolfson and [3]Kaplan Hospitals
 ISRAEL.

INTRODUCTION

The pathophysiological signs of anaphylaxis result from the production of a wide array of mediators released from antigen-activated cells, which are present or infiltrate into various tissues. Leukotrienes and platelet-activating factor (PAF) are largely responsible for sustaining the symptoms of anaphylaxis, particularly the potentially lethal airway constriction. We now bring evidence that nitric oxide (NO) may also be an important participant in the anaphylactic reaction.

Under normal physiological conditions endothelial NO is associated with maintenance of the vasomotor tone (Kelm et al., 1991; Schulz and Triggle, 1994). In pathological states such as inflammation local hormones, including acetylcholine and bradykinin, or inflammatory agents such as lipopolysaccharide (LPS), can stimulate NO production from the neutrophils and macrophages which accumulate at the site (Moncada, 1991). NO is implicated as one of the agents which increase vascular permeability in inflammation (Ialenti et al., 1992; Oyanagui et al., 1993; Ferreira, 1993). Anaphylaxis bears a remarkable resemblance to inflammation with respect to recruitment of cells and the various mediators which are generated. So, as in inflammation, it might be expected that NO be generated during anaphylaxis. An enhanced release within the vascular arterial system could lower vasomotor tone and lead to the hypotension which, together with bronchoconstriction, is a characteristic cause of death in anaphylactic shock.

As well as anaphylactic shock in the whole animal, we have been studying cardiac anaphylaxis in the isolated perfused (Langendorff) guinea pig heart. This system offers more controlled conditions for examining the biochemical pathways of anaphylaxis, and also serves as a useful model for myocardial ischemia-myocardial infarction (Ashkenazy et al., 1990; Moshonov et al., 1986). A major characteristic of cardiac anaphylaxis is the sustained increase in coronary arterial resistance, due to release of leukotriene D_4 and PAF.

Drugs were administered which interfere with or mimic NO, and we measured the ensuing changes in coronary arterial resistance in the anaphylactic heart, or noted the incidence of mortality in guinea pigs sensitized to ovalbumin or bee venom. As a result of these observations we conclude that NO is generated during anaphylaxis and, like the other mediators, has a modulating effect on the response at the local level and on the whole body reaction.

Biochemical, Pharmacological, and Clinical Aspects of Nitric Oxide
Edited by B. A. Weissman *et al.*, Plenum Press, New York, 1995

METHODS AND MATERIALS

Materials

Diphenylene iodonium sulfate (DPI; inhibitor of NO synthase) was kindly prepared for us by Dr. Tuvia Berkovitz, Dept. of Membrane Research, Weizmann Institute of Science. Ovalbumin grade III, L-arginine, sodium nitroprusside (SNP; chemical source of exogenous NO) and N-methylarginine (NMA; specific inhibitor of NO synthesis) were purchased from Sigma, St.Louis. K252a (protein kinase C inhibitor) was a gift from Dr. H. Kase, Kyowa Hakko Kogyo Co., Japan. GF 109203X (specific protein kinase C inhibitor) was a gift from Glaxo, France. Bee venom was purchased from Carmon Handassa, Mazur, Israel.

Methods

Active immunization of guinea pigs. Male, pathogen-free 5 to 6-week old DH guinea pigs were sensitized on Day 1 with 5 mg ovalbumin in 0.5 ml alum, given intraperitoneally (i.p.). On Days 3 and 5 they received a booster of 1 mg ovalbumin in 0.5 ml saline. The antigen challenge was given between Days 15 and 23, when the animals respond maximally: 5-10 mg ovalbumin in 0.5 ml saline i.p. was given in *in vivo* experiments, and 1-2 mg in 0.1ml physiological fluid (Tyrode) in *in vitro* experiments. Some guinea pigs (those treated with GF 109203X) were sensitized with 800µg/kg bee venom instead of ovalbumin: Sensitization was boosted twice with 400µg/kg bee venom in saline.

Pretreatment with PKC inhibitor or DPI in vivo. Between five and ten minutes before Ag challenge, guinea pigs were injected i.p. with the protein kinase C inhibitor 10µg//kg K252a (20µg/ml in saline), or 400µg/kg GF 109203X (400µg/ml in saline), or with the NO synthase inhibitor 200µg/kg DPI (200µg/ml in saline). The behaviour and state of health of the animals was observed for the next 120 minutes (groups treated with K252a or DPI), with an assessment of intensity of anaphylaxis being made at 15 min intervals. The anaphylactic score, compounded from the observations of the working group, ranged from 0, no signs of anaphylaxis, to 4, death from anaphylactic shock (Paz et al., 1991). In animals treated with GF 109203X, mortality was noted at 2h, 6h and 20h after challenge.

Isolated perfused heart (Langendorff) preparation. Hearts were rapidly removed from the guinea pigs 2-3 weeks after sensitization with ovalbumin and immediately suspended, following retrograde aortic cannulation, in a warmed organ chamber and perfused through the coronary arteries with an oxygenated Tyrode solution, maintained at 37°C (Langendorff heart). Once the heart had stabilized (about 10 min) the drugs were introduced by adding them to the perfusion fluid reservoir. The heart was left to re-stabilize (about 10 min), before injecting the Ag challenge directly into the fluid entering the heart. Each heart could be used for only one drug or pair of drugs. The perfusate was collected and its volume measured at 1 min interval for 7 min after challenge, and then at 3 min intervals until the experiment was terminated at 15-20 min. The coronary flow rate (CFR) was measured in all experiments as a gauge of coronary arterial resistance. The following drugs were used: K252a 150 ng/ml; DPI 2µg/ml; L-arginine 2mM, NO synthase substrate; sodium nitroprusside (SNP) 1µM; SNP is very light-sensitive so whenever it was used all the tubing was covered with aluminium foil; N-methylarginine (NMA) 100µM.

RESULTS

The influence of drugs affecting NO or PKC on coronary arterial resistance during cardiac anaphylaxis.

In the absence of any drug, antigen (ovalbumin) challenge causes an immediate decrease in CFR reaching a nadir, 56±4% of the control (14.4±1.6ml/min; n=16) at 2 min. The effect is sustained, and 15 min later is still only 64±5% of the control value. The antigen-induced fall in CFR at 2 min in the presence of the various drugs is shown in Figures 1 and 2.

DPI in a dose-dependent manner, exacerbated the effects of antigen challenge, with maximum effect at 2μg/ml, the CFR falling to 13±3% of the control value (p<0.0001; Fig. 2). Higher concentrations (5μg/ml) were toxic. Even before challenge, 2μg/ml DPI reduced the CFR to 85±4% (n=3) of the control. The effect of DPI and over the whole time spectrum can be seen in Figure 1. About 7 min after challenge a generalized system failure began to set in, evident as a decrease in heart rate and contractility, along with a large increase in CFR, indicating the inability of coronary arteries to maintain vascular tone. Meaningful results are therefore presented up to 6 min after antigen challenge.

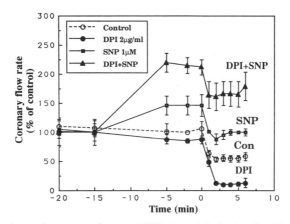

Figure 1. Percent changes in coronary flow rate (CFR) through isolated perfused hearts from ovalbumin-sensitized guinea pigs induced by sodium nitroprusside (SNP) and diphenylene iodonium (DPI). Drugs were added to the perfusion fluid between 10 to 15 min (at time -15 to -10 min) before antigen challenge (at time 0 min). Con = control CFR. Each point represents the mean ± s.e.m. of 3 (DPI; SNP), 4 (DPI+SNP) or 12 (Con) experiments. Statistical significance of differences was estimated according to Student's t-test, using the Statview program: comparing DPI with Control - p<0.05 from 2 to 7 mins; comparing SNP with DPI+SNP - p≤0.05 from -5 to 6 min (except at 1min).

Sodium nitroprusside (1μM) caused a large increase, 146±19% (n=3), in the basal CFR. It attenuated but did not abolish the antigen-induced drop, and the maximum fall still only reached 88±10% of the control CFR (Fig. 1).

Given in combination, DPI had the remarkable effect of almost doubling the changes in CFR in response to SNP (basal CFR 220±16%, n=4, Fig. 1). As with SNP alone, the reduction in CFR following antigen challenge was not abolished by SNP+DPI, the nadir (16.4±2.4 ml/min, n=4), notwithstanding, still being some 60% higher than the basal CFR (10.1±2.2 ml/min, n=4). As with DPI alone, toxic effects began to appear about 7 min after antigen challenge, so results are presented up to 6 min after challenge.

Arginine (2mM) did not significantly affect either the basal CFR or antigen-reduced CFR, though it did blunt its fall immediately after challenge (Fig. 2). Simultaneous administration of arginine and DPI did not affect the basal CFR (13.1±3.0 ml/min in the absence, and 13.1±3.3 ml/min, n=7 in the presence of arginine+DPI). The anaphylactic CFR appeared to be an additive response of each individual drug, the drop being about 59% (Fig. 2).

Unlike DPI, N-methylarginine did not alter the basal CFR, 10.0±0.7 ml/min before and 9.9±1.0 ml/min (n=4) after adding NMA to the perfusion fluid. Following induction of cardiac anaphylaxis the maximum drop in CFR, at 2 min, increased from 56.0±4.3% (n=16) to 36.6±2.9% (n=4) of control (p<0.05; Fig. 2).

The effect of inhibiting PKC activity on coronary arterial resistance during cardiac anaphylaxis.

The PKC inhibitor, K252a 150ng/ml, increased the basal (pre-challenge) CFR by 42%, and then entirely prevented the antigen-induced drop in CFR (p<0.005; Fig. 3). It has not yet been examined in the presence of an NO synthase inhibitor such as NMA or DPI.

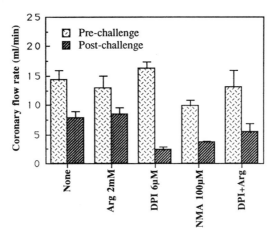

Figure 2 Effect of antigen challenge on coronary arterial flow through isolated perfused hearts from ovalbumin-sensitized guinea pigs in the presence of inhibitors of NO synthase (DPI; N-methylarginine = NMA) and NO-precursor, L-arginine (Arg). Each drug group comprised between 4 and 7 hearts; control group comprised 16 hearts. Measurements ± s.e.m. are taken at 2 min after challenge.

The influence of drugs which inhibit protein kinase C activity on mortality from anaphylactic shock.

Within 45 minutes of i.p injection of ovalbumin or bee venom the guinea pigs began to respond to the challenge. Signs of anaphylaxis ranged from mild apathy to severe respiratory distress. K252a, GF 109203X and DPI, given 10 minutes before challenge, all significantly reduced the incidence of anaphylactic shock and mortality in guinea pigs. The results are shown in Figure 4.

DISCUSSION

We have been manipulating NO pharmacologically in two models of anaphylaxis in order to find out whether it is generated in and plays a role in the expression of anaphylactic shock. The anaphylactic response itself is highly complex involving stimulation of a variety of agents which mediate multi-system reactions. In the isolated perfused heart preparation cardiac anaphylaxis is still a complex process, but here a single aspect of a well-documented local response can be measured - i.e. changes in flow rate through the coronary arteries (CFR), which directly reflects changes in coronary arterial resistance.

A major characteristic of cardiac anaphylaxis is the marked drop in CFR, induced largely by formation and release of vasospastic lipid mediators from cells within the coronary arterial walls.

A relatively low concentration of exogenous NO, 1μM SNP, had a powerful effect, significantly raising both the basal and anaphylactic CFR. However, in its presence antigen challenge was still able to increase the arterial resistance, implying that NO does not prevent the formation and release of the vasospastic mediators, but behaves as a

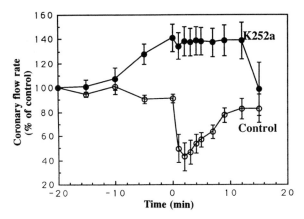

Figure 3. Effect of protein kinase C inhibitor, K252a, on coronary arterial flow through isolated perfused hearts from ovalbumin-sensitized guinea pigs (n=11 for K252a and n=10 for control hearts). Results are shown as percent of control CFR ± s.e.m. The drug was added to perfusion fluid at -10 min, and antigen challenge was at 0 min.

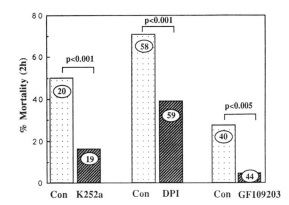

Figure 4. Reduction in mortality of anaphylactic guinea pigs treated with PKC inhibitors, K252a 10 μg/kg and GF 109203 400μg/kg, or with NOS/NOX inhibitor DPI 200μg/kg. K252a and DPI were administered i.p. to animals sensitized with ovalbumin, and GF 109203X to animals sensitized with bee venom 10 min before challenge. Incidence of mortality was noted 2 h after challenge. Numbers inside columns indicate number of guinea pigs in each group. Statistics were calculated using Chi-square test with Statview program.

physiological antagonist and attenuates their activity. Obviously, this should be confirmed by direct measurement of the mediators, particularly since NO was found to prevent histamine release from ischemic hearts (Masini et al., 1991).

This study shows that NO is released during cardiac anaphylaxis, since blocking its production, by DPI or the specific inhibitor NMA, exacerbated the antigen-induced decrease in CFR. A slight increase in coronary arterial resistance on perfusing with DPI was also observed before challenge with the antigen. This indicates a state where NO is continuously produced, presumably from constitutive NO synthase in the endothelium, which is in line with the notion that the vasodilatory action of NO is one of the regulators of coronary blood flow and of vasomotor tone in the intact animal (Jones and Brody, 1992). Our work thus confirms earlier reports that isolated hearts from naive guinea pigs, rats and rabbits produce NO, which helps regulate the basal coronary vascular tone (Kelm et al., 1988; Masini et al., 1991; Bouma et al., 1992; Berti et al., 1993).

Inducible NO synthase may be stimulated and NO generated from the endothelium, macrophages, smooth vascular muscle cells, ventricular myocytes and neutrophils (Salter et al., 1991; Bernhardt et al., 1991). Thus during cardiac anaphylaxis, which is akin to an inflammatory state, any or all of these cells may be producing NO. In the whole animal, neutrophils and macrophages are recruited during anaphylaxis; in the isolated heart which is perfused with a physiological salt solution, neutrophils are unlikely to be found since sensitization alone does not cause cell migration (unpublished observations). Macrophages however may well be present in the heart and its vascular tissue. We have already noted that antigen-induced ischemia and reperfusion which comprise the aspect of cardiac anaphylaxis which we have been measuring, closely parallels the classic coronary arterial ischemia-reperfusion which precede an acute myocardial infarction (AMI; Ashkenazy et al., 1990; Moshonov et al., 1986). Therefore we suggest by extrapolation that in addition to release of the vasospastic, platelet-aggregating phospholipid mediators prior to an AMI, vasorelaxing, aggregation-inhibiting NO is also produced. There have not appeared, to our knowledge, reports of an increase in NO release associated with AMI, but exogenous NO did reduce myocardial injury in anesthetized dogs (Lefer et al., 1993). Concomitant release of NO could moderate the ischemic-reperfusion damage.

In the isolated guinea pig heart the effects on the antigen-induced reduction in CFR of L-arginine ("endogenous" NO) and SNP (exogenous NO) when combined with DPI were astonishingly different. L-arginine + DPI produced a logical, essentially additive response, with the final change in CFR (42% of the control) being closer to the change induced by the Ag alone (56% of the control). However, the effect of SNP which by itself raised the basal CFR to $146\pm17\%$ (n=3) was potentiated by DPI, and now raised it to $220\pm16\%$ (n=4).

The explanation for this phenomenon may lie in the dual action of DPI, which in addition to inhibiting NO synthase, also inhibits NADPH oxidase (Cross and Jones, 1986). This enzyme catalyzes production of superoxide, a free oxygen radical which is also the precursor of other reactive oxygen species. The Langendorff heart releases superoxide, especially during ischemia and reperfusion (Prasad et al., 1992; Goldhaber and Weiss, 1992). Reactive oxygen species interact with NO molecules converting them to peroxynitrates in which form they are no longer vasodilatory. This means that both before and after antigen challenge there is a steady state in which the amount of available NO is determined by the rate of inactivation by superoxide. Since exogenous NO (SNP) will also be subject to attack by superoxide, the vasodilatory effect of SNP cannot actually reach its full potential until production of these molecules is curtailed by DPI. The amount of exogenous NO is so much greater than the endogenous NO as to render inactivation of the endogenous NO irrelevant.

The generation of excessive quantities of NO is now believed to be a major factor in the dangerous hypotension of endotoxemia, septic shock and hemorrhagic shock (Thiemermann et al., 1993; Moncada et al., 1991). Since the pathophysiology of shock is similar regardless of the cause, it should not be surprising if NO is generated during immune shock (anaphylaxis), and contributes to the severe hypotension. In this case the reduction in mortality by DPI could be directly attributed to its prevention of the NO-induced fall in blood pressure. However, death in anaphylaxis, particularly in guinea pigs, is equally attributed to bronchoconstriction (which we observed as respiratory distress), and NO has smooth muscle relaxant properties which oppose antigen-induced bronchoconstriction (Persson et al., 1993). However, reactive oxygen species are also generated by antigens in the respiratory system and they cause bronchoconstriction (Ikuta et al., 1992; Lansing et al., 1993). Therefore, at least part of the life-saving action of DPI on anaphylactic guinea pigs may well be due to its superoxide-inhibitory activity.

Finally we shall assess briefly the effect of PKC in cardiac and whole animal anaphylaxis with respect to its relationship with NO. PKC clearly has a vital role in anaphylaxis since its inhibition totally abolishes the antigen-induced fall in CFR in the isolated heart, and significantly reduces the incidence of anaphylactic mortality. Inhibiting PKC also caused an immediate increase in the basal CFR, indicating neutralization of one or more local vasoconstrictor elements which regulate the vasomotor tone. NO release from endothelial cells contributes to maintenance of the tonus, and PKC may be restricting its production, as found in human and pig endothelial cells (Tsukahara et al., 1993; Hecker et al., 1993). Unlike the antigen-induced response in the presence of exogenous NO (SNP),

186

antigen challenge caused absolutely no increase in coronary arterial resistance when PKC was inhibited. The difference between the two responses probably lies in the fact that PKC inhibition also interferes with production of the vasospastic mediators (Goldman et al., 1992).

If NO formation in endothelial cells also rises *in vivo* when PKC activity is suppressed, then PKC inhibitors would promote hypotension, and worsen the anaphylactic shock. However, in other cells, macrophages and microglia, inhibition of PKC activity has been associated with a decrease in NO production (Severn et al., 1993; Hortelano et al., 1993). Thus, the relationship between PKC and NO is far from clear, the powerful action of PKC inhibitors against anaphylaxis *in vivo* or *in vitro* cannot, at the moment , be explained in terms of modulating NO synthase activity.

Acknowledgements

U.Z. is an incumbent of the W.B. Graham Chair in Pharmacology.

REFERENCES

Ashkenazy, Y., S. Moshonov, G. Fischer, D. Feigel, A. Caspi, F. Kusniec, B.-A. Sela, and U. Zor, 1990, Magnesium-deficient diet aggravates anaphylactic shock and promotes cardiac myolysis in guinea pigs, Magnesium Trace Elements 9, 283.

Bernhardt, J., M.R. Tschudi, Y. Dohi, I. Gut, B. Urwyler, F.R. Bühler, and T.F. Lüscher, 1991, Release of nitric oxide from human vascular smooth muscle cells, Biochem. Biophys. Res. Commun. 180, 907.

Berti, F., G. Rossoni, D. Della Bella, L.M. Villa, A. Buschi, F. Trento, and M. Berti, 1993, Nitric oxide and prostacyclin influence coronary vasomotor tone in perfused rabbit heart and modulate endothelin-1 activity, J. Cardiovasc. Pharmacol. 22, 321.

Bouma, P., P. Ferdinandy, P. Sipkema, C.P. Allaart, and N. Westerhof, 1992, Nitric oxide is an important determinant of coronary flow in the isolated blood perfused rat heart, Basic Res. Cardiol. 87, 570.

Cross, A.R., and T.G. Jones, 1986, The effect of the inhibitor diphenylene iodonium on the superoxide-generating system of neutrophils. Specific labelling of a component polypeptide of the oxidase, Biochem. J. 237, 111.

Ferreira, S.H., 1993, The role of interleukins and nitric oxide in the mediation of inflammatory pain and its control by peripheral analgesics, Drugs 46, 1.

Goldhaber, J.I., and J.N. Weiss, 1992, Oxygen free radicals and cardiac reperfusion abnormalities, Hypertension 20, 118.

Goldman, R., E. Ferber, and U. Zor, 1992, Reactive oxygen species are involved in the activation of cellular phospholipase A2, FEBS Letts. 309, 190.

Hecker, M., A. Luckhoff, and R. Busse, 1993, Modulation of endothelial autacoid release by protein kinase C: feedback inhibition or non-specific attenuation of receptor-dependent cell activation?, J. Cell Physiol. 156, 571.

Ialenti, A., A. Ianaro, S. Moncada, and M. Di Rosa, 1992, Modulation of acute inflammation by endogenous nitric oxide, Eur. J. Pharmacol. 211, 177.

Ikuta, N., S. Sugiyama, K. Takagi, T. Satake, and T. Ozawa, 1992, Implication of oxygen radicals on airway hyperresponsiveness after ovalbumin challenge in guinea pigs, Am. Rev. Respir. Dis. 145, 561.

Jones, L.F., and M.J. Brody, 1992, Coronary blood flow in rats is dependent on the release of vascular nitric oxide, J. Pharmacol. Exp. Therap. 260, 627.

Kelm, M., and J. Schrader, 1988, Nitric oxide release from the isolated guinea pig heart, Eur. J. Pharmacol. 155, 317.

Kelm, M., M. Feelisch, A. Deussen, B.E. Strauer, and J. Schrader, 1991, Release of endothelium derived nitric oxide in relation to pressure and flow, Cardiovasc. Res. 25, 831.

Lansing, M.W., A. Ahmed, A. Cortes, M.W. Sielczak, A. Wanner, and W.M. Abraham, 1993, Oxygen radicals contribute to antigen-induced airway hyperresponsiveness in conscious sheep, Am. Rev.

Respir. Dis. 147, 321.

Lefer, D.J., K. Nakanishi, W.E. Johnston, and J. Venten-Johansen, 1993, Antineutrophil and myocardial protecting actions of a novel nitric oxide donor after acute myocardial ischemia and reperfusion of dogs, Circulation 88, 2337.

Masini, E., S. Bianchi, L. Mugnai, F. Gambassi, M. Lupini, A. Pistelli, and P.F. Mannaioni, 1991, The effect of nitric oxide generators on ischemia reperfusion injury and histamine release in isolated perfused guinea-pig heart, Agents and Actions 33, 53.

Moncada, S., R.M.J. Palmer, and E.A. Higgs, 1991, Nitric oxide: Physiology, pathophysiology, and pharmacology, Pharmacol. Rev. 43, 109.

Moshonov, S., Y. Ashkenazy, A. Meshorer, N. Hurwitz, N. Kauli, and U. Zor, 1986, Immunological challenge with virus initiates leukotriene C4 production in the heart and induces cardiomyolysis in guinea pigs, Prostaglandins Leukotrienes and Medicine 25, 17.

Oyanagui, Y., and S. Sato, 1993, Histamine paw edema of mice was increased and became H2-antagonist sensitive by co-injection of nitric oxide forming agents, but serotonin paw edema was decreased, Life Sci. 52, 159.

Paz, O., Y. Ashkenazy, S. Moshonov, G. Fischer, D. Feigel, F. Kusniec, D. Geltner, and U. Zor, 1992, Attenuation of anaphylactic shock and related mortality in guinea pigs after administration of a potent protein kinase inhibitor, K252a, J. Basic Clin. Physiol. Pharm. 2, 287.

Persson, M.G., S.G. Friberg, P. Hedqvist, and L.E. Gustafsson, 1993, Endogenous nitric oxide counteracts antigen-induced bronchoconstriction, Eur. J. Pharmacol. 249, R7.

Prasad, K., P. Lee, S.V. Mantha, J. Kalra, M. Prasad, and J.B. Gupta, 1992, Detection of ischemia-reperfusion cardiac injury by cardiac muscle chemiluminescence, Mol. Cell. Biochem. 115, 49.

Salter, M., R.G. Knowles, and S. Moncada, 1991, Widespread tissue distribution, species distribution and changes in activity of Ca^{2+}-dependent and Ca^{2+}-independent nitric oxide synthases, FEBS nnLetts. 1, 145.

Schulz, R., and C.R. Triggle, 1994, Role of NO in vascular smooth muscle and cardiac muscle function, TIPS 15, 255.

Severn, A., M.J. Wakelam, and F.Y. Liew, 1992, The role of protein kinase C in the induction of nitric oxide synthesis by murine macrophages, Biochem. Biophys. Res. Commun. 188, 997.

Thiemermann, C., C. Szabo, J.A. Mitchell, and J.R. Vane, 1993, Vascular hyporeactivity to vasoconstrictor agents and hemodynamic decompensation in hemorrhagic shock is mediated by nitric oxide, Proc. Natl. Acad. Sci. U.S.A. 90, 267.

Tsukahara, H., D.V. Cordienko, and M.S. Goligorsky, 1993, Continuous monitoring of nitric oxide release from human umbilical vein endothelial cells, Biochem. Biophys. Res. Commun. 193, 722.

NITRIC OXIDE AND CEREBROVASCULAR REGULATION

Turgay Dalkara and Michael A. Moskowitz

Stroke Research Laboratory
Massachusetts General Hospital and
Harvard Medical School
Boston, MA 02114, USA

Nitric oxide (NO), a ubiquitous molecule in mammalian tissues, or a related nitroso-compound is generally accepted as the endothelium-dependent relaxing factor (Palmer et al., 1987, 1988). In the brain, NO has been proposed as a mediator of cerebral blood flow regulation, hypercapnic hyperemia, flow-metabolism coupling and of various pathological processes including cerebral ischemia (Snyder, 1993; Pelligrino, 1993; Iadecola et al., 1994). NO is synthesized from the guanidino nitrogen of L-arginine and molecular oxygen (Knowles et al., 1989; Nathan, 1992). The reaction requires NADPH and produces citrulline and NO following a five electron-oxidation of L-arginine. Flavins, tetrahydrobiopterin are additional cofactors. At least three isoforms of nitric oxide synthase (NOS) have been identified: constitutive neuronal and endothelial isoforms and an inducible isoform originally isolated from macrophages (Marletta, 1993). The constitutive isoforms are calcium / calmodulin dependent. The inducible isoform is calcium-insensitive and is stimulated by endotoxins and cytokines, a process that leads to a slower but longer lasting NO increase compared to calcium-dependent NO synthesis. In the brain, constitutive NOS exists in neurons (Bredt et al., 1990), astrocytes (very low levels of expression, Murphy et al., 1993), perivascular nerves and cerebrovascular endothelium (Nozaki et al., 1993) and, the inducible form in astrocytes and microglia (Murphy et al., 1993), vascular smooth muscle (Knowles et al., 1990) and endothelial cells (Gross et al., 1991).

Effects of L-arginine

Synthesis from the constitutively expressed protein is enhanced by raising intracellular calcium (Nathan, 1992). Providing more cofactor does not affect the rate of synthesis nor does providing additional substrate. For example, free intracellular L-arginine [300-800 μM (Baydoun et al., 1990, Mitchell et al., 1990)] is greater than the K_m derived for bovine endothelial NOS (2.9 μM, Pollock et al., 1991) or rat cerebellar NOS (2 μM, Bredt and Snyder, 1990). Despite these considerations, we observed that intravenous

Biochemical, Pharmacological, and Clinical Aspects of Nitric Oxide
Edited by B. A. Weissman *et al.*, Plenum Press, New York, 1995

189

infusion of L-arginine causes dose-dependent and sustained increases in pial arteriolar diameter and regional cerebral blood flow (rCBF) in anesthetized rats (Morikawa et al., 1992a, 1994). A possible role for nitric oxide was suggested by the potency of the L- but not the D- amino acid isomer and by the inhibition of the vasodilator response by L-arginine methyl ester (L-NAME). We speculate that the sustained effects of a 10-min infusion relate to continued endothelial NO production from L-arginine and perhaps NO sequestered in plasma combined to proteins as an S-nitroso adduct (Stamler et al., 1992). We remain intrigued by the apparent specificity of the response to the cerebrovasculature (no changes in systemic arterial pressure was observed after L-arginine) and by the suggestion that within this compartment, nitric oxide synthase remains unsaturated with substrate.

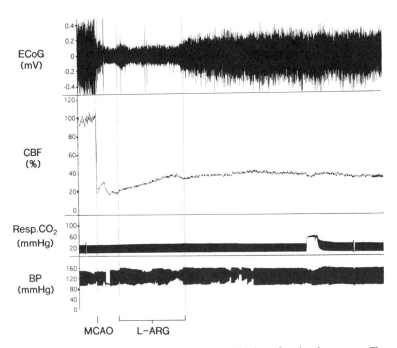

Figure 1. L-arginine infusion increases ischemic rCBF and leads to functional recovery. The computer print-out of a one-hour recording illustrates ECoG and rCBF recorded from the same cortical gray matter sample in the penumbral region of dorsolateral cortex distal to an occluded MCA. End-tidal CO_2 and arterial blood pressure are also displayed. rCBF fell to 20% of the preischemic level upon clipping the MCA. Intravenous L-arginine (300 mg/kg i.v., over 10 min) starting 5 minutes after the occlusion increased rCBF. An improvement in ECoG began 5.5 minutes after rCBF exceeded 30% of baseline and sustained along with the increase in rCBF. No rCBF response to hypercapnia was observed during ischemia although a hyperemic response had been recorded before ischemia (not shown).

The rCBF response to L-arginine was also present in ischemic brain distal to an occluded middle cerebral artery. rCBF increased within dorsolateral cortex to "penumbral" values (from 20% to >30% of preischemic baseline) within 10 mins, and this increase sustained for at least 2 hours (Morikawa et al., 1992a, 1994) (Fig. 1). Findings using dynamic susceptibility contrast MRI are in agreement with the above (Hamberg et al., 1993). In those experiments, L-arginine infusion was accompanied by increases in indices of both cerebral blood volume and flow within the ischemic brain of Spontaneously Hypertensive rats (SHR) after middle cerebral (MCA) / carotid artery occlusion as well as by an apparent decrease in the volume of unperfused tissue.

We also demonstrated that L-arginine infusion given prior to or immediately after ischemia reduced infarct size in 2 models of focal cerebral ischemia (Morikawa et al., 1992b, 1994). We think that the mechanism of protection probably relates to vasodilation and increases in brain blood flow mediated by enhanced nitric oxide synthesis. This is an interesting observation in view of the lack of prior convincing data suggesting a role for vasodilators in the treatment of ischemia (Grotta, 1987). The difference may be that most drugs decrease resistance in other vascular beds as well, thereby reducing perfusion pressure or like hypercapnia, cause rCBF increases but not within penumbral tissue. The importance of blood flow to tissue survival is underscored by the data showing that L-arginine infusion leads to electrical recovery if blood flow enhancement exceeds the functional flow threshold of approximately 30% of pre-ischemic flow (Dalkara et al., 1994). The functional recovery, as detected by a glass microelectrode placed within cortex immediately subjacent to the laser-Doppler flow probe, followed the increase in flow within minutes but never vice versa in 7 rats studied (Fig. 1).

L-arginine (300 mg/kg) does not induce the heat shock protein as a potential mechanism for improving survival [assessed by immunohistochemistry 24 hrs after MCA occlusion (unpublished)]. Since the heat shock response is a sensitive index of tissue injury, this finding may also suggest that L-arginine is not "toxic" to normal brain tissue. NO has been implicated in the pathophysiology of focal cerebral ischemia based on its actions as a mediator of neuronal injury (Beckman, 1991; Dawson et al., 1992). L-arginine infusion may not have been toxic because the neuronal enzyme is normally saturated with substrate and hence the availability of more L-arginine would not enhance NO production. The heat shock protein results would support this conclusion.

There are several disadvantages to the use of L-arginine in focal ischemia. For example, synthesis of nitric oxide is dependent upon a complex enzymatic reaction which may not sustain within ischemic endothelium, as found recently for brain NOS activity and NO levels (Malinski et al., 1993; Kader et al., 1993). Decreases in enzyme activity over time may account for preliminary findings showing that L-arginine treatment begun at one hour after MCA occlusion failed to both increase blood flow or reduce infarct size (unpublished).

To our knowledge, the results with L-arginine are the first to demonstrate that enhancing blood flow to the ischemic penumbra may be associated with greater tissue survival in focal ischemia. Of note, administering NO donors has recently been shown to reduce infarct volume as well (Zhang and Iadecola, 1993). Having said this however, we have not excluded the possibility that L-arginine merely slowed the evolution of infarction without affecting its eventual outcome (e.g., after 1 week). Additional experiments will be needed to clarify this point. Taken together these findings suggest that cerebral blood vessels possess unique features of nitric oxide synthesis which suggest unique strategies for improving blood flow to the brain.

NO and flow-metabolism coupling

It is also likely that NO could participate in rCBF increases elicited by neural activity. A study from our laboratory found that topical application of nitro-L-arginine (L-NA, 1 mM) by superfusion in a cranial window preparation, inhibited whisker stimulation-induced rCBF increase by 40% in anesthetized rats (Irikura et al., 1994a) (Fig. 2). This finding is in contrast to some other studies reporting no significant changes with NOS inhibitors in flow enhancements evoked by neuronal activation (for review,

Iadecola et al., 1994). One possibility that may account for the apparent contradictions in the literature is the degree of enzyme inhibition obtained by administration of NOS inhibitors using different routes and protocols. Measuring brain NOS activity after topical or intravenous L-arginine analogs provides useful information which can reduce the possibility of invalid conclusions. This is illustrated by our study in which the regional rCBF response to whisker stimulation was correlated with the degree of NOS inhibition within the underlying cortex following topical L-NAME or L-NA (Irikura et al., 1994a). Significant inhibition of the physiological response was achieved only at 30 minutes or longer or until at least 50% of enzyme activity was inhibited after topical L-NA application. Had these experiments ended at 15 rather than at 30 or 60 min, incorrect conclusions would have been reached. In all likelihood, the level of enzyme inhibition

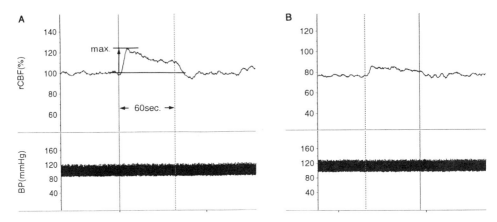

Figure 2. rCBF response recorded over the cortical barrel fields to vibrissal stimulation (2-3 Hz manual deflection for 1 min) by laser-Doppler flowmetry in anesthetized rats. A: Before L-NA (1 mM, 60 min), B: After L-NA, the maximum increase and total response (integral, shaded area) are depressed.

depends upon the route, dosage and time of administration and differs for each cell and tissue source. On the other hand, local application of high concentrations of these agents for prolonged periods of time increase the likelihood of non-specific effects. More detailed studies will be needed to clarify these issues. Transgenic mice lacking neuronal or endothelial NOS expression or selective inhibitors of the two isoforms of constitutive NOS may help to elucidate the role of NO in metabolic-vascular coupling and also the related tissue compartment generating NO.

NO and hypercapnic hyperemia

The role of NO in hypercapnic hyperemic response is also controversial. Studies using NOS inhibitors have given contradictory results (for review, Iadecola et al., 1994). We found that topical application of L-NA for 30 or 60 min inhibited the hypercapnic response in parallel to the degree of enzyme inhibition achieved in the underlying cortex (Irikura et al., 1994b) (Fig. 3). At least 40% enzyme inhibition was required to see any attenuation of the physiological rCBF response.

Since L-NA inhibition of the vascular response to acetylcholine was complete in 15 min, involvement of neuronal rather than endothelial NOS appeared to be more relevant to the hypercapnic response. However, our recent studies on transgenic mice in which neuronal NOS was selectively knocked-out (Huang et al., 1993), demonstrated a robust hypercapnic response which was not significantly different than the response in the Wild type.

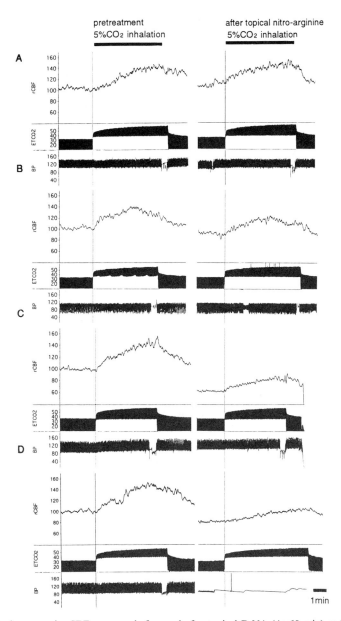

Figure 3. The hypercapnic rCBF response before and after topical D-NA (A: 60 min) and L-NA (B: 15 min, C: 30 min, D: 60 min) in 4 representative rats. rCBF (laser-Doppler flowmetry through a closed cranial window), end-tidal CO_2 (ETCO2) and aystemic arterial pressure (BP) were monitored during 5% CO_2 inhalation before and after topical administration of 1 mM L-NA. Time-dependent and stereospecific inhibition of the rCBF response to hypercapnia were demonstrated.

Acknowledgments

Some of the studies described herein were supported by NIH grant NS10828, the MGH Interdepartmental Stroke Program Project, and NS 26361.

REFERENCES

Baydoun AR, Emery PW, Pearson JD, Mann GE (1990) Substrate-dependent regulation of intracellular amino acid concentrations in cultured bovine aortic endothelial cells. Biochem Biophys Res Commun 173: 940-948

Beckman JS (1991) The double-edged role of nitric oxide in the brain function and superoxide-mediated injury. J Dev Physiol 15: 53-59

Bredt DS, Hwang PM, Snyder SH (1990) Localization of nitric oxide synthase indicating a neural role for nitric oxide. Nature 347: 768-770

Bredt DS, Snyder SH (1990) Isolation of nitric oxide synthase, a calmodulin-requiring enzyme. Proc Natl Acad Sci USA 87: 682-685

Dalkara T, Morikawa H, Moskowitz MA, Panahian N (1994) L-arginine infusion induces functional recovery in a rat model of cerebral ischemia. Am J Physiol (in press).

Dawson TM, Dawson VL, Snyder SH (1992) A novel neuronal messenger in brain: the free radical, nitric oxide. Ann Neurol 32: 297-311

Gross SS, Jaffe EA, Levi R, Kilbourn RG (1991) Cytokine-activated endothelial cells express an isotype of nitric oxide synthase which is tetrahydrobiopterin-dependent, calmodulin-independent and inhibited by arginine analogs with a rank-order potency characteristic of activated macrophages. Biochem Biophys Res Commun 178: 823-829

Grotta JC (1987) Can raising cerebral blood flow improve outcome after acute cerebral infarction. Stroke 18: 264-267

Hamberg LM, Huang Z, Hunter GJ, Caramia F, Moskowitz MA, Rosen BR (1993) Time effects of L-arginine on cerebral hemodynamics and ischemic volume during acute focal ischemia demonstrated by dynamic MRI. Proceedings of the Society of Magnetic Resonance in Medicine, 12th annual scientific meeting, August 1993, New York, 1: 397

Huang PL, Dawson TM, Bredt DS, Snyder SH, Fishman MC (1993) Targeted disruption of the neuronal nitric oxide synthase gene. Cell 75: 1273-1276

Iadecola C, Pelligrino DA, Moskowitz MA, Lassen NA (1994) Nitric oxide synthase inhibition and cerebrovascular regulation. J Cereb Blood Flow Metab 14: 175-192

Irikura K, Maynard KI, Moskowitz MA (1994a) The importance of nitric oxide synthase inhibition to the attenuated vascular responses induced by topical L-nitroarginine during vibrissae stimulation. J Cereb Blood Flow Metab 14: 45-48

Irikura K, Maynard KI, Lee WS, Moskowitz MA (1994b) L-nitroarginine decreases cortical hyperemia and brain cGMP levels following CO_2 inhalation in Sprauge-Dawley rats. Am J Physiol (in press)

Kader A, Frazzini VI, Solomon RA, Trifiletti RR (1993) Nitric oxide production during focal cerebral ischemia. Stroke 24: 1709-1716

Knowles RG, Palacios M, Palmer RMJ, Moncada S (1989) Formation of nitric oxide from L-arginine in the central nervous system: a transduction mechanism for stimulation of the soluble guanylate cyclase. Proc Natl Acad Sci USA 86: 5159-5162

Knowles RG, Salter M, Brooks SL, Moncada S (1990) Anti-inflammatory glucocorticoids inhibit the induction by endotoxin of nitric oxide synthase in the lung, liver and aorta of the rat. Biochem Biophys Res Commun 172: 1042-1048

Malinski T, Bailey F, Zhang ZG, Chopp M (1993) Nitric oxide measured by a porphyrinic microsensor in rat brain after transient middle cerebral artery occlusion. J Cereb Blood Flow Metab 13: 355-358

Marletta MA (1993) Nitric oxide synthase structure and mechanism. J Biol Chem 268: 12231-12234

Mitchell JA, Hecker M, Anggard EE, Vane JR (1990) Cultured endothelial cells maintain their L-arginine level despite the continuous release of EDRF. Eur J Pharmacol 182: 573-576

Morikawa E, Huang Z, Moskowitz MA (1992b) L-arginine decreases infarct size caused by middle cerebral arterial occlusion in SHR. Am J Physiol 263: H1632-H1635

Morikawa E, Moskowitz MA, Huang Z, Yoshida T, Irikura K, Dalkara T (1994) L-arginine infusion promotes nitric oxide -dependent vasodilatation, increases regional cerebral blood flow, and reduces infarction volume in the rat. Stroke in press

MULTIPARAMETRIC RESPONSES TO CORTICAL SPREADING DEPRESSION UNDER NITRIC OXIDE SYNTHESIS INHIBITION

Sigal Meilin[1], Nili Zarchin[1], Avraham Mayevsky[1], and Shlomo Shapira[2]

[1] Department of Life Sciences
 Bar-Ilan University
 Ramat Gan 52900
[2] Israel Institute for Biological Research
 Ness Ziona, Israel

INTRODUCTION

Cortical spreading depression (SD) described initially by Leao (1944a) is a multifactorial event affecting the electrical, ionic, metabolic and hemodynamic activities in the brain (Vyskocil *et al.*, 1972; Mayevsky *et al.*, 1974; Bures *et al.* 1974; Mayevsky and Weiss, 1991). Due to disturbances in the ion homeostasis, the Na^+K^+-ATPase activity and energy metabolism are stimulated in order to restore the normal extracellular ion levels (Mayevsky *et al.*, 1974; Hansen, 1985; Mayevsky and Weiss, 1991). The hemodynamic response to SD was a challenge to many investigators since the initial observation of dilation of pial vessels (Leao, 1944b). He concluded that the vascular responses are secondary to the local changes in the activity of neural elements. The changes in cerebral blood flow (CBF) just before, during and after the depolarization wave of SD were described by various investigators (Van Harreveld and Stamm, 1952; Van Harreveld and Ochs, 1957; Burevsova, 1957; Hansen *et al.*, 1980; Lauritzen *et al.*, 1982; Mies and Paschen, 1984; Lauritzen, 1984; Lauritzen and Diemer, 1986) and have been reviewed by Lauritzen (1987a,b). In all studies, a large increase in cerebral blood flow was recorded during the wave. Lauritzen and collaborators descried a post-spreading depression wave hypoperfusion, while a preceding vasoconstriction (immediately before the wave) was not established or proved. The mechanism behind the changes in CBF due to the SD wave is not clear although recently nitric oxide NO was proposed to be involved (Goadsby *et al.*, 1992; Duckrow 1993). NO was suggested as an important factor in CBF regulation (Beckman *et al.*, 1991; Iadecola *et al.*, 1994; Irikura *et al.*, 1994) as well as having direct effects on neuronal elements (Culotta and Koshland 1992; Mayer *et al.*, 1992). In order to clarify the role of NO in this multifactorial event (SD) we adopted the multiparametric monitoring system (MPA) by which the hemodynamic, metabolic, ionic and electrical activities were measured simultaneously from the surface of the brain (Mayevsky *et al.*, 1992). Energy state and metabolism were evaluated by monitoring the cerebral blood flow and volume (Laser Doppler flowmetry) as well as intramitochondrial redox state (surface NADH fluorometry reflectometry). Ion homeostasis was evaluated by the extracellular K^+,

Biochemical, Pharmacological, and Clinical Aspects of Nitric Oxide
Edited by B. A. Weissman *et al.*, Plenum Press, New York, 1995

Ca^{2+} and H^+ levels (surface mini-electrodes). Electrical activities were assessed by the spontaneous electrocortical activity - ECoG as well as by DC steady potential.

METHODS

Multiprobe Assembly - MPA

In order to monitor all the required parameters from the same cortical tissue we used a multiprobe assembly that we have developed during the last 10 years (Fig. 1). Hemodynamic responses were monitored with Laser Doppler flowmetry, which allows real-time and continuous monitoring. The metabolic state of the brain was evaluated by monitoring the intramitochondrial redox state using NADH surface fluorometry reflectometry (Chance & Williams, 1955). Ionic homeostasis was measured by real-time monitoring of extracellular levels of K^+, Ca^{2+} and H^+. The electrical status of the cortex was measured by electrocortiography (ECoG) and direct current (DC) steady potential.

Local Cerebral Blood Flow

In order to measure in real-time the CBF from the same cortical area as the MPA location, we used the Laser Doppler flow meter (LDF) technique (Dirnagl et al., 1989; Haberl et al., 1989; Wadhwani and Rapoport, 1990). The LDF measures relative flow changes, and readings have been shown to correlate with relative changes in CBF measured by the two other quantitative approaches (for review see Wadhwani and Rapoport, 1990).

The run signal is analyzed by a complicated algorithm developed by the manufacturers and the results are presented in percent of a full scale (0-100%), providing relative flow values. The change in the total back-scattered light is an indirect measure of the blood volume in the sampled tissue.

NADH Redox State Fluorometry

The principle of NADH monitoring from the surface of the brain is that excitation light (366 nm) is passed from the fluorometer to the brain via a bundle of optical fibers made of quartz. The emitted light (450 nm), together with the reflected light at the excitation wavelength, is transferred to the fluorometer via another bundle of fibers. The changes in the reflected light are correlated to changes in tissue blood volume and also serve to correct for hemodynamic artifacts appearing in the NADH measurement. The changes in fluorescence and reflectance signals are calculated relative to the calibrated signals under normoxic conditions. More details on this technique have been published by our group (Mayevsky, 1976,1984; Mayevsky and Chance 1975,1982). The combination of NADH and Laser Doppler flowmetry techniques has been in routine use in our laboratory for the past 4 years.

Ion selective electrodes

In order to monitor extracellular levels of K^+, Ca^{2+} and H^+ we used special design mini-electrodes made by WPI (Sarasota, Florida, USA). The sensitivity of the electrodes to the specific ion was close to the Nernstian value namely 50-60 mv/decade for K^+ and H^+ or 25-30 mv/decade for Ca^{2+}.

DC steady potential electrode

DC potential was measured concentrically around the ion selective electrodes (K^+, Ca^{2+}, Na^+, H^+). Each electrode had a saline bath around its perimeter and an Ag/AgCl electrode (WPI) was connected to it.

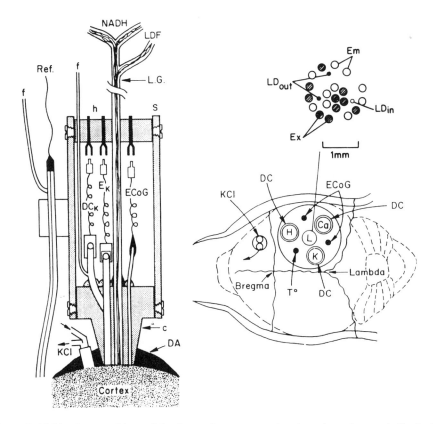

Figure 1: Multiprobe assembly used in the awake rat to monitor hemodynamic, metabolic, ionic and electrical activities from the brain. The left side shows a longitudinal section. In the right part the location of the MPA and the skull is shown.

C - Plexiglas probe holder; DA - dental acrylic cement; KCl - push pull cannula for KCl; ECoG - Electrocortical electrodes; K, Ca, H - ion specific electrodes; DC - area of DC steady potential monitoring; NADH - 2 arms of NADH monitoring light guide; h - connectors holder; s - aluminum sleeve; Ref - reference electrode; f - feeling tube of the reference or the other DC electrodes; T° - termistor for local temperature measurement; E_x, E_m.- Excitation and Emission fibers for NADH monitoring; LD_{in}, LD_{out} - optical fibers for monitoring blood flow and volume.

Reference electrode

An Ag/AgCl electrode connected via a saline bridge to the neck area of the animal was used as the reference electrode. A polyethylene tubing, stuffed with a cotton string that expanded when wet, was inserted into the electrode holder (WPI) and glued with 5 minute epoxy.

Electrocorticography

Spontaneous electrical activity of brain surface was measured by two polished stainless steel rods or silver wire inserted into the multiprobe assembly (MPA).

Animal preparation

Experimental protocols were approved by the Institutional Animal Care and Use Committee of Bar-Ilan University.

Experiments were performed using adult rats (180-200 g). Each rat was anesthetized by an intraperitoneal injection (0.3 ml/100g) of Equithesin (each ml contains: pentobarbital 9.72 mg, chloral hydrate 42.51 mg, magnesium sulfate 21.25 mg, propylene glycol 44.34% w/v, alcohol 11.5% and water). The skull was exposed and a 6 mm hole was drilled in the parietal bone (right or left). The dura mater was gently removed and the MPA was located on the brain so that pressure on the brain was avoided. The cannula and screws were cemented to the skull with dental acrylic in 2-4 different locations. In order to elicit a SD wave, a special push-pull cannula (2 mm diameter) was located epidurally 2-3 mm anterior to the monitored area. The rat was kept slightly anesthetized during the entire experiment. Two hours of recovery from the operation are given and then the rat was exposed to SD by epidural application of KCl solution (0.1-0.5 M). IP injection of N^{ω}-nitro-L-arginine methyl ester (L-NAME) was given (50 mg/Kg) 90 minutes later. The second SD wave was induced 30-60 minutes after the injection of the drug.

RESULTS

Figures 2 and 3 show the typical responses to SD (induced by KCl application) before (A) and after injection of L-NAME (B). As seen, extracellular K^+ level increased while Ca^{2+} decreased. The pH response was toward acidification. The metabolic responses are seen in the oxidation of NADH (decrease CF) and the hyperperfusion of the tissue (increase in CBF). Also, the reflectance trace (R) showed a biphasic response correlated to the changes in blood volume (CBV).

As seen in Figures 2 and 3 inhibition of NO synthesis led to changes only in the hemodynamic and metabolic responses. Figure 4 demonstrates the changes in the responses to SD before and after L-NAME injection. All other parameters that were analyzed did not respond to treatment by L-NAME.

Due to variations in the control responses to SD between rats, it was necessary to quantitate the changes and statistically analyze the responses to NO inhibition. In each of the responses two values were calculated namely the Vmin and Vmax representing minimal and maximal levels of the signal in terms of amplitude. The duration of the responses was also affected by L-NAME treatment but the statistical analysis was done using the amplitude change. The main effect of L-NAME on the blood flow response seen as an initial hypoperfusion phase (Vmin) which was not detectable in the control rats. In the NADH trace the typical oxidation wave was changed into a biphasic wave, namely, an initial increase in NADH followed by an oxidation wave. Changes in blood volume characterized by the reflectance trace (using fluorometry) and the blood volume calculated by the Laser Doppler flowmeter were also affected by L-NAME injection. Statistical analyses of the two groups of rats are shown in Figs. 5-8. The effect of L-NAME on the response in CBF to SD wave is shown in Fig. 5. As seen the values of Vmin after L-NAME treatment (2) were significantly lower, namely that a phase of hypoperfusion was created. The Vmax values namely the large hyperperfusion was not affected by the injection of L-NAME. The typical response of the NADH signal to SD, a wave of oxidation (decrease in NADH), was changed into a biphasic wave (Fig. 6). The changes in the reflectance and blood volume (CBV) are shown in Figs. 7 and 8. The initial increase phase of the reflectance was significantly higher (Vmax) while the decrease phase (Vmin) almost disappeared (Fig. 7). As seen in the control animals the 2 waves led to the same changes in Vmax and Vmin. The same type of changes were recorded by the Cerebral blood volume signal (CBV) shown in Fig. 8. The Vmin showed a larger decrease in wave 2 but was not statistically significant.

The Vmax was significantly smaller after the L-NAME treatment. In order to show the effect of L-NAME on the baseline levels of CBF during the duration of the experiment Figure 9 is presented. The traces are averages of 7 rats in each group. As seen the CBF was very stable in the control rats (open circles) while a significant decrease in CBF was recorded after L-NAME injection. The two L-NAME treated groups were very similar in their responses although one of them was exposed to SD waves.

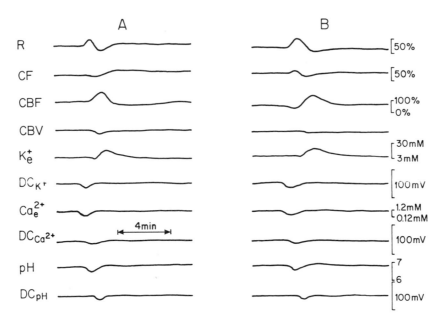

Figure 2: Hemodynamic, Metabolic, ionic and electrical responses to spreading depression before (A) and after (B) IP injection of L-NAME (NO synthetase inhibitor).
R, CF - reflectance and corrected NADH fluorescence; CBF, CBV - cerebral blood flow and volume; K^+_e, Ca^{2+}_e, pH - extracellular levels of potassium, calcium and hydrogen; DC_{K^+}, $DC_{Ca^{2+}}$, DC_{pH}. Direct current steady potential measured concentric to each of the ion specific electrode.

DISCUSSION

The involvement of NO in CBF regulation and especially under metabolic activated state is not clear. In the present study we adopted the multiparametric monitoring approach to test the involvement of NO in various brain activities under spreading depression. According to our results, we could conclude that inhibition of NO synthesis by L-NAME injection did affect significantly the resting CBF level without any detectable change in mitochondrial redox state, extracellular levels of ions or electrical activities. As shown in Fig. 9 injection of L-NAME led to 20-30% decrease in CBF although NADH levels were unaffected (not shown in the figure). One possible explanation to the uncoupling between CBF and NADH is that O_2 extraction was increased gradually to compensate for the decrease in CBF. The fact that extracellular K^+ levels were unaffected suggests that energy availability was unchanged as indicated by the stable NADH redox state. We have showed in the past that ischemia induced decrease in CBF was accompanied by an increase in NADH and an increase in extracellular K^+ (Mayevsky, 1990).

When the brain was exposed to a spreading depression wave, changes were recorded in all parameters monitored (Figs. 2 and 3) using the system. It was hard to analyze the responses to SD in terms of sequence of events. In other studies performed in our laboratory (Sonn and Mayevsky, unpublished results) we were able to analyze the sequence of CBF, NADH, K^+ and DC potential responses to SD wave. According to those studies we conclude that the initial changes were in extracellular K^+ and DC potential. The responses

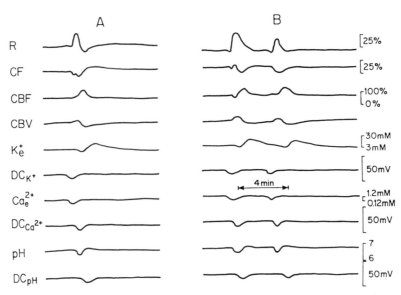

Figure 3: Responses to SD wave before (A) and after (B) L-NAME injection measured in a second rat shown in Fig. 1. All abbreviations are the same. In this rat two waves were recorded after L-NAME injection.

of NADH and CBF were recorded later on. This result, for the first time, approved the coupling between the , stimulated Na⁺-K⁺-ATPase activity and the metabolic and hemodynamic responses. Therefore, it is possible to conclude that most of the events recorded under SD wave are coupled to each other.

There are three main phases of the SD wave that required discussion in terms of CBF response and other changes:

I.   Initial depolarization phase.
II. Metabolic and hemodynamic compensation phase.
III. Post wave period.

According to the results of the present study, the leakage of K⁺ and changes in DC potential were not affected by inhibition of NO synthesis suggesting that NO is not part of the initiation of the SD wave. The fact that an initial hypoperfusion was recorded during the initial phase due to NO-inhibition (Figs. 2, 3 and 5) suggest that NO may play a role during this period. It is documented that during depolarization (extracellular increase in K⁺ and decrease in Ca²⁺) blood vessels constrict (Betz *et al.*, 1975; Pickard, 1987). The suggestion of Duckrow (1993) that this constriction is balanced by dilation due to NO release is confirmed in the present study. During the second phase NO inhibition was not effective and the large hyperperfusion due to the increased metabolic demand was recorded and was similar to the control wave. We were unable to confirm the findings of Goadsby *et al.* (1992) who were able to block the hyperfusion response induced by the SD wave. This may suggest that NO is not a major factor in the regulation of CBF during the recovery phase from the SD wave. This finding cannot confirm the findings of Duckrow (1993) who showed that NO inhibition by L-NAME led to a smaller hyperperfusion (although he claimed that it was not statistically significant). Therefore we are suggesting that the hyperperfusion phase of the SD wave is tightly coupled to the increased energetic demand created by the high K⁺ levels in the extracellular space. Since NO inhibition did not affect the leakage of K⁺ during the SD wave one could expect that the same hyperperfusion response is needed to compensate for the same metabolic need.

200

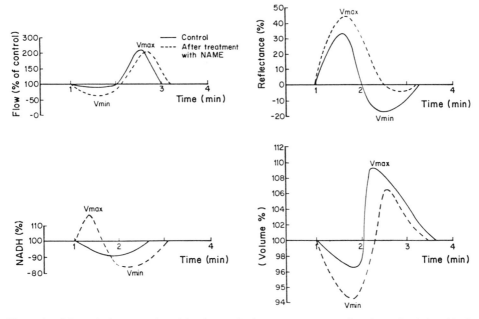

Figure 4: Schematic demonstration of the changes in the responses to spreading depression induced by L-NAME injection. The changes presented in the figure are the average of all the rats (n=7) used in each group. Vmin, Vmax - minimal and maximal values of average amplitudes calculated for the various parameters, in the control and L-NAME treated rats

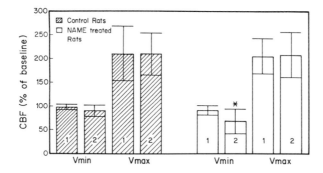

Figure 5: Effects of L-NAME Treatment on the cerebral blood flow (CBF) responses to spreading depression. The numbers 1 and 2 represent the wave before and after treatment on the same interval of time in the control animals.

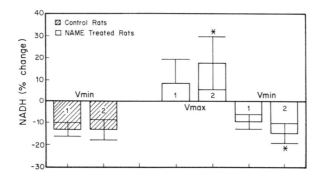

Figure 6: Effects of L-NAME Treatment on the NADH responses to spreading depression. The numbers 1 and 2 represent the wave before and after treatment on the same interval of time in the control animals.

201

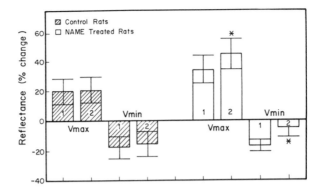

Figure 7: Effects of L-NAME Treatment on the reflectance responses to spreading depression. The numbers 1 and 2 represent the wave before and after treatment on the same interval of time in the control animals.

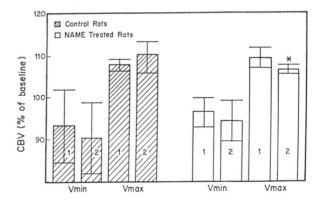

Figure 8: Effects of L-NAME Treatment on the cerebral blood volume (CBV) responses to spreading depression. The numbers 1 and 2 represent the wave before and after treatment on the same interval of time in the control animals.

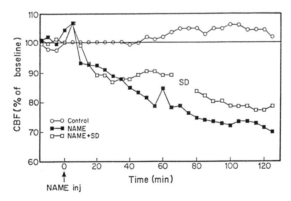

Figure 9: Changes in resting levels of CBF in controls or due to L-NAME injection with and without SD wave. Each line represents an average of 7 rats.

An important finding of the present study is the significant correlation between the changes in CBF and the NADH redox state.

Under normal conditions SD led to an oxidation cycle correlated to the hyperperfusion phase. During the initial phase NADH was not changed in the control cycle but did show a clear increase phase (less energy) correlated with the initial hypoperfusion seen in the CBF trace. We were unable to confirm the existence of any significant post wave hypoperfusion described previously (Lauritzen, 1984; Duckrow, 1993). In the present study the resting CBF as well as NADH were the same after the wave. Also, L-NAME treatment did not change the resting CBF and NADH after the wave compared to the pre wave CBF.

We conclude that NO may play a role during the initial phase of SD namely during the depolarization phase. The NO dilation effect is needed to balance the vasoconstriction effect created by the high extracellular K^+ levels. Later on in the SD event NO may not play any significant role.

Acknowledgement

This work was supported by a grant from the Committee for Research and Prevention in Occupational Safety and Health, Ministry of Labour and Social Affairs, Israel, the Chief Scientist's Office, Ministry of Health, and by Grant from the Research Committee at Bar-Ilan University.

REFERENCES

Beckman, J.S., Conger, K.A., Chen, J., Ten, M.J. and Halsey, J.H. 1991, Nitric oxide helps regulate cerebral blood flow. *J. Cerebral Blood Flow Metab.* 11:S629.

Betz. E., Enzenross, H.G. and Vlahov, V. 1975 Interactions of ionic mechanisms in the regulation of the resistance of pial vessels. *in*: "Cerebral Circulation and MEtabolism", T.W. Langfitt, L.C. McHenry, M. Reivich, and H. Wollman, eds., Spriger, New York.

Bures, J., Buresova, O. and Krivanek, J. (Eds.) 1974 "The Mechanisms and Application of Leao's Spreading-Depression of Electroencephalographic Activity". Academic Press, New York and London.

Buresova, O. 1957. Changes in cerebral circulation in rats during spreading EEG depression. *Physiol. Bohemoslov.* 6:1.

Chance B., and G. R. Williams. 1955, Respiratory enzymes in oxidative phosphorylation. I. Kinetics of oxygen utilization. *J. Biol. Chem.* 217:383.

Culotta, E. and Koshland, D.E. 1992, No news is good news. *Science* 258:1862.

Dirnagl, U., B. Kaplan, M. Jacewicz, and W. Pulsinelli. 1989, Continuous measurement of cerebral cortical blood flow by Laser-Doppler Flowmetry with a rat stroke model. *J. CBF and Metabol.* 9:589.

Duckrow, B. 1993, A brief hypoperfusion precedes spreading depression if nitric oxide synthesis is inhibited. *Brain Res.* 618:190.

Goadsby, P.J., Kaube, H. and Hoskin, K.L. 1992, Nitric oxide synthesis couples cerebral blood flow and metabolism. *Brain Res.* 595:167.

Haberl, R. L., M. L. Heizer, A. Marmarou, and E. F. Ellis. 1989, Laser Doppler assessment of brain microcirculation: Effect of systemic alterations. *Am. J. Physiol.* 256:H1247.

Hansen, A.J. 1985. Effect of anoxia on ion distribution in the brain. *Physiol. Rev.* 65:101.

Hansen, A.J., Quistorff, B. and Gjedde, A. 1980. Relationship between local changes in cortical blood flow and extracellular K^+ during spreading depression. *Acta Physiol. Scan.* 109:1.

Iadecola, C., Pelligrino, D.A., Moskowitz, M.A. and Lassen, N.A. 1994, Nitric oxide synthase inhibition and cerebrovascular regulator. *J. Cereb. Blood Flow Metab.* 14:175.

Irikura, K., Maynard, K.I. and Moskowitz, M.A. 1994. Importance of nitric oxide synthase inhibition to the attenuated vascular responses induced by topical L-Nitroarginine during vibrissal stimulation. J. Cereb. Blood. Flow Metab. 14:45.

Lauritzen, M. 1984. Long-lasting reduction of cortical blood flow of the rat brain after spreading depression with preserved autoregulation and impaired CO_2 response. *J. CBF and Metab.* 4:546.

Lauritzen, M. 1987a Cortical spreading depression as a putative migraine mechanism. *Trends Neurosci.* 10:8.

Lauritzen, M. 1987b. Cerebral blood flow in migraine and cortical spreading depression. *Acta Neurol. Scand.* 76 (Suppl 113):1.

Lauritzen, M. and Diemer, N.H. (1986) Uncoupling of cerebral blood and metabolism after single episodes of cortical spreading depression in the rat brain. *Brain Res.* 370:405.

Lauritzen, M., Balslev Jorgensen, M., Diemer, N.H., Gjedde, A. and Hansen, A.J. 1982. Persistent oligemia of rat cerebral cortex in the wake of spreading depression. *Ann. Neurol.* 12:469.

Leao, A.A.P. 1944a Spreading depression of activity in cerebral cortex. *J. Neurophysiol.* 7:359.

Leao, A.A.P. 1944b. Pial circulation and spreading depression of activity in the cerebral cortex. *J. Neurophysiol.* 7:391.

Mayer, B., Klatt, P., Bohme, E. and Schmidt, K. 1992, Regulation of neuronal nitric oxide and cyclic GMP formation by Ca^{2+}. *J. Neurochem.* 59:2024.

Mayevsky, A. 1976, Brain energy metabolism of the conscious rat exposed to various physiological and pathological situations. *Brain Res.* 113:327.

Mayevsky, A. 1984. Brain NADH redox state monitored in vivo by fiber optic surface fluorometry. *Brain Res. Rev.* 7:49.

Mayevsky, A. 1990 Level of ischemia and brain functions in the Mongolian gerbil *in vivo. Brain Res.*, 524:1.

Mayevsky, A., and Chance, B. 1975, Metabolic responses of the awake cerebral cortex to anoxia hypoxia spreading depression and epileptiform activity. *Brain Res.* 98:149.

Mayevsky, A., and Chance, B. 1982, Intracellular oxidation reduction state measured in situ by a multichannel fiber-optic-surface fluorometer. *Science* 217:537.

Mayevsky, A. and Weiss, H.R. 1991 Cerebral blood flow and oxygen consumption in cortical spreading depression. *J. CBF and Metabol.* 11:829.

Mayevsky, A., Zeuthen, T. and Chance, B. 1974 Measurements of extracellular potassium, ECoG and pyridine nucleotide levels during cortical spreading depression in rats. *Brain Res.* 76:347.

Mayevsky, A., Frank, K., Muck, M., Nioka, S., Kessler, M. and Chance, B. 1992 Multiparametric evaluation of brain functions in the Mongolian gerbil *in vivo. J. Basic & Clinical Physiol & Pharmacol.* 3:323.

Mies, G., Paschen, W. 1984. Regional changes of blood flow, glucose and ATP content determined on the brain sections during a single passage of spreading depression in the rat brain cortex. *Exp. Neurol.* 84:249.

Pickard, J.D. 1987, Ionic and eicosanoid regulation of cerebrevascular Smooth Muscle Contraction , in: "Cerebral Blood Flow: Physiological and Clinical Aspects" J.H. Wood, ed., McGraw Hill Book Company, New York.

Van Harreveld, A. and Ochs, S. 1957. Electrical and vascular concomitants of spreading depression. *Am. J. Physiol.* 189:159.

Van Harreveld, A. and Stamm, J.S. 1952. Vascular concommitants of spreading cortical depression. *J. Neurophysiol.* 15:487.

Vyskocil, F., Kriz, N., Bures, J. (1972) Potassium-selective microelectrodes used for measuring brain potassium during spreading depression and anoxic depolarization in rats. *Brain Res.* 39: 255-259.

Wadhwani, K. C., and S. I. Rapoport. 1990, Blood flow in the central and peripheral nervous systems. in: "Laser-Doppler Blood Flowmetry", A.P. Shepherd and P.A. Oberg , eds., Kluwer Academic Pub., Boston

THE EFFECTS OF SODIUM NITROPRUSSIDE AND L-GLUTAMATE ON THE REGULATION OF THE CYTOSKELETAL ASSOCIATED PROTEIN TAU IN PRIMARY CULTURED NEURONS FROM RAT

J. Chen, H. Wang, Y. Ying, L. Juarez, L. Binder, H. Ghanbari and
F. Murad

Molecular Geriatrics Corporation
Lake Bluff, Illinois 60044, USA

INTRODUCTION

Some of the hallmarks of neurodegenerative diseases such as Alzheimer's Disease are the presence of paired helical filaments (PHF) associated with neurofibrillary tangles and neuritic plaques in histological sections of brains of patients with Alzheimer's Disease (1). Tau is a neuronal protein that associates with microtubules, i.e., microtubule associated protein or MAP (2). Tau promotes microtubule assembly and its phosphorylation may be important for axonal growth during development. However, hyperphosphorylated tau may polymerize and lead to aggregated forms that are associated with paired helical filaments (3). It is believed that hyperphosphorylated tau may participate in the pathogenesis of Alzheimer's Disease and, perhaps, other neurodegenerative processes.

In other neurodegenerative processes such as that associated with stroke, it is thought that excess L-glutamate production and release occurs. This causes, through the N-methyl-D-aspartate (NMDA) receptor, increased neuronal calcium and cyclic GMP that are associated in some manner to the degenerative process. In neurons and many other cell types, an increase in cytosolic calcium leads to nitric oxide synthase activation, increased nitric oxide production, guanylyl cyclase activation and cyclic GMP increases (see review by Murad in this monograph). It is not known which of the events in this cascade is associated with the neurodegenerative process.

In this study with primary rat neuronal cultures, we examined the effects of L-glutamate and the nitric oxide donor compound, sodium nitroprusside (SNP), on the presence of phospho- and dephospho-forms of tau and neurodegeneration. Neurodegeneration was determined histologically and by the release of iactic dehydrogenase into the culture media. The abundance of tau and its phospho- and dephospo- forms in cell extracts was determined with immunoblots using antibodies selective for the phosphorylated and dephosphorylated forms of tau.

Biochemical, Pharmacological, and Clinical Aspects of Nitric Oxide
Edited by B. A. Weissman *et al.*, Plenum Press, New York, 1995

MATERIALS AND METHODS

Preparation of Neurons. Pregnant rats (15-16 days of gestation) were used to prepare neurons. Cortical, striatal, hippocampal, and the raphe nucleus areas were dissected under a stereomicroscope while the meninges and vascular structures were carefully removed. Cells were dissociated by passing several times through fire bored pasture pipets. The cells were then counted with a hemacytometer and cell viability was determined by trypan blue exclusion. Cells at $1\text{-}2 \times 10^5$ cells/cm^2 were cultured onto poly-D-lysine coated tissue culture plates in DMEM containing 10 mM HEPES, 100 units/ml each of penicillin and streptomycin, 20 µg/ml of insulin and transferrin, 10 ng of sodium selenite, and with or without 5% Hyclone fetal bovine serum. For those cultures with serum, araC at 10 µM was added between 4 to 5 days after the seeding of the cells to eliminate proliferating cells. Neurons were used typically between 6 to 8 days after culturing. At the 7th day, the cultured cells were 90-95% neurons as determined by neurofilament and GFAP immunostains.

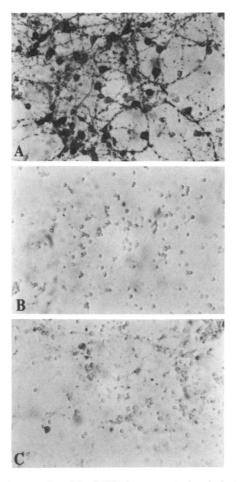

Figure 1. Neurodegeneration monitored by PHF1 immunocytochemical staining. SNP-induced or L-glutamate-induced neurodegeneration was performed as described in Methods. The samples were then immunostained with PHF1. (A) Control striatal neurons without treatment. (B) SNP (30µM) treatment. (C) L-Glu (lmM) treatment.

SNP or L-glutamate-induced neuronal degeneration

Neuronal degeneration experiments were done in buffer A (20 mM HEPES at pH7.00, 140 mM NaCl, 2 mM MgCl2, 1.2 mM CaCl2, 5.6 mM KCl, and 0.45% D-glucose). For SNP-induced neuronal degeneration, neurons in lml of buffer A were incubated with various amounts of SNP at 37°C overnight, unless otherwise indicated. For L-glutamate-induced neuronal degeneration, lmM L-glutamate was added to the neurons and incubated at room temperature for 15 minutes, and the cultures were then replenished with condition medium and incubated at 37°C overnight. Neuronal degeneration was monitored by morphological changes, lactic dehydrogenase activity in the media and Western immunoblots.

Immunocytochemical Staining

Neurons were prepared and treated to cause degeneration as described above. At the end of the experiments, neurons were fixed with 3% paraformaldehyde for 15 minutes at room temperature followed by washing in PBS and PBS-1% glycine. Neurons were permeabilized with PBS-0.5% Triton X-100 for 15 minutes, and blocked with PBS-1% normal goat serum-0.05% Tween 20. Neurons were then incubated with primary antibody (PHFl) for 1 hour at room temperature. After three washes, goat anti-mouse IgG peroxidase conjugate was added and allowed to react for 1 hour at room temperature. After washing, diaminobenzidine tetrahydrochloride at 0.66 mg/ml with stable hydrogen peroxide substrate (Pierce) was added and color development was observed under a Leica inverted microscope. The samples were then washed and mounted for photography.

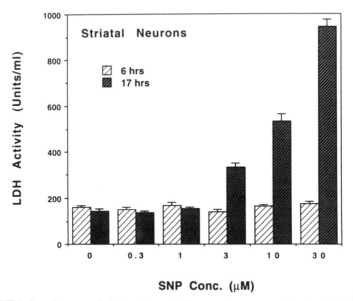

Figure 2. SNP-induced neuronal death. Neuronal degeneration was monitored with LDH activities present in the culture supernatant fractions. LDH assay kit was obtained from Sigma Chemicals. After 6 hours of 30μM SNP treatment, LDH release was not obvious, while after 17 hours LDH activity released into the supernatant fractions was several fold higher than that of the controls.

SDS-PAGE and Western Blots

SNP-induced neuronal degeneration was performed as described above. At the end of the neuronal degeneration experiments, the neuronal cultures were harvested by centrifugation at 7000 rpm for 4 minutes at 4°C. The resulting pellets were extracted with 100 μl of TBS containing Triton X-100, sodium deoxycholate and protease inhibitors. The samples were centrifuged again at 12,000 rpm for 5 minutes and the supernatant fractions were collected. Protein concentrations were determined with Pierce commassie plus protein assay reagent. The samples, containing 20μg protein, were boiled for 5 minutes and loaded on to 10% SDS PAGE and electophoresed in an ISS (Integrated Separated System) Mini plus gel electrophoresis apparatus. At the end of electrophoresis, proteins were transferred on to PDVF membranes with a Fisher Semi dry electric transfer apparatus. The membranes were blocked with TBS-5% non-fat milk-0.1% Tween 20, washed and stained with appropriate antibodies (Tau 1, PHFl, T46.1 and Tujl [a tubulin specific monoclonal antibody]) in the same buffer for 1 hour at room temperature. After washing, goat anti-mouse IgG-peroxidase was added and allowed to react for 1 hour at room temperature. After four washes, the membranes were treated with Amersham ECL reaction mixture for 1 minute and then exposed to Kodak X-omat AR film. The films were developed in Kodak GBX developer and fixer.

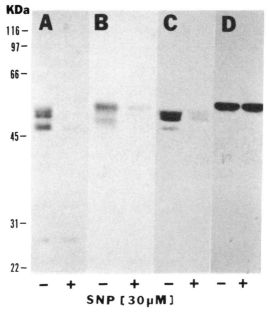

Figure 3. Attenuation of phosphorylated tau during NSP-induced neuronal degeneration. SNP-induced neuronal degeneration and Western immunoblots were performed as described in Methods. Samples without or with 30 μM SNP treatment, at 20μg protein per lane, were immunoblotted with Tau 1 (A), PHF1 (B), T46.1 (C), and TUj 1 (D), respectively.

The antibodies used for immunocytochemistry and Western immunoblots were Tau 1, T46.1 and PHF1 and were prepared and used as described previously (4). Tau 1 is selective for nonphosphorylated tau, while PHF1 recognizes only phosphorylated tau and T46.1 recognizes both nonphosphorylated and phosphorylated tau. As an internal standard levels of ton immunoblots using Tuj 1.

RESULTS

The cultured neurons showed intensive staining with PHF1 antibody and the stain was distributed throughout the axons (Figure 1A). Both SNP and L-glutamate resulted in neurodegeneration and decreases in PHF1 staining (Figures 1B and 1C). The decrease in PHF1 staining with SNP was concentration dependent and was also time dependent. Degeneration was not observed at 6 hours, but required a 17 hour incubation as summarized in Figure 2 with LDH release. The effects of SNP were observed with as little as 3 to 10μM SNP. Figure 3A & 3B show the immunoblots of cell extracts using antibodies selective for the dephospho- (Tau 1) and phosphoforms of tau (PHF1). Antibody T46.1 recognized both the phospho- and dephosphoforms of tau (Figure 3C). As an internal standard, we also examined the amount of tubulin in samples which was unchanged as measured by TuJl immunostain (Figure 3D). Similar immunoblot patterns were seen with L-glutamate treated cell extracts as shown in Figure 4.

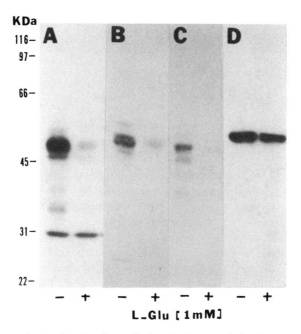

Figure 4. Decrease of phosphorylated tau during L-glutamate-induced neuronal degeneration. L-Glutamate-induced neuronal degeneration, SDS-PAGE and Western Blots were performed as described in Methods. Samples without or with 1 mM L-glutamate treatment, at 20μg protein per lane, were immunoblotted with Tau 1 (A), PHF1 (B), T46.1 (C), or Tuj 1 (D).

We have previously reported that SNP increases cyclic GMP accumulation in these primary neuronal cultures (5). However, the effects of SNP on degeneration were not mimicked or altered with 8-bromocyclic GMP in the absence or presence of SNP (Figures 5 and 6). These results indicate that the neurodegenerative effects of Lglutamate and SNP were presumably due to nitric oxide formation and not cyclic GMP accumulation. The roles for cyclic GMP, if any, in this system are presently unknown.

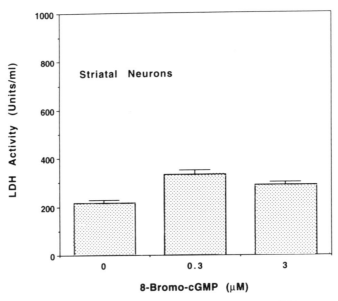

Figure 5. 8-Bromo-cGMP did not degenerate neurons. 8-Bromo-cGMP, an active and less hydrolyzable analog of cGMP, was added to striatal neurons at 37°C overnight (17 hours). LDH activity in the culture supernatant fractions was assayed using LDH assay kit (Sigma Chemical).

DISCUSSION

As reported by us and others previously, L-glutamate and nitric oxide donor compounds or prodrugs such as sodium nitroprusside cause neurotoxicity in several neuronal cell culture model systems. It is thought that L-glutamate, through its NMDA receptor, results in calcium entry that initiates the cytotoxic event. Nitric oxide synthase has several isoforms, some of which are calciumcalmodulin dependent as summarized by Murad in a review article in this monograph (6). This enzyme converts L-arginine to nitric oxide and citrulline through a complex oxidation of the guanidino amino group on arginine. Presumably, the increased formation of nitric oxide from either L-glutamate treatment or the addition of sodium nitroprusside mediates the cytotoxicity through, as yet, undetermined mechanisms. Interestingly, the neurotoxicity of sodium nitroprusside which was observed with as little as 3μM is about one to two orders of magnitude less than the concentrations used by other laboratories. While nitric oxide can activate guanylyl cyclase and increase cyclic GMP formation it may have additional effects as well. Older studies have suggested that nitric oxide can form complexes with a variety of thiol groups to form nitroso thiols (7). More recent studies have also demonstrated that nitric oxide can interact with superoxide anion to form peroxynitrite which is also a very reactive species (8).

Thus, cytotoxicity could be associated with one or more of the effects or fates of nitric oxide. We have found in these studies that the neurodegenerative effects of sodium nitroprusside can not be mimicked with 8-bromocyclic GMP either in the absence or presence of sodium nitroprusside. Presumably the cytotoxic effects of L-glutamate and sodium nitroprusside must be mediated through other nitric oxide pathways.

While hyperphosphorylation of tau has been thought to participate in some neurodegenerative processes such as Alzheimer's Disease, this does not appear to be the

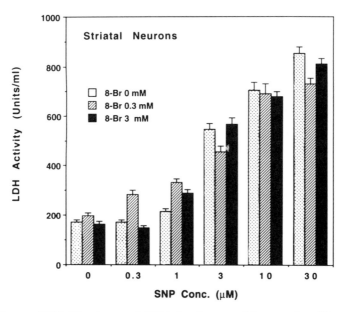

Figure 6. 8-Bromo-cGMP did not prevent SNP-induced neuronal degeneration. 8Bromo-cGMP was added to striatal neurons prior to the addition of SNP. The neurons were then incubated at 37°C for overnight (17 hours). LDH activity was determined using LDH assay kit (Sigma Chemical).

case with L-glutatmate- or sodium nitroprusside-induced neurodegeneration in this cell culture model system. We, and others, have found transient increase of phosphorylated tau during L-glutamate treatment (9). With short treatment of L-glutamate (30 seconds to 5 minutes), PHFl staining increased as determined by immunocytochemical studies (data not shown), yet neurons did not degenerate. When neurons started to degenerate, we observed that axons retract, and PHFl immunostaining decreases. Both L-glutamate and sodium nitroprusside caused decreased levels of both tau and phosphorylated tau in these cell cultures as determined by several antibodies that are selective for non-phosphorylated or phosphorylated forms of tau. In agreement with other laboratories, we have also found phosphorylated forms of tau in embryonic cultured neurons from rat.

The mechanisms of nitric oxide-induced neurotoxicity and the interrelationships, if any, with tau and its phosphorylation obviously require additional studies.

REFERENCES

1. Alzheimer Disease. Eds., Terry, R.D., Katzman, R., and Bick, K.L. Raven Press, New York, NewYork, pp 198, 1994.
2. Cleveland, D.W., Hwo, S.Y., and Kirschner, M.W.: Purification of tau, a microtubule-associated protein that induces assembly of microtubules from purified tubulin. J. Mole. Biol., 116:207-225, 1977.
3. Wolozin, B.L., Pruchnick, A., Dickson, D.W., and Davies, P. A neuronal antigen in the brain of Alzheimer patients. Science, 232:648-650, 1986.
4. Kosik, K.S., Orecchi, L.D., Binder, L.I., Trojanowski, J., Lee, V., and Lee, G. Epitopes that span the tau molecule are shared with paired helical filaments. Neuron, 1:817-825, 1988.
5. Chen, J., Chang, B., William, M., and Murad, F. Sodium nitroprusside de~enerates cultured rat striatal neurons. NeuroReport, 2(3):121-123, 1991.
6. Murad, F. The nitric oxide signal transduction system (chapter in this monograph).

7. Ignarro, L.J., Lippton, H., Edward, J.D., Baricos, W.H., Hyman, A.L., Kadowitz, P.J., and Gruetter, C.A. Mechanism of vascular smooth muscle relaxation by organic nitrates, nitrites, nitroprusside and nitric oxide: Evidence for the involvement of S-nitrosothiols as active intermediates. J. Pharmacol. Exp. Ther., 218:739-749, 1981.

8. Beckman, J.S., Beckman, T.W., Chen, J., Marshall, P.A., and Freeman, B.A. Apparent hydroxyl radical production by peroxynitrite: Implications for endothelial injury from nitric oxide and superoxide. Proc. Natl. Acad. Sci. USA, 87:1620-1624, 1990.

9. Sindou, P., Lesort, M., Couratier, P., Yardin, C., Esclaire, F., and Hugon, J. Glutamate increases tau phosphorylation in primary neuronal cultures from fetal rat cerebral cortex. Brain Res., 646:124-128, 1994.

BRAIN LESION AND NITRIC OXIDE SYNTHASE/NADPH-DIAPHORASE: A LIGHT AND ELECTRON MICROSCOPICAL STUDY

Gerald Wolf, Werner Schmidt, Jaroslaw Calka, Gabriele Henschke, and Sabine Würdig

Institute of Medical Neurobiology
University of Magdeburg
Erich-Weinert-Str. 3
D-39112 Magdeburg, Germany

INTRODUCTION

The role of nitric oxide (NO) in the pathogenesis of cerebral disorders is poorly understood (Bruhwyler et al., 1993; Choi, 1993). Many reports suggest that brain damage caused by excessive release of excitatory amino acids is mediated by NO formation (Dawson et al., 1991; Nowicki et al., 1991; Buisson et al., 1993). But there are conflicting findings which show that NO can function rather as a protective agent (Yamamoto et al., 1992; Weissmann et al., 1992). Moreover, the contribution of glial cells to the NO production in intact and damaged brain tissue is quite unclear. Choi (1993) has recently summarized the current discussion concluding that "a plethora of variables and the inherent complexity of NO biology hinder present efforts to define the effects of NO upon the injured brain".

In order to elucidate morphological aspects of the NO pathology in relation to neurodegenerative processes we localized NO synthase (NOS), the enzyme for the biosynthesis of NO, at the light and electron microscopical level in degenerating brain tissue. NOS was identified by the NADPH-diaphorase (NADPH-d) reaction, which is, if aldehyde-fixation is used, widely accepted to be a staining procedure of high specificity (Hope et al., 1991; Matsumoto et al., 1993). Exposure to quinolinic acid (QUIN) was used as a model for glutamate-mediated brain damage.

MATERIALS AND METHODS

Adult Wistar rats anestetized by hexobarbital sodium were injected with 1 or 0.5 µmol QUIN (Sigma) intracerebroventricularly (for hippocampal degeneration, 6 animals) or, locally into the striatum, with 120 nmol QUIN [2 µl, diluted in phosphate (0.1 M)

Biochemical, Pharmacological, and Clinical Aspects of Nitric Oxide
Edited by B. A. Weissman *et al.*, Plenum Press, New York, 1995

213

buffered saline, PBS; 1 µl/min; 20 animals]. After a survival time of four days experimental as well as control (n = 20, PBS injected) and untreated (n = 8) rats were transcardially perfused for 20 min with 400 ml of a fixative consisting of 4% paraformaldehyde, 0.4% glutaraldehyde and 2% sucrose in PBS.

For *light microscopical NADPH-d staining* tissue blocks containing the hippocampus or the striatum were stored in 15% sucrose (in PBS) at 4°C overnight, frozen, and cut into 20-µm cryostat sections. The incubation of the sections was performed freely floating in 0.1 M phosphate buffer, pH 8.0, containing 0.8% Triton X-100, 1.2 mM NADPH (Serva, Heidelberg) and 0.8 mM Nitroblue tetrazolium chloride (NBT, Serva) at 37°C for 90 min.

In some cases *double staining* was carried out after NADPH-d histochemistry to identify astroglial and microglial cells. Monoclonal antibodies against glial fibrillary acid protein (GFAP; Boehringer, Mannheim) were used as astroglia marker and isolectin B4 (*from Griphonia simplicifolia*, Sigma; recognizes α-D-galactose residues), as an established marker for microglial/macrophagic cells (Streit and Kreutzberg, 1987; Marty et al., 1991). Both compounds were peroxidase conjugated and routinely visualized by the diaminobenzidine reaction.

For *electron microscopy*, 50-µm vibratome sections of tissue blocks were incubated freely floating at 37 °C for 90 min in a solution containing 1.2 mM NADPH and 1.2 mM 2-(2'-benzothiazolyl)-5-styryl-3-(4'-phthalhydrazidyl)tetrazolium chloride (BSPT; Sigma, St. Louis), diluted in 0.1 M phosphate buffer (pH 8.0). BSPT was used for the ultrastructural NADPH-d identification in place of NBT to yield an osmiophilic formazan precipitation (for more details, see Wolf et al., 1992, 1993). After washing in PBS, areas of interest were cut out, osmicated in 1% OsO_4 (1 h) and processed to 70% alcohol. After block-contrasting in 0.5% uranyl acetate in 70% ethanol (1 h) and dehydration in 100% ethanol sections were embedded in a drop of Durcupan between acetate foils for ultrathin sectioning.

Selected sections were additionally stained for GFAP or isolectin B4. In that case, vibratome sections were processed for the second cytochemical procedure immediately following the incubation with BSPT. After extensive rinsing sections were treated as described above for light microscopy, followed by osmication, block-contrasting in uranyl acetate, and ultrathin-sectioning.

RESULTS

Exposure to QUIN led to a massive loss of neuronal cells in the hippocampus (CA3-, CA1-, and CA4-region) and the striatum as being observed by light and electron microscopical inspection. Most neurons underwent a pale, edematous type of necrosis. Electron microscopically, their cytoplasm was rich in microvacuoles, distended membrane-limited cisternae, and electron-dense bodies, filled with floccular material („moth-eaten appearance"; Fig. 1). In other cases shrinking of the perikarya was observed characterized by a dark cytoplasm and clumping of chromatin.

Single neurons were seen in the lesioned area which apparently survived the QUIN administration. They were surrounded by cell debris and surviving glial cells. But even in such neurons swelling of the endoplasmic reticulum was visible, and their cytoplasm showed some microvacuoles. NADPH-staining resulted in an electron-dense reaction product, BSPT-formazan, which was deposited distinctly at endomembranes, predominantly those of the endoplasmic reticulum, including the nuclear envelope (Fig. 2).

In neuron-depleted areas a striking proliferation of astro- and microglial cells was seen. The morphological identity was confirmed by selective staining for GFAP and IB4 (Fig. 3). Whereas quiescent glia in normal striatal and hippocampal tissue displayed only, if any, a tiny NBT-formazan staining and, electron microscopically, small portions of membrane-bound BSPT-formazan deposits (mostly perinuclear membranes), reactive glial cells revealed a quite different feature: As visible under the light microscope, the staining intensity for IB4 and GFAP increased dramatically, and the NADPH-d reaction of glial cells of the lesion focus (needle tract) was also enhanced. In particular the electron microscopically demonstrable labeling of endomembranes with BSPT-formazan was markedly extended, mainly to those of cytoplasmic areas (Fig. 4), sometimes to membranes of the Golgi apparatus and of mitochondria. As seen in striatal lesioned areas around the needle tract a number of IB4-positive cells showed globular shape and were, by light microscopy, heavily stained for NADPH-d (Fig. 5). Ultrastructurally, such cells were rich in phagocytotic debris and the labeling of membranes including parts of the plasmalemma as well as in cisternae filled with electron-dense formazan puncta indicating the presence of (inducible ?) NOS containing vacuoles (Fig. 6,7). Other IB4-stained cells belonged to the ramified type and were, easily seen, larger than quiescent microglia. But their NADPH-d reaction tended to be rather moderate. GFAP-stained cells were also noticeably enlarged, when compared with normal tissue. The NADPH-d reaction was markedly increased in that case, but did not reach the intensity of globular IB4-cells.

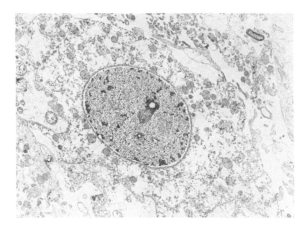

Figure 1. Electron micrograph of a degenerated cell in the hippocampal CA3-region. The degeneration is characterized by clumping of chromatin and by swelling and disruption of organelles (x 6,500).

DISCUSSION

The present study has shown that, apart from neurons, astro- and microglial cells contain NADPH-d activities, which are thought to be identical with NOS. Adapting the NADPH-d histochemistry to the electron microscopical level by using the tetrazolium salt BSPT we have demonstrated that there is a strict correlation between the light microscopical staining intensity (NBT-formazan) and the extent of labeled endomembranes (BSPT-formazan; Wolf et al., 1992, 1993). However, up to now no definite conclusion have reached on the question of specificity of the NADPH-d staining for NOS. There are many other enzymes in brain tissue, which utilize NADPH as a coenzyme to be displayed as NADPH-d activity (Kuonen et al., 1988; Tracey et al., 1993). Matsumoto et al. (1993) have demonstrated that aldehyde fixation, as used in the present study, is crucial for excluding NADPH-d staining that is unrelated to NOS. Moreover, the attachment of NOS/NADPH-d to endomembranes as described in the present as well as in preceding papers (Hope and Vincent, 1989; Wolf et al., 1992, 1993, 1994) is in apparent contradiction to biochemical findings, by which merely the inducible mf NADPH-d we were able to demonstrate that the neuronal form is primarily bound to membranes, but can easily be detached (Wolf et al., 1994). isoform of NOS is shown to be particulate, whereas the neuronal (constitutive) NOS is suggested to be a soluble protein (Frstermann et al., 1991; Tracey et al., 1993). As opposed to this, by testing the influence of the detergent Triton X-100 on the localization

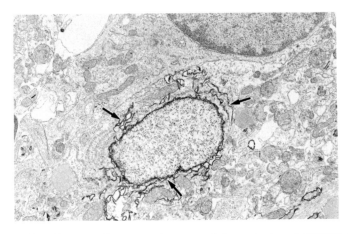

Figure 2a. A surviving hippocampal neuron: ultrastructural demonstration of NADPH-diaphorase by membrane-bound deposits of electron-dense BSPT-formazan (arrows). Predominantly membranes of the perinuclear endoplasmic reticulum and those of endoplasmic cisternae are labeled (x 10,200).

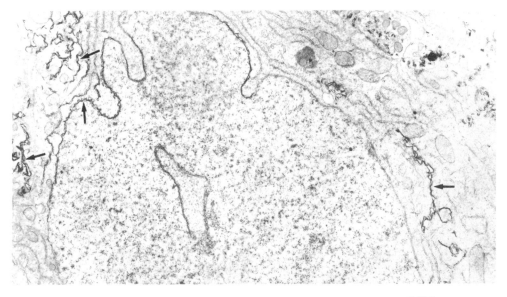

Figure 2b. A normal, heavily BSPT-stained (arrows) hippocampal neuron (x 10,800).

Our results demonstrate that glial cells may exhibit NADPH-d activity even under normal conditions. Indications for a potential 'nitrinergic' role for glia are favored by the observation that there is an increase in number and extent of labeled membranes due to QUIN exposure. However, little information is available on the function of glia-derived

216

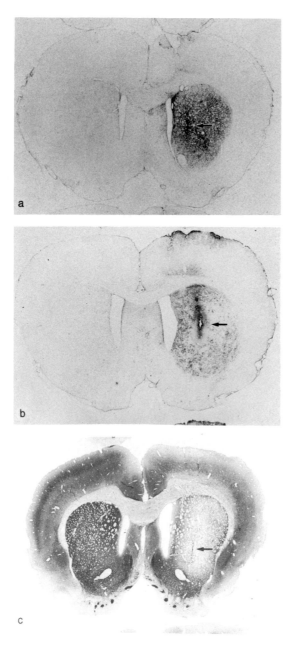

Figure 3. Coronal sections through a frontal rat brain four days after local injection of quinolinic acid into the right striatum. GFAP-immunostaining (a) and isolectin-B4 staining (b) reveal an intense proliferation of astro- and microglia at the lesion side. The section in (c) demonstrates a striking loss of NADPH-diaphorase stained (NBT- formazan) structures at the same side. Arrow indicates needle tract.

NO, induced or constitutive, in the degeneration process. Increased NO production in damaged nervous tissue, possibly induced by cytokinins (Merrill et al., 1993; Lee et al., 1993), may enhance cerebral blood flow and may contribute to the inflammatory response. Also, numerous data are available to demonstrate that NO, if produced from glia or not, may cause cell death (Chao et al., 1992), or, on the contrary, can have a beneficial effect by

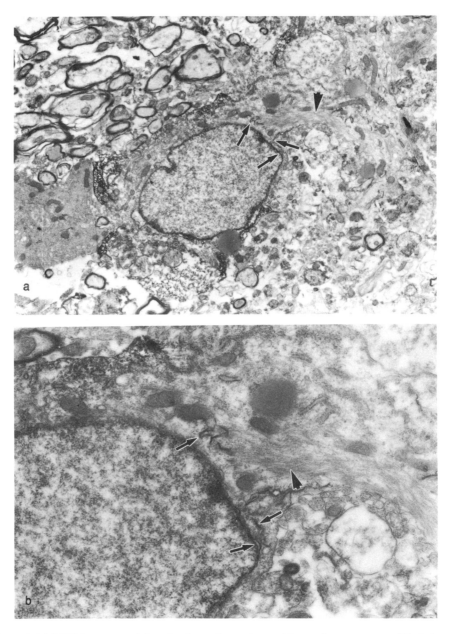

Figure 4. (a) BSPT-formazan staining of endomembranes (arrows) is seen in an astrocyte wihin lesioned striatal tissue. Arrowhead: glial filaments (x 9,600) **(b)** At higher magnification (x 26,400).

protecting nerve cells from excitotoxic damage (Manzoni et al., 1992) and from reactive oxygen species (Wink et al., 1993). In any case, the morphological approach by studying the precise distribution patterns of the NO-producing capacity of the different glial cell types in combination with those of neurons is suggested to be an important way to elucidate the role of NO under various physiological and pathological conditions.

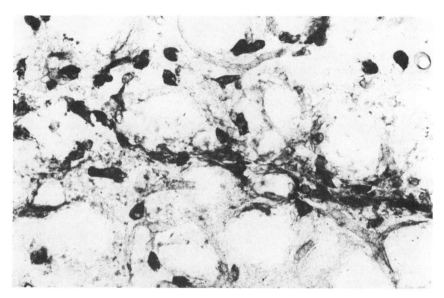

Figure 5. Intense NBT-formazan reaction in globular-type microglial cells/macrophages around the needle tract in damaged striatal tissue (x 1,500).

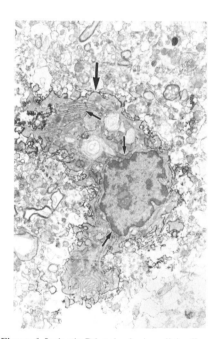

Figure 6. Isolectin B4-stained microglial cell (activated) micro-(labeling of plasmalemma, arrow) within damaged striatal tissue. Little arrows show BSPT-formazan deposits at endomembranes (x 5,800).

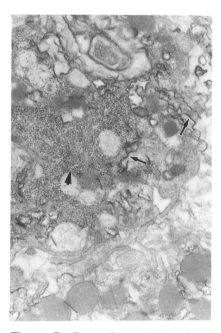

Figure 7. Part of a globular-shaped glial cell/macrophage. NADPH-diaphorase reactive endomembranes and plasmalemma are visible (arrows), moreover vacuoles filled with electron-dense formazan puncta (arrowheads) (x 15,800).

Acknowledgments

We thank Mrs. J. Czerney, Mrs. K. Klingenberg, and Mrs. M. Mckel for expert technical assistance.

219

REFERENCES

Bruhwyler, J., Chleide, E., Ligeois, J.F., and Carreer, F., 1993, Nitric oxide: a new messenger in the brain, *Neurosci. Biobehav. Rev.* 17:373-384.

Buisson, A., Margaill, I., Callebert, J., Plotkine, M., and Boulu, R.G., 1993, Mechanisms involved in the neuroprotective activity of a nitric oxide synthase inhibitor, *J. Neurochem.* 61:690-696.

Chao, C.C., Hu, S., Molitor, T.W., Shaskan, E.G., and Peterson, P.K., 1992, Activated microglia mediate neuronal cell injury via a nitric oxide mechanism, *J. Immunol.* 149: 2736-2741.

Choi, D.W., 1993, Nitric oxide: foe or friend to the injured brain?, *Proc. Natl. Acad. Sci. USA* 90:9741-9743.

Dawson, V.L., Dawson, T.M., London, E.D., Bredt, D.S., and Snyder, S.H., 1991, Nitric oxide mediates glutamate neurotoxicity in primary cortical cultures, *Proc. Natl. Acad. Sci. USA* 88:6368-6371.

Frstermann, U., Schmidt, H.H.H.W., Pollock, J.S., Sheng, H., Mitchell, J.A., Warner, T.D., Nakane, M., and Murad, F., 1991, Isoforms of nitric oxide synthase. Characterization and purification from different cell types, *Biochem. Pharmacol.* 42:1849-1857.

Hope, B.T., and Vincent, S.R., 1989, Histochemical characterization of neuronal NADPH-diaphorase, *J. Histochem. Cytochem.* 37:653-661.

Hope, B.T., Michael., G.J., Knigge, K.M. and Vincent, S.R., 1991, Neuronal NADPH diaphorase is a nitric oxide synthase, Proc. Natl. Acad. Sci. USA 88:2811-2814.

Hope, B.T., Michael, G.J., Knigge, K.M., and Vincent, S.R., 1991, Neuronal NADPH diaphorase is a nitric oxide synthase, Proc. Natl. Acad. Sci. USA 88:2811-2814.

Kuonen, D.R., Kemp, M.C., and Roberts, P.J., 1988, Demonstration and biochemical characterization of rat brain. NADPH-dependent diaphorase, J. Neurochem. 50:1017-1025.

Lee, S.C., Dickson, D.W., Liu, W., and Brosnan, C.F., 1993, Induction of nitric oxide synthase activity in human astrocytes by interleukin-1ß and interferon-γ, J. Neuroimmunol. 46:19-24.

Manzoni, O., Prezeau, L., Marin, P., Deshager, S., Bockaert, J., and Fagni, L., 1992, Nitric oxide-induced blockade of NMDA receptors, Neuron 8:653-662.

Marty, S., Dusart, I. and Peschanski, M., 1991, Glial changes following an excitotoxic lesion in the cns-I. Microglia/macrophages, Neuroscience 45:529-539.

Matsumoto, T., Nakane, M., Pollock, J.S., Kuk, J.E.,and Förstermann, U., 1993, A correlation between soluble brain nitric oxide synthase and NADPH-diaphorase activity is only seen after exposure of the tissue to fixative, Neurosci. Lett. 155:61-64.

Merrill, J.E., Ignarro, L.J., Sherman, M.P., Melinek, J., and Lane, T.E., 1993, Microglial cell cytotoxicity of oligodendrocytes is mediated through nitric oxide, J. Immunol. 151:2132-2141.

Nowicki, J.P., Duval, D., Poignet, H., and Scatton, B., 1991, Nitric oxide mediates neuronal death after focal cerebral ischemia in the mouse, Eur. J. Pharmacol. 204:339-340.

Streit, W.J. and Kreutzberg, G.W., 1987, Lectin binding by resting and reactive microglia, J. Neurocytol. 16:249-260.

Tracey, W.R., Nakane, M., Pollock, J.S., and Firstermann, U., 1993, Nitric oxide synthase in neuronal cells, macrophages and endothelium are NADPH diaphorase, but represent only a fraction of total cellular NADPH diaphorase activity, Biochem. Biophys. Res. Comm. 195: 1035-1040.

Weissman, B.A., Kader, T., Brandeis, R., and Shapira, S., 1992, N^G-nitro-L-arginine enhances neuronal death following transient forebrain ischemia in gerbils, Neurosci. Lett. 146:139-142.

Wink, D.A., Hanbauer, I., Krishna, M.C., DeGraff, W., Gamson, J., and Mitchell, J.B., 1993, Nitric oxide protects against cellular damage and cytotoxicity from reactive oxygen species, Proc. Natl. Acad. Sci. USA 90:9813-9817.

Wolf, G., Würdig, S., and Schünzel, G., 1992, Nitric oxide synthase in rat brain is predominantly located at neuronal endoplasmic reticulum: an electron microscopic demonstration of NADPH-diaphorase activity, Neurosci. Lett., 147:63-66.

Wolf, G., Henschke, G. and Würdig, S., 1993, Glutamate agonist-induced hippocampal lesion and nitric oxide synthase/NADPH-diaphorase: a light and electron microscopical study in the rat, Neurosci. Lett. 161:49-52.

Wolf, G., Würdig, S., and Henschke, G., 1994, Nitric oxide synthase in the brain: light and electron microscopical findings based on the NADPH-diaphorase reaction, J. Neural. Transm. (in press)

Yamamoto, S., Golanov, E.V., Berger, S.B., and Reis, D.J., 1992, Inhibition of nitric oxide synthesis increases focal ischemic infarction in rat, J. Cereb. Blood Flow Metab. 12:717-726.

DOSE-DEPENDENT EFFECTS OF NITRIC OXIDE ON IN VIVO AND IN VITRO NEURONAL FUNCTIONS

Shlomo Shapira[1], Shira Chapman[1], Tamar Kadar[1], Ben Avi Weissman[1], and Eli Heldman[2]

[1]Department of Pharmacology
[2]Department of Organic Chemistry
 Israel Institute for Biological Research
 Ness-Ziona IL-74048, Israel.

INTRODUCTION

The role of nitric oxide (NO) in mediating ischemia-induced processes is being extensively investigated. Nonetheless, there is still a considerable dispute about the question whether or not NO is cytoprotective or cytotoxic (Choi, 1993), substantiated by a great deal of evidence. On one hand, a vast amount of data attribute a distinct toxic role to NO following ischemia, both *in vitro* (Dawson et al., 1991), as well as *in vivo* (Nowicki et al., 1991; Buisson et al., 1992). On the other hand, equally large body of evidence suggest just the opposite both *in vivo* and *in vitro* (Sancesario et al., 1994; Pauwels and Lysen, 1992; Demerele-Pallardy et al., 1991). In accord with these recent publications, we observed (Weissman et al., 1992) an enhancement of neuronal death following a 5 min forebrain ischemia in gerbils pretreated with a single high-dose (50 mg/kg, i.p.) of the specific NO synthase (NOS) inhibitor, N^G-nitro-L-arginine (NARG). A wide variety of NOS inhibitors was used in the different studies, as well as miscellaneous animal species and various models of brain ischemia (e.g.: focal vs forebrain ischemia; permanent vs transient cessation of blood supply). However, there is very little information on the dose-dependent effect of gradual NOS inhibition on neurophysiological parameters like behavior and histologic-morphometric changes.

One of the most important homeostatic mechanisms in all cells, especially those of excitable tissues, is the Na^+/K^+-ATPase. Na^+/K^+-ATPase (sodium pump; EC 3.6.1.3) is a membrane associated enzyme whose activity is energy-dependent, and is modulated by intracellular condition such as Na^+ concentration ($[Na^+]_i$), as well as by a series of endogenous effectors, like insulin (Resh et al., 1980) or biogenic amines (Clausen and Flatman, 1980). As a result of brain ischemia, there is a rapid decrease of available energy sources and a resulting derangement of Na^+/K^+-ATPase activity (Ekholm et al., 1993), and other energy-dependent processes (Madl and Burgesser, 1993). This insult is an early and severe event following brain ischemia (Nagafuji et al., 1992), and is followed by a sequence

Biochemical, Pharmacological, and Clinical Aspects of Nitric Oxide
Edited by B. A. Weissman *et al.*, Plenum Press, New York, 1995

221

of progressive pathological processes, resulting in a permanent neuronal cell damage and cell death (Pulsinelli, 1992; Scheinberg, 1991). Moreover, pharmacological manipulation leading to a partial recovery of Na^+/K^+-ATPase activity was proven effective in treating brain ischemia (Nagafuji et al., 1992).

The present study was designed to shed some more light on the role that NO plays at the central nervous system (CNS) following transient ischemia, and to unfold a possible mechanism whereby NO affect ischemic brain tissue. The study is devided into two parts. In the first *in vivo* study, administration of increasing doses of NARG to gerbils was followed by a 5 min forebrain ischemia. Followup was based on behavioral and histologic-morphometric evaluation of the gerbils. In the second, *in vitro* study, the change in Na^+/K^+-ATPase activity was assessed in PC12 pheochromocytoma cells and C6 glioma cells, in response to a series of stimuli that either increase or inhibit NO production. We chose to use NARG, since it is a specific and powerful inhibitor of NOS (Klatt et al., 1994) and does not posses nonspecific characteristics, like some of the other NOS inhibitors (Buxton et al., 1993). Furthermore, it was shown to produce dose-dependent NOS inhibition, both *in vivo* and *in vitro* (Dwyer et al., 1991).

PC12 pheochromocytoma cells carry most of the features of neuronal cells (Nakae, 1991; Eherngruber et al., 1993) and were shown to posses both NO-induced cyclic GMP (cGMP) activity (Haby et al., 1994), and Na^+/K^+-ATPase activity (Kurihara et al., 1994). C6 glioma cells represent a distinct component of the CNS, and contain a different type of NOS (Murphy et al., 1993), which is induced, among other factors, by lipopolysaccharide (LPS) to produce NO, resulting in large cGMP output (Simmons and Murphy, 1992).

MATERIALS AND METHODS

In vivo Experiment

Male mongolian gerbils (58-66 g) housed (5 per cage) in a temperature (21±2°C) and light (12 h light/dark cycle) controlled room, with free access to water and food. Groups of gerbils were injected (i.p.) with either 5 (N=5), 10 (N=5), 25(N=5) or 50 (N=4) mg/kg of N^G-nitro-L-arginine (Sigma). Four h later the gerbils were operated under halothane (2%)/oxygen anesthesia and their carotid arteries were exposed on both sides, and bilaterally occluded for 5 min, during which time the anesthesia was shut off. Cessation of blood flow distal to the occlusion site during the ischemia, as well as reperfusion, were confirmed visually. Control ischemia group (N=5) underwent 5 min ischemia without NARG pretreatment. Control NARG group (N=5) received NARG (50 mg/kg) and was subjected to sham operation. NARG (50 mg/kg, i.p.) followed by a sham operation was shown in our experience to have no effect on behavior and brain morphology (Weissman et al., 1992), and was considered as normal control. Assessment of spontaneous activity was performed on days 1, 2, 4 and 6 post ischemia, in a 30x36x15 cm cage, using an electronic activity monitor (Selective Activity Meter model 2S, Columbus Instruments, Columbus, OH). At the same time points, body weights were monitored. On the 6th post ischemia day, under deep pentobarbital anesthesia, the gerbils were transcardially perfused (0.9% NaCl followed by 4% buffered paraformaldehyde), their brains removed, further fixed and processed routinely for paraffin embedding. Serial coronal sections (6 μm thick) were cut, and selected sections were stained with hematoxylin and eosin (H&E) for histological evaluation. The histologic quantitative evaluation was based on a scoring system (Weissman et al., 1992) as follows: 0 - normal brain tissue; 1 - damage confined to CA1 hippocampal cells; 2 - damage to CA1 and other hippocampal structures; 3 - damage to striatum and/or cortex, in addition to hippocampal injury. Cells containing clear rounded nucleus and a visible nucleolus were considered normal, whereas damaged cells were shrunken with dark-colored nucleus and without visible nucleoli.

Morphometric analysis was carried out utilizing a computerized image analyzer system (CUE-3, Galai, Israel), and was based on differential (normal versus damaged) cell count of CA1 cells at the dorsal hippocampus in sections corresponding to plate 32 of the rat brain atlas of Paxinos and Watson (1986). Cell count was performed bilaterally, within a 0.04 mm^2 frame using a x25 objective magnification, on two serial sections from each gerbil.

Results are expressed as mean ± S.E.M. Non-parametric Kolmogorov-Smirnov Two Sample Test was used to asses the quantitative histologic evaluation. Repeated measures analysis of variance (ANOVA) was used to calculate statistical significance (at p<0.05) in all other experiments.

In vitro Experiment

PC12 pheochromocytoma cells were grown in RPMI 1640 supplemented with 2mM glutamine, 10% heat-inactivated horse serum and 5% fetal calf serum. C6 glioma cells were grown in DMEM supplemented with 2mM glutamine and 10% fetal calf serum. The growth media for both cell lines contained penicillin (100 IU/ml) and streptomycin (100 µg/ml). Two days before each assay, either PC12 cells or C6 cells were seeded into 24 well plates and Na^+/K^+-ATPase activity was assessed by a previously described method of ^{86}Rb influx (Gupta et al, 1991). At the beginning of the experiment the growth medium was replaced and the cells were washed with 1 ml of Krebs buffer containing (mM): NaCl (118), KCl (5), $CaCl_2$ (1.9), $MgCl_2$ (2), glucose (10) and Tris-HCl (25), in pH 7.4 at 25°C. Cells were then preincubated at 25°C for 8min in 0.5 ml of medium with or without ei, L-arg or sodium nitroprusside (SNP). Each treatment was repeated in the presence or absence of ouabain (1 mM). Then ^{86}Rb (0.5-1.0 µCi/well) was added and the cells were incubated at 25°C for additional 8min. The reaction was stopped by washing the cells three times with ice-cold Krebs buffer. The cellular content of radioactivity was assessed after lysis by freezing in DDW with 5% acetic acid, and radioactivity was assessed in a scintillation counter without a scintillation liquid. The ouabain-sensitive ^{86}Rb influx was calculated by subtracting the ouabain insensitive influx from the total influx, and served as a measure of the Na^+/K^+-ATPase activity (Akera et al, 1981). The effect of K^+-free medium or LPS were studied by incubating cells at 37°C for 1.5 hr with K^+-free Krebs, or 4 hrs with LPS, respectively, and adding normal Krebs during the incubation with the ^{86}Rb.

The following materials were tested: N^G-nitro-L-arginine (NARG) 0.1-20µM; L-arginine (L-arg) 300 µM, sodium nitroprusside (SNP) 100 µM and lipopolysaccharide (LPS) 100µg/ml. All the materials were purchased from Sigma (St. Louis, MO, USA). ^{86}Rb was purchased from New-England Nuclear (MA, USA) with a specific activity of 1mCi/ml.

Ouabain-sensitive ^{86}Rb influx was calculated as described above, and the effect of each of the materials tested on ouabain-sensitive ^{86}Rb influx is displayed as percent of control, untreated cells.

RESULTS

In vivo Experiment

Figure 1 displays the changes in body weights in the various experimental groups. There is a significant (p<0.05) decrease in body-weight in all groups that underwent ischemia, starting on day 1 post ischemia, and a delayed weight-gain in the control NARG group. The control ischemis and 5 mg/kg groups show a milder weight loss, as compared to the higher dose groups.

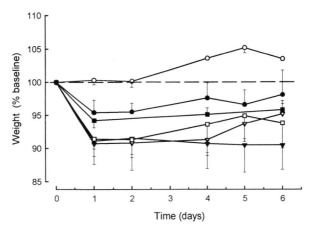

Figure 1. Time course of body weights of gerbils injected (ip) with various doses of NARG, 4 h before 5 min of bilateral carotid artery occlusion. ○ - Control-NARG group (NARG, 50 mg/kg, without ischemia); ■ - Control-ischemia group (5 min ischemia without NARG pretreatment); ●- 5 mg/kg; ▽- 10 mg/kg; ▼ - 25 mg/kg; - 50 mg/kg of NARG (N=4-5 per group). There was a significant (p<0.05) weight loss from day 1 in all groups that underwent ischemia, as compared to control-NARG (N=4-5 per group).

Twenty four and 48 h following ischemia, spontaneous hyperactivity was observed in all gerbils exposed to ischemia. At 24 h, the normal habituation pattern observed in control NARG group (a decrease to 68±7% in spontaneous activity, compared to pre-ischemia baseline activity) was absent in all ischemia groups, and there was a dose-dependent increase of spontaneous activity to 117±5%, 134±27%, 139±13%, 191±24%, 196±14% of baseline activity, in the control-ischemia, and 5, 10, 25 and 50 mg/kg groups, respectively (Fig. 2). At 48 h, the pattern of mild hyperactivity (126-135% of baseline activity) was observed in all ischemia groups, except the 25 mg/kg group which displayed a prominent increase of activity to 176% of baseline (Fig. 2).

Damaged CA1 hippocampal cells were evident in all gerbils subjected to ischemia. Injured cells were scattered among a variable number of normal neurons, and were in various stages of degeneration, ranging from acidophilic, shrunken cells, to complete disappearance of cellular structures, which were then replaced by vacuoles. A quantitative evaluation of the histopathology (Fig. 3) revealed a pattern of injury whereby the 25 mg/kg group demonstrated the highest degree of degeneration which was significantly (p<0.01) worse than either control ischemia or 5 mg/kg group. The 5 mg/kg animals showed a degree of damage similar to, but less distinct than control-ischemia group, and less than each of the other dose groups.

Morphometric analysis confirmed the above findings, with a dose-dependent increase in the number of damaged cells, and a decrease in the number of normal cells, in control-ischemia and in all NARG-ischemia groups of 10 mg/kg and above (Fig. 4). The 5 mg/kg group was outstanding: It was not different from control-NARG, and it was statistically better than control-ischemia.

Spontaneous hyperactivity was closely associated with the histological findings. A significant correlation could be found between the decline in normal cell count and the hyperactivity at 24 h (R=-0.61, p<0.01), and at 48 h (R=-0.51, p<0.05), and between the increase in damaged cell count and hyperactivity at 24 h (R=0.45, p<0.05).

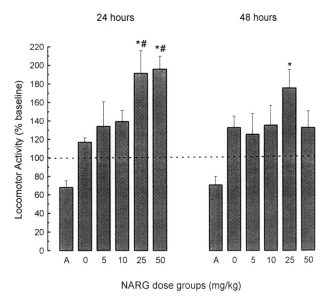

Figure 2. Changes in spontaneous locomotor activity of gerbils 24 and 48 h after administration (ip) of different doses of NARG and implementation of 5 min forebrain ischemia. Spontaneous activity was measured in a 30x36x15 cm cage, in 10 min sessions, using electronic activity meter. A - Control-NARG; 0 - Control-ischemia. * p<0.01 compared to control-NARG; # p<0.01 compared to control-ischemia. (N=4-5 per group)

In vitro Experiments

Incubation of PC12 cells with increasing concentrations of NARG resulted in a dose-dependent inhibition of ouabain-sensitive ^{86}Rb influx (Fig. 5). Non-linear regression yielded an IC50 of 9.7μM.

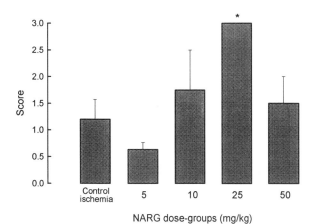

Figure 3. Quantitative histopathological evaluation. Gerbils were pretreated with various doses of NARG and 4 h later were subjected to 5 min forebrain ischemia. Assessment was based on a scoring system where: 0 - normal brain; 1 - damage which is confined to CA1 cells; 2 - damage that has extended also to other hippocampal structures; 3 - damage which is observed at the cortex and striatum, in addition to the hippocampus. * p<0.01 compared to control-ischemia and 5 mg/kg groups (N=4-5 per group).

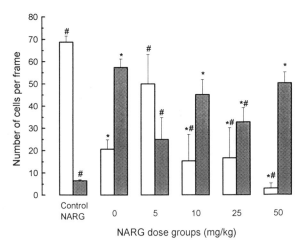

Figure 4. Differential morphometric analysis of CA1 hippocampal cells 6 days after a 5 min forebrain ischemia. Ischemia was performed 4 h following administration (ip) of NARG at various doses. Data are presented as number of cells in a frame area of 0.04 mm^2, on both hemispheres, two serial sections from each gerbil, with a x25 objective magnification. Evaluation was performed on coronal sections corresponding to plate number 32 in the rat brain atlas of Paxinos and Watson (1986). ▭ normal cells; ▨ damaged cells. * p<0.01 compared to control-NARG; # p<0.01 compared to control-ischemia (N=4-5 per group).

In PC12 cells, L-arg (300µM) reversed the NARG (10µM)-inhibited influx from 58±14% (mean ± SD) of control, to 83%, while L-arg alone enhanced the ouabain-sensitive influx (153±4% of control), and the addition of NARG (10µM) to L-arg (300µM) attenuated the increased ^{86}Rb influx from 153±4% to 83% of control (Fig. 6).

Similar results were obtained in C6 cells, where L-arg (300µM) induced an increase of ouabain-sensitive ^{86}Rb influx to 121% of control, and NARG (10µM) inhibited the L-arg (300µM) induced uncrease of ^{86}Rb influx from 121% to 81% of control (Fig. 6).

LPS was shown, among other factors, to induce substantial NOS activity in cells of the CNS (Simmons and Murphy, 1992). In PC12 cells, LPS (100µg/ml) caused an increase of ouabain-sensitive ^{86}Rb influx to 150% of control, whereas NARG (10µM) attenuated this increase by 27% (Fig. 7). A strong activator of the Na$^+$/K$^+$-ATPase is an increased. [Na$^+$]$_i$. Incubation of PC12 cells in a K+-free medium for 1.5 h which is known to increase the [Na$^+$]$_i$, caused, as expected an augmentation of ouabain-sensitive ^{86}Rb influx to 189±26% of control cells which were incubated in normal-K$^+$ medium. Yet under these circumstances, NARG (10µM), displayed a similar (60%) inhibition of ouabain-sensitive ^{86}Rb influx (Fig.7). An 8 min incubation of either PC12 or C6 cells with the NO donor SNP, caused a 5% increase in ouabain-sensitive ^{86}Rb influx in both cell-lines.

DISCUSSION

The main findings in the present study were the bidirectional, dose-depof NOS inhibition on brain pathophysiology, and the dose-dependent association between NO and Na$^+$/K$^+$-ATPase activity in neuronal cells.

The effect of NARG on brain histopathology was inverted as the dose changed from 5 to 10 mg/kg, with the 5 mg/kg dose having a significant protective effect, whereas higher doses had a deleterious effect, as compared to control-ischemia. This phenomenon may

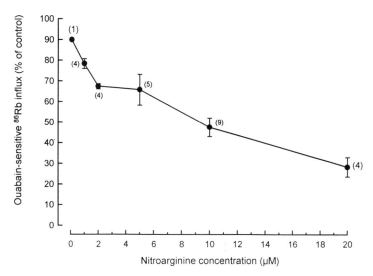

Figure 5. Effect of NARG on ouabain-sensitive ^{86}Rb influx in PC12 cells. Cells werepreincubated for 8 min at 25°C with various doses of NARG, then [86]Rb (0.5-1μCi/well) was added and the cells were incubated for an additional 8 min. After washing, the cells were lysed by freezing in DDW with 5% acetic acid, and radioactivity was measured by a scintillation counter. Ouabain-sensitive ^{86}Rb influx was calculated by subtracting the ouabain-insensitive ^{86}Rb influx from the total ^{86}Rb influx. The points (mean±SD with the number of repetitions in parentheses) represent ^{86}Rb influx as percent of control (untreated) cells. There is a distinct dose-dependent inhibition of ouabain-sensitive ^{86}Rb influx.

represent either a true stepwise response or a uniform dose-response curve, but since doses between 0 and 5, and between 5 and 10 mg/kg of NARG were not used, no definite conclusion can be drawn at this stage. The discrepancy between the protective effect of 5 mg/kg NARG on histopathology, and the lack of protection on behavioral parameters, may be accounted for by the fact that histopathology is more sensitive than behavior, or by the

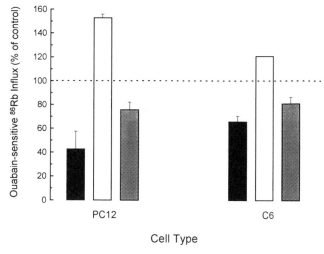

Figure 6. The effect of L-arg and NARG on ouabain-sensitive ^{86}Rb influx in PC12 and C6 cells. Experimental design is described in Fig. 5. Preincubation time was 8 min for either L-arg, NARG and the combination of both. L-arg (300μM) enhanced the ouabain-sensitive ^{86}Rb influx in both cell-lines with strong inhibiting effect of NARG (10μM). Both stimulating and inhibition effects were more effective in PC12. ▄ NARG (10μm); ☐ L-arg (300μM); ▨ L-arg (300μM)+NARG (10μm)

227

fact that other, more specific or more demanding behavioral tests would reveal subtle beneficial effect at the 5 mg/kg group. The results of the *in vivo* study are in accord with a body of recently published data (Haberny et al., 1992; Lerner-Natoli et al., 1992; Pauwels and Leysen, 1992; Weissman et al., 1992; Yamamoto et al., 1992) showing either no effect or aggrevating the effect of brain ischemia by inhibition of NO synthesis. In addition, in an experimental setting similar to ours, a narrow therapeutic range (3 mg/kg, i.p., repeated administrations) of NARG was found to be beneficial following a 10 min bilateral carotid occlusion in gerbils (Nagafuji et al., 1993).

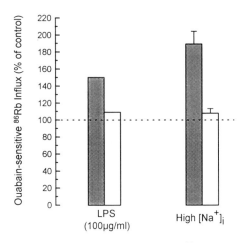

Figure 7. The effect of LPS and high [Na$^+$]$_i$ on ouabain-sensitive ^{86}Rb influx in PC12 cells. Experimental design is described in Fig. 5. Incubation time for LPS (100µg/ml) was 4 hr at 37°C; high [Na$^+$]$_i$ was achieved by incubating the cells in a K$^+$-free medium for 1.5 hr. In both experiments NARG (10µm) was added at the last 8 min of the incubation. ▭ with NARG; ▥ without NARG.

The main finding in the in vitro study was the dependence of Na$^+$/K$^+$-ATPase activity on NO production. All factors which were shown to increase NO production (e.g.: L-arg, LPS, and SNP), increased also Na$^+$/K$^+$-ATPase activity, and NARG which is an efficacious NOS inhibitor, inhibited Na$^+$/K$^+$-ATPase activity in a dose-dependent manner. The exact mode of interaction between Na$^+$/K$^+$-ATPase and NO was not fully clarified in the present study, although it was clearly shown that NO does not act through changes in the [Na$^+$]$_i$, since a given dose of NARG (10µM) caused similar degree of inhibition at high and at normal [Na$^+$]$_i$ (60% vs 50.3%, respectively).

Several attampts were made to explain the contradictory effects of NO on neuronal tissue in various experimental setups. Moskowitz (1994) observed a differential effect to the inhibition of endothelial NOS causing a decrease in CBF and enhancing the damage of ischemic neuronal tissue, while inhibition of neuronal NOS prevent the toxic, neurodegenerative effect of NO radical on ischemic brain tissue. Thus, he claimed that borderline ischemic brain tissue may be salvaged with the use of specific inhibitors of neuronal NOS, like 7-nitro indazole (Moore et al., 1993). Another attempt to explain the variable effect of NO on brain tissue was through its variable redox potential (Lipton et al., 1993), with either NO• radicals reacting with superoxide ions, creating the highly toxic peroxynitrite ions, or NO$^+$ which binds and downregulates the NMDA receptor's redox modulatory site, thereby inhibiting the Ca$^+$ influx and reducing the NMDA-induced neurotoxicity.

Based on the data presented, we suggest a different model to the paradoxical effect of NO on ischemic brain tissue. Most of the endogenously produced NO is utilized by beneficial processes, such as: Increase in cerebral blood flow (Zhang and Iadecola, 1993; Iadecola et al., 1994), and scavenging of free radicals (Wink et al., 1993). The present study points to an additional NO-regulated process, namely, enhancing the Na$^+$/K$^+$-ATPase activity. All these processes are favorable to the ischemic nervous tissue. When those processes are fully activated, excess amount of NO may then exert a neurotoxic effects, by acting as a free radical and causing membrane peroxidation. Thus, Inhibition of this excessive NO proves beneficial, whereas inhibition of a more substantial amount of NO is detrimental to the ischemic brain tissue by preventing the above-mentioned favorable responses.

REFERENCES

Akera, T., S. Yamamoto, K. Temma, D. Kim and T.A. Brody, 1981, Is ouabain-sensitive rubidium or potassium uptake a measure of sodium pump activity in isolated cardiac muscle. Biochim Biophys Acta 640:779-790.

Buisson, A., M. Plotkine and R.G. Boulu, 1992, The neuroprotective effect of a nitric oxide inhibitor in a rat model of brain ischemia. Br J Pharmacol 106:766-767.

Buxton, I.L.O., D.J. Cheek, D. Eckman, D.P. Westfall, K.M. Sanders and D. Keef, 1993, N^G-nitro L-arginine methyl ester and other alkyl esters of arginine are muscarinic receptor antagonists. Circ Res 72:387-395.

Choi, D.W., 1993, Nitric oxide: Foe or friend to the injured brain? Proc Natl Acad Sci USA 90:9741-9743.

Clausen, T. and J.A. Flatman, 1980, β_2-Adrenoceptor mediates the stimulating effect of adrenaline on active electrogenic Na-K-transport in rat soleus muscle. Br J Pharmacol 68:749-755.

Dawson, V.L., T.M. Dawson, E.D. London, D.S. Bredt and S.H. Snyder, 1991, Nitric oxide mediates glutamate neurotoxicity in primary cortical cultures. Proc Natl Acad Sci USA 88:6368-6371.

Demerele-Pallardy, C., M-O. Lonchampt, P-E. Chabrier, P. Braquet, 1991, Absence of implication of L-arginine/nitric oxide pathway on neuronal cell injury induced by L-glutamate or hypoxia. Biochem Biophys Res Comm 181:456-464.

Dwyer, M.A., D.S. Bredt, and S.H. Snyder, 1991, Nitric oxide synthase: irreversible inhibition by L-N^G-nitroarginine in vitro and in vivo. Biochem Biophys Res Commun 176:1136-1141.

Ehrengruber, M.U., D.A. Deranleau, C. Kempf, P. Zahler and M. Lanzrein, 1993, Arachidonic acid and other unsaturated fatty acids alter membrane potential in PC12 and bovine adrenal chromaphin cells. J Neurochem 60:282-288

Ekholm A, Katsura K and Siesjo B, 1993, Coupling of energy failure and dissipative K$^+$ flux during ischemia: Role of preischemic plasma glucose concentration. J Cereb Blood Flow Metab 13:193-200,

Gupta S., N.B. Ruderman, E.J. Cragoe and I. Sussman, 1991, Endothelin stimulates Na$^+$/K$^+$-ATPase activity by protein kinase C-dependent pathway in arabbit aorta. Am J Physiol 261(Heart Circ Physiol 30):H38-H45.

Haberny, K.A., S. Pou and C.U. Eccles, 1992, Potentiation of quinolonate-induced hippocampal lesions by inhibition of NO synthesis. NeurosciLett 146:187-190.

Haby,C., F. Lisovoski, D. Aunis and J. Zwiler, 1994, Stimulaof the cyclic GMP pathway by NO induces expression of the immediate early genes c-*fos* and *jun* B in PC12 cells. J Neurochem 62:496-501.

Iadecola, C., D.A. Palligrino, M.A. Moskowitz and N.A. Lassen, 1994, Nitric oxide synthase inhibition and cerebrovascular regulation. J Cereb Blood Flow Metab 14:175-192.

Klatt, P., K. Schmidt, F. Brunner and B. Mayer, 1994, Inhibitors of brain nitric oxide synthase. J Biol Chem 269:1674-1680.

Kurihara, K., K. Hosoi, T. Ueha and S. Yamada, 1994, Effects of nerve growth factor and dexamethasone on Na$^+$,K$^+$-ATPase of cultured PC12 cells. Hormone Metabol Res 26:14-18.

Lerner-Natoli, M., G. Rondouin, F. de Bock and J. Bockaert, 1992, Chronic NO synthase inhibition fails to protect hippocampal neurons against NMDA toxicity. Neuroreport 3:1109-1112.

Lipton, S.A, Y.B. Choi, Z.H. Pan, S.Z. Lei, H.S. Chen, N.J. Sucher, J. Loscalzo, D.J. Singel and S.J. Stamler, 1993, A redox based mechanism for the neuroprotective and neurodestructive effects of nitric oxide and related nitroso-compounds. Nature 364(6438):626-632.

Madl, J.E. and K. Burgesser, 1993, Adenosine triphosphate depletion reverses sodium-dependent neural uptake of glutamate in rat hippocampal slices. J Neurosci 13:4429-4444.

Moore, P.K., R.C. Babbedge, P. Wallace, Z.A. Gaffen and S.L. Hart, 1993, 7-Nitro indazole, an inhibitor of nitric oxide synthase, exhibits an anti-nocipetive activity in the mouse without increasing blood pressure. Br J Pharmacol 108:296-297.

Moskowitz, M.A. and members of the Stroke Research Laboratory, 1994, The comlex role of nitric oxide in the physiology of the cerebral circulation and cerebral ischemia. Proc 38th Oholo Conference, April 17-21, Eilat, Israel

Murphy, S., M.L. Simmons, L. Agullo, A. Garcia, D.L. Feinstein, E. Galea, D.J. Reis, D. Minc-Golomb and J.P. Schwartz, 1993, Synthesis of nitric oxide in CNS glial cells. Trends Neurol Sci 16:323-328.

Nagafuji, T., M. Sugiyama, T. Matsui and T. Koide, 1993, A narrow therapeutical window of nitric oxide synthase inhibitor against transient ischemic brain injury. Eur J Pharmacol 248:325-328.

Nagafuji, T, T. Koide and M. Takado, 1992, Neurochemical correlates of selective neuronal loss following cerebral ischemia: role of decreased Na^+,K^+-ATPase activity. Brain Res 571:265-271.

Nakae, H., 1991, Morphological differentiation of rat pheochromocytoma cells (PC12 cells) by electric stimulation. Brain Res 558:348-352.

Nowicki, J.P., D. Duval, H. Poignet and B. Scatton, 1991, Nitric oxide mediates neuronal death after focal cerebral ischemia in the mouse. Eur J Pharmacol 204:339-340.

Pauwels, P.J. and J.E. Leysen, 1992, Blockade of nitric oxide formation does not prevent glutamate-induced neurotoxicity in neuronal cultures from rat hippocampus. Neurosci Lett 143:27-30.

Paxinos, G. and C. Watson, 1986, The rat brain in stereotaxic coordinates, second edition (Academic Press Inc., San-Diego, CA 92101).

Pulsinelli, W., 1992, Pathophysiology of acute ischaemic stroke. Lancet 339:533-536.

Resh, M.D., R.A. Nemenoff and G. Guidotti, 1980, Insulin stimulation of (Na^+,K^+)-adenosine triphosphatase-dependent $^{86}Rb^+$ uptake in rat adipocytes. J Biol Chem 255:10938-10945.

Sancesario, G., M. Iannone, M. Morello, G. Nistico and G. Bernardi, 1994, Nitric oxide inhibition aggrevates ischemic damage of hippocampal but not of NADPH neurons in gerbils. Stroke 25:436-444.

Scheinberg, P., 1991, The biologic basis for the treatment of acute stroke. Neurology 41:1867-1873.

Simmons, M.L. and S. Murphy, 1992, Induction of nitric oxide synthase in glial cells. J Neurochem 59:897-905.

Weissman, B.A., T. Kadar, R. Brandeis and S. Shapira, 1992, N^G-nitro-L-arginine enhances neuronal death following transient forebrain ischemia in gerbils. Neurosci Lett 146:139-142.

Wink, D.A., I. Hanbauer, M.C. Krishna, W. DeGraff, J. Gamson, and J.B. Mitchell, 1993, Nitric oxide protects against cellular damage and cytotoxicity from reactive oxygen species. Proc Natl Acad Sci USA 90:9813-9817.

Yamamoto, S., E.V. Golanov, S.B. Berger, and D.J. Reis, 1992, Inhibition of nitric oxide synthesis increases focal ischemic infarction in rat. J Cereb Blood Flow Metab 12:717-726.

Zhang, F. and C. Iadecola, 1993, Nitroprusside improves blood flow and reduces brain damage after focal ischemia. Neuroreport 4:559-562.

INHIBITION OF NITRIC OXIDE PRODUCTION IMPAIRS SPECIFIC COGNITIVE PROCESSES IN RATS

Rachel Brandeis, Michal Sapir, Eti Stein and Ben Avi Weissman

Pharmacology Department
Israel Institute for Biological Research
P.O.B. 19
Ness Ziona 70450, ISRAEL

INTRODUCTION

Recent evidence suggests that nitric oxide (NO) may act as a novel intercellular messenger in the central nervous system (Southam and Garthwaite, 1991). In particular, NO has been implicated in the induction of long-term potentiation (LTP) in the hippocampus (Schuman and Madison, 1991) an important model of synaptic plasticity and a cellular model of learning and memory (Collingridge and Lester, 1989). For example, it has been demonstrated that NO synthase (NOS) activity and NO are necessary for the production of LTP (Schuman and Madison, 1991) and that inhibitors of NOS can block LTP (Bohme et al., 1991; O'Dell et al., 1991; Schuman and Madison, 1991). However, the role played by NO in learning and memory processes is not clear. A few behavioral studies concerning the involvement of NO synthesis in learning and memory functions have been published.

N[G]-nitro-L-arginine (L-NNA), a potent and selective NOS inhibitor, injected i.c.v., impaired passive avoidance retention in rats and mice while L-arginine, also injected i.c.v., antagonized this amnesia (Schindler et al, 1992). L-NNA (Schindler et al., 1992; Bohme et al., 1993), injected i.p., had no significant effect on passive avoidance retention in these animals. N[G]-nitro-L-arginine methyl ester (L-NAME), injected i.p., significantly reduced learning of a shuttle-box active avoidance test in mice, while i.p., injected L-arginine reversed these amnesic effects (Schindler et al., 1992).

Bilateral intrahippocampal injections of L-NAME significantly impaired working-memory (WM) evaluated with a three-panel runway task (Ohno et al., 1993). Reference-memory (RM) was not affected by L-NAME on the same task. L-arginine attenuated the WM impairment induced by L-NAME.

A slowing down of WM-based spatial learning (Bohme et al., 1993) was observed also following treatment with L-NNA, using the radial eight arm maze (RAM). However, in this study, L-NNA was administered at very high doses: 100 mg/kg i.p., twice daily, for

Biochemical, Pharmacological, and Clinical Aspects of Nitric Oxide
Edited by B. A. Weissman *et al.*, Plenum Press, New York, 1995

231

4 days preceding the experiment, followed by 100 mg/kg i.p., daily for the 12-days experiment. In spite of the high dose administered the deficit in learning disappeared after 10 days.

The effect of L-NAME was studied also using a place navigation task, (Morris, 1984), the Morris Water Maze (MWM). In one study (Estall et al., 1993) acquisition of RM-based spatial learning was impaired in a dose-dependent manner for a limited period of time, while memory was not tested. In another study (Chapman et al., 1992) L-NAME impaired the acquisition of spatial learning on the seventh day of training and spatial RM tested immediately after the end of training. However, L-NAME did not impair the retention of a well-acquired spatial learning under normal conditions. L-arginine reversed the L-NAME-induced acquisition impairment.

The behavioral results mentioned above indicate that the effect of inhibition of NOS on learning and memory is a result of an interaction of many variables like route of administration, the dose of the NO inhibitor, the behavioral test used and the cognitive process evaluated. The present study examined the effects of L-NNA on specific cognitive processes, spatial learning, memory and reversal learning, using the MWM which is considered to be most sensitive to hippocampal manipulations (Morris et al., 1982; Brandeis et al., 1989) and to suppression of LTP (Morris et al., 1986).

MATERIALS AND METHODS

Subjects

Male Sprague-Dawley rats (3 months old, weighing about 300g), obtained from Charles River Breeding Laboratories, UK, were housed 5 per cage, in a temperature-controlled environment ($22\pm1°C$) with a 12-h normal light/dark cycle. The rats had ad lib access to food and drinking water. Behavioral testing was carried out between 0800 and 1300 h, five days a week.

Drug Administration

Rats were randomly divided into 5 treatment groups (n = 9). Groups 1-4 were treated with N^G-nitro-L-arginine (Sigma), (L-NNA) at doses of 4, 10, 25 and 62.5 mg/kg i.p. in a volume of 1 ml/kg, while group 5 (control group) was treated with saline (pH = 10.5). L-NNA and saline were administered daily for 5 days, 60 min before testing.

Apparatus

Rats were tested in a circular metal water maze (diameter: 1.4 m, height: 50 cm) that was painted white and was filled to a height of 25 cm with water ($26\pm1°C$) in which powdered milk was dissolved. A white metal platform (12x12 cm) covered by wire mesh was present inside the pool; its top surface was 20 mm below the surface of the water, thus making it invisible to a viewer inside the pool. The platform was placed midway between the center and rim of the pool in any of its four equal quadrants.

The maze was brightly lit and surrounded by well-lit, salient objects, which were held constant throughout testing. Performance in the maze was monitored by a tracking system consisting of an overhead video camera linked to a TV monitor and an image analyzer coupled to a micro copmputer (Galai-Migdal Ha-Emek, Israel).

Procedure

Each rat was trained for four consecutive days, four trials (one block) per day, in which the platform position remained constant. Within each block of four trials, each rat started at each of the starting locations, but the sequence of locations was randomly selected. The rat had to find the platform during a period of 120 sec. The inter-trial-interval was 60 sec, during which the rat remained on the platform. Escape latency, path length and speed were recorded on each trial.

Transfer test: Three min following the last training trial, the platform was entirely removed from the pool. In this probe trial (trial 17), the rat was placed into the water for a limited period of 60 sec, and its spatial bias was measured by recording the relative distribution of escape latency and path length over the four quadrants of the pool.

Reversal test: During trials 18-21, on the fifth day, the platform position was changed to a place opposite the training quadrant. Thus, during reversal learning, the platform location was moved relative to the configuration of objects within the room. Testing of rats and measures taken were the same as in training.

RESULTS

Training

For each rat, the escape latency, path length and swimming speed of every four trials, in each of the training days, were grouped into blocks (one block for each day). The scores of the three measures were analyzed by a 2-way ANOVA (5x4) with one repeated variable (days) and one non repeated variable (treatment - various doses of L-NNA). Specific comparisons were performed, using the scheffe contrasts or the simple main effects contrasts analysis, which is specifically suited for testing significant interactions.

For both measures, escape latency and path length, the interaction between treatment x days was found statistically significant [$F(12/120) = 2.66$, $p<0.005$ and $F(12/120) = 3.29$, $p<0.001$ for the escape latency and path length measures, respectively]. L-NNA at a dose of 4 mg/kg did not result in any change in behavior. L-NNA at a dose of 10 mg/kg impaired the rats' performance during the second day of training only ($p<0.05$, see Fig. 1). L-NNA at a dose of 25 mg/kg impaired performance during the first ($p<0.01$) and second ($p<0.05$) days of training (see Figs 1 and 2). A dose of 62.5 mg/kg impaired performance during the first three days of training ($p<0.05$ - $p<0.001$, depending on day and measure, see Fig. 2). A characteristic computer depiction of the paths travelled by L-NNA-treated and control rats is illustrated in Fig. 3.

No significant differences between the swimming speeds of the control group and the different L-NNA-treated groups were found (see Fig. 4).

Transfer trial

The escape latency and path length measures for the transfer trial were analyzed by a 2-way ANOVA (5x4) with one repeated variable (quadrant in the pool) and one non repeated variable (treatment - various doses of L-NNA).

L-NNA had no significant effect on the relative distribution of escape latency or path length over the four quadrants of the pool (see Figs. 5-6). L-NNA -treated rats displayed a considerable spatial bias, similar to the control animals [$F(3/120) = 68.77$, $p<0.001$ and $F(3/120) = 73.83$, $p<0.001$, for the escape latency and path length, respectively]. Thus, all rats spent more time and swam a longer distance in the training quadrant than in the three other quadrants of the pool ($p<0.001$).

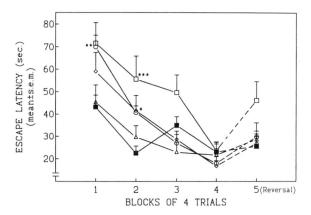

Figure 1: Escape latency of L-NNA treated rats. Filled squares: saline (1 ml/kg); Triangles: L-NNA 4 mg/kg; diamonds: 10 mg/kg; circles: 25 mg/kg; open squares: 62.5 mg/kg. * p<0.05 **p<0.01 *** p<0.001 compared to saline.

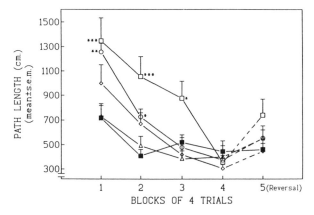

Figure 2: Path length of L-NNA treated rats. Filled squares: saline (1ml/kg); triangles: L-NNA 4 mg/kg; diamonds: 10 mg/kg; circles: 25 mg/kg; open squares: 62.5 mg/kg. * p<0.05, ** p<0.01, *** p<0.001 compared to saline.

Reversal test

For each rat, the escape latency, path length and swimming speed of the reversal test (trials 18-21) were grouped into one block. All three measures were analyzed by a one-way ANOVA, for the treatment-variable effect.

L-NNA impaired reversal-learning performance at the dose of 62.5 mg/kg compared to control group (see Fig. 1); however, this difference was not statistically significant (p<0.1). Swimming speed was not affected by L-NNA during reversal test.

DISCUSSION

Specific cognitive functions in rats were significantly impaired in our study following i.p. administration of L-NNA, a selective NOS inhibitor. Spatial learning was impaired in a dose-related manner and for a limited period of time. The deficit in acquisition was firstly observed following the administration of a dose of 10 mg/kg, and the severity and duration of the impairment increased with the increase in the dose of L-NNA. However, place learning was not eventually prevented, and on the fourth day of training all L-NNA-treated animals performed the task as well as control rats. The transient effect of L-NNA on learning is consistent with the results of other studies (Estall et al., 1993; Bohme et al., 1993).

According to the literature (Dwyer et al, 1991), a maximum of 95% inhibition of NOS is achieved in the cerebellum after either 4 or 7 days administration of L-NNA (50 mg/kg i.p., twice a day). Furthermore, doses of 100 mg/kg i.p. of L-NNA were reported to be necessary to block LTP in the CA1 area of the hippocampus (Bohme et al., 1993). The doses of L-NNA administered in our study, during the four days of training, were lower (62.5 mg/kg i.p.), and the percent inhibition of NOS in the hippocampus (and thus the level of LTP blocking) is not known. Therefore, the recovery of the learning deficit with time might be explained either by the residual level of NOS activity or on the basis of a compensatory effect produced by a different neural mechanism.

A deficit in reversal learning was observed in our study, following the administration of L-NNA- (62.5 mg/kg i.p.), although the effect was not statistically significant. Reversal learning, as an expression of the ability to shift strategies to task demands (Smith, 1988), had not yet been evaluated in the context of NOS inhibition. This complex, higher level

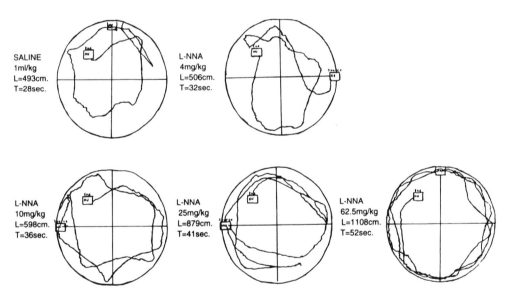

SALINE
1ml/kg
L=493cm.
T=28sec.

L-NNA
4mg/kg
L=506cm.
T=32sec.

L-NNA
10mg/kg
L=598cm.
T=36sec.

L-NNA
25mg/kg
L=879cm.
T=41sec.

L-NNA
62.5mg/kg
L=1108cm.
T=52sec.

Figure 3: A characteristic computer depiction of the path length travelled by L-NNA treated rats.

cognitive function, is very sensitive to hippocampal lesions (Morris et al., 1986; Brandeis et al., 1989). It was shown previously that NOS inhibitors can block hippocampal LTP (Bohme et al; 1991; O'Dell et al., 1991; Schuman and Madison, 1991) which is hypothesized to be important in spatial learning (Morris et al., 1986). Our results suggest that L-NNA may produce the deterioration in reversal learning by a similar neural mechanism.

Spatial memory tested 3 min after the end of training was not affected by L-NNA administration in our study. In contrast, an impairment in the same cognitive function was reported elsewhere (Chapman et al., 1992) following the administration of L-NAME - 75 mg/kg i.p. In that respect it should be noted that in our study **learning recovered** before memory was tested, while in the other study **learning was still impaired** on the day before memory testing. It was mentioned before (Chapman et al., 1992) that NOS inhibitors block the induction of hippocampal LTP, but do not affect its magnitude or duration once established. In that context it was found that L-NAME injections did not impair the retention of a well-acquired spatial learning. Thus, we assume that once learning was established in our study, the structure of LTP was produced in the hippocampus, resulting in the conservation of the memory process.

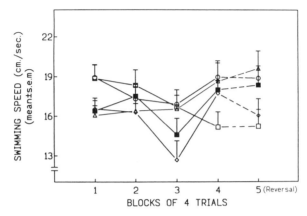

Figure 4: Swimming speed of L-NNA treated rats. Filled squares: saline (1 ml/kg); triangles L-NNA 4 mg/kg; diamonds: 10 mg/kg; circles: 25 mg/kg; open squares: 62.5 mg/kg.

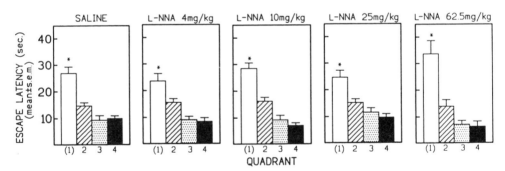

Figure 5: Distribution of escape latency during transfer trial for L-NNA treated rats. * $p<0.001$ compared to quadrant no. 1 in the respective group.

The effect of L-NAME, an NOS inhibitor, on the acquisition of spatial learning was suggested to be similar (Estall et al., 1993) to that of AP5 [N-methyl-D-aspartate (NMDA) receptor antagonist; aminophosphonovaleric acid] in a similar place navigation learning task (Morris et al., 1986). Furthermore, both L-NAME (Chapman et al, 1992) and AP5 (Morris, 1989) impaired acquisition rather then recall of spatial memory. The similarity in results was supported by the notion that NMDA receptors are also necessary for both the induction of LTP (Collingridge et al., 1983; Harris et al., 1984) and for learning in the MWM (Morris et al., 1986).

Since it was proposed that NMDA receptors initiate NO synthesis (Garthwaite et al., 1989) it was concluded that these results support the hypothesis linking NMDA receptor activation to induction of NO synthesis during learning. A systematic comparison

Chapman et al., 1992) and AP5 (Morris et al., 1986 Morris, 1989) in the MWM, shows that the latter are stronger, more consistent and last for a longer period of time, whether in acquisition, spatial memory as measured by a transfer test or reversal learning

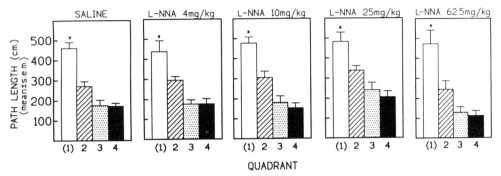

Figure 6: Distribution of path length during transfer trial for L-NNA treated rats. * p<0.001 compared to quadrant no. 1 in the respective group.

However, since NOS inhibitors had not been studied thoroughly and systematically in relation to their behavioral effects, the differences could have been attributed to differences in administered doses or the different compounds concerned.

Nonspecific motor coordination effects could not explain the behavioral deficits displayed by L-NNA-treated rats, since no such effects were demonstrated in the swimming ability of the rats. These findings are in accordance with these of other studies (Estall et al., 1993; Chapman et al., 1992; Bohme et al., 1993) which showed that L-NAME or L-NNA had no effect on sensorimotor and motivational processes. These results suggest that NOS inhibitors interfere with the ability of rats to image the platform location or the association of extra-maze cues with these images (Estall et al., 1993), cognitive functions which are based on central nervous system processes.

In conclusion, results shown here support the concept that NO is involved in some specific cognitive processes. The dissociative effect of NOS inhibitors on cognition might be a result of the administered doses or the different inhibitors involved, differentially interfering with the induction of hippocampal LTP.

REFERENCES

Bohme, G.A.; Bon, C.; Lemaire, M.; Reibund, M.; Piot, O.; Stutzmann, J.M.; Doble, A.; Blanchard, J.C. Altered synaptic plasticity and memory formation in nitric oxide synthase inhibitor-treated rats. Proc. Natl. Acad. Sci. U.S.A., 90, 9191-9194, 1993.

Bohme, G.A.; Bon, C.; Stutzmann, J.M.; Doble, A.; Blanchard, J.C. Possible involvement of nitric oxide in long-term potentiation. Eur. J. Pharmacol., 199, 379-381, 1991.

Brandeis, R.; Brandys, Y.; Yehuda, S. The use of the Morris water maze in the study of memory and learning. Int. J Neurosci.; 48, 29-69, 1989.

Chapman, P.F.; Atkins, C.M.; Todd Allen, M.; Haley, J.E.; Steinmetz, J.E. Inhibition of nitric oxide synthesis impairs two different forms of learning. Neuro Report, 3, 567-570, 1992.

Collingridge, G.L.; Kehl, S.J.; McLennan, H. The antagonism of amino acid-induced excitations of rat hippocampal CA1 neurons in vitro. J. Physiol., 334, 19-31, 1983.

Collingridge, G.L.; Lester, R.A.J. Excitatory amine acid receptors in the vertebrate central nervous system. Pharmacol. Rev., 41, 143-210, 1989.

Dwyer, M.A.; Bredt, D.S.; Snyder, S.H. Nitric oxide synthase: Irreversible inhibition by L-N^G-nitroarginine in brain in vitro and in vivo. Biochem. Biophys. Res. Commun., 176, 1136-1141, 1991.

Estall, L.B.; Grant, S.J.; Cicala, G.A. Inhibition of nitric oxide (NO) production selectively impairs learning and memory in the rat. Pharmacol. Biochem. Behav., 46, 959-962, 1993.

Garthwaite, J.; Garthwaite, G.; Palmer, R.M.J.; Moncada, S. NMDA receptor activation induces nitric oxide synthesis from arginine in rat brain slices. Eur. J. Pharmacol., 172, 412-416, 1989.

Harris, E.W.; Ganong, A.H.; Cotman, C.W. Long-term potentiation in the hippocampus involves activation of N-methyl-D-aspartate receptors. Brain Res., 323, 132-137, 1984.

Morris, R.G.M. Developments of a water-maze procedure for studying spatial learning in the rat. J. Neurosci. Meth., 11, 47-60, 1984.

Morris, R.G.M. Synaptic plasticity and learning: Selective impairment of learning in rats and blockade of long-term potentiation in vivo by the N-Methyl-D-Aspartate receptor antagonist AP5. J. Neurosci, 9, 3040-3057, 1989.

Morris, R.G.M.; Anderson, E.; Lynch, G.S.; Baudry, M. Selective impairment of learning and blockade of long-term potentiation by an N-methyl-D-aspartate receptor antagonist, AP5. Nature, 319, 774-776, 1986.

Morris, R.G.M.; Garrud, P.; Rawlins, J.N.P.; O'Keefe, J. Place navigation impaired in rats with hippocampal lesions. Nature, 197, 681-683, 1982.

O'Dell, T.J.; Hawkins, R.D.; Kandel, E.R.; Arancio, O. Tests of the roles of two diffusible substances in long-term potentiation: Evidence for nitric oxide as a possible early retrograde messenger. Proc. Natl. Acad. Sci. U.S.A., 88, 11285-11289, 1991.

Ohno, M.; Yamamoto, T.; Watanabe, S. Deficits in working memory following inhibition of hippocampal nitric oxide synthesis in the rat. Brain Res., 632, 36-40, 1993.

Schindler, U., Libri, V.; Nistico, G. Inhibitors of nitric oxide synthase impair passive and active avoidance learning in rodents. Symposium Proceedings of the meeting "Nitric oxide: brain and immune system" (Paraelios, Calabria - Italy, 16-18 September, 1992).

Schuman, E.M.; Madison, D.V. A requirement for the intercellular messenger nitric oxide in long-term potentiation. Science, 254, 1503-1506, 1991.

Smith, G. Animal models of Alzheimer's disease: Experimental holinergic denervation. Brain Res. Rev., 13, 103-118, 1988.

Southam, E.; Garthwaite, J. Intercellular action of nitric oxide in adult rat cerebellar slices. Neuro Report, 2, 658-660, 1991.

Teyler, T.J.; DiScenna, P. Long-term potentiation. Ann. Rev. Neurosci., 10, 131-161, 1987.

THE EFFECT OF AGING ON NOS ACTIVITY IN THE RAT HIPPOCAMPUS AND ITS RELATION TO COGNITIVE FUNCTIONS

Shira Chapman, Ettie Grauer and Tamar Kadar

Department of Pharmacology
Israel Institute for Biological Research
Ness-Ziona 70450, ISRAEL

INTRODUCTION

The role of the central cholinergic system, particulary the hippocampus, in cognitive functions including learning and memory is now well established (Kadar et al., 1990). In aged rats, morphological alterations as well as impaired hippocampal synaptic plasticity have been shown to correlate well with learning deficits (Kadar et al., 1990; Levy et al., 1994). Recently, it has been suggested that nitric oxide (NO), a neuronal messenger, may play a role in the process of learning through facilitation of long-term potentiation (Bon et al., 1992). Thus, changes in NO activity may be associated with modifications in learning and memory. In spite of the elaborative study of the interaction between NO and cognitive functions, little is known about the age-related changes in NOS activity. The aim of the present study was to explore the age-related changes in the activity and distribution of NO synthase (NOS), the synthesizing enzyme for NO in the hippocampus, and to relate them to the cognitive impairment observed in normal aging. For this purpose, young and old Sprague Dawely rats, were tested for their performance in the Morris water maze (MWM), after which their brains were processed for histochemical evaluation of NOS activity by the NADPH-diaphorase reaction. There is evidence for neuronal NADPH-diaphorase being a NOS in the brain (Bredt et al., 1991).

METHODS

Animals

Male Sprague Dawely rats (Charles River, U.K.) at the ages of 3 and 24 months were used. The animals were maintained on a 12 hr light-dark cycle and were provided with rat purina chow and water ad libitum.

Biochemical, Pharmacological, and Clinical Aspects of Nitric Oxide
Edited by B. A. Weissman *et al.*, Plenum Press, New York, 1995

239

Behavior

The MWM task enables the testing of rats for their spatial reference memory performance, by following their ability to learn the location of an escape platform, submerged in opaque water. Rats were trained and tested in a black circular water maze measuring 140 cm in diameter and 50 cm high, filled to a depth of 25 cm with water at 24 °C. A black platform was placed 2 cm beneath the water. The pool surface was divided into four imaginary quadrants of equal area and four equally spaced points around the edge of the pool were used as starting positions. Performance in the maze was monitored by a tracking system, consisted on an overhead video camera linked to a computerized analysis system (HVS, England). Each rat was given four training trials (120 sec each) per day on four consecutive days, and escape latencies (the time to find the platform) were recorded. For each rat, the platform position remained constant throughout the four training days. On day 5 (24 hr after the final training day), the "reversal ability" of the rat was tested. Rats were tested as in the training sessions except that the platform position was changed. Reversal testing continued for 4 trials, similarly to each training day. The first day of training was considered as an habituation day and was omitted from the statistical analysis.

Histochemistry

At the termination of the behavioral study, the animals were sacrificed by decapitation, their brains were removed, fixed in 4% paraformaldehyde in phosphate buffer for 18 hr, cryoprotected in 30% sucrose for 24 hr and stored at -80°C until use. Frozen sections, 20µm thick, were cut at the coronal plane through the dorsal hippocampus and were attached to gelatin-coated slides.

NOS staining was performed by NADPH-diaphorase histochemistry (Matsumoto et al., 1993). Sections were dried in room temperature for 15 min, then washed in Tris buffer (50 mM, pH 7.4) and incubated for one hour in a mixture containing: 1% Triton, 0.5mM NBT and 1mM NADPH in Tris buffer at 37°C. The reaction was terminated by two washes (1 min each) in Tris buffer. Sections were dehydrated through graded alcohols and xylene and permounted with mounting media (Lipshaw).

Morphometry

Quantitative evaluation of the histochemical reaction was based on: 1. Measurements of the number of NADPH-diaphorase positive cells within various hippocampal sub-fields. Counting was performed on whole area of each subfield in the coronal section. 2. Semi-quantitative analysis of the intensity of the reaction in the brain utilizing an arbitrary score scale ranging from 0 for weak reaction to 4 for intensive staining. These data were used for morpho-behavioral correlation.

Data Analysis

Two-way analysis of variance (ANOVA) with repeated measures on days was performed across age groups on the behavioral data. One way ANOVA was carried out for the morphometric data. The relationship between the behavioral data and the histochemical findings was determined using the Pearson's correlation coefficients.

RESULTS

Behavior

Figure 1 presents the escape latencies of the four trials of each day, grouped into daily blocks. A significant difference was found between the scores of old vs young animals, when comparing the escape latencies, $F(1,8)=7.67$, $P<0.025$, (two way ANOVA; groups x days with repeated measure on the last three days). When the reversal ability was tested (changing the place of the platform on the fifth day) there was a tendency towards a difference between the two groups, but this failed to reach statistical significance (Fig. 1). There was no difference in swimming speed between old and young rats.

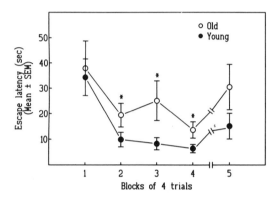

Figure 1. Escape latency (mean ± SEM) of 3 months (young) and 24 months (old) Sprague Dawely rats, during training sessions and reversal test, as explained in the text.

Histochemistry

In the hippocampus of young animals, the highest densities of NADPH-diaphorase were observed in the CA1 pyramidal layer and the dentate gyrus. Figure 2 illustrates the NADPH-diaphorase histochemical reaction in the hippocampus of young (A,B,E) and old (C,D) rats. As can be seen, a remarkable decline in the activity of the enzyme was found in brains of 24 months old rats. The decline was prominent in the hippocampus in most of its subfields (Fig. 2-C).

Table 1 illustrates the number of positive NADPH-diaphorase cells in discrete regions of the hippocampus in young and old rats. A general decrease (23-55%) in the number of NADPH-diaphorase positive cells was observed in all hippocampal subfields. Statistical analysis revealed a significant decline in the number of positive cells in CA1 and in the upper granular layer of the dentate gyrus in brains of old rats.

Morpho-behavioral correlation. Fig. 3 depicts the correlation between the intensity of the enzymatic reaction and the individual behavioral scores (escape latencies of days 3 and 4). A significant correlation was found between the escape latency score and the intensity of the staining ($r=-0.84$, $P<0.002$).

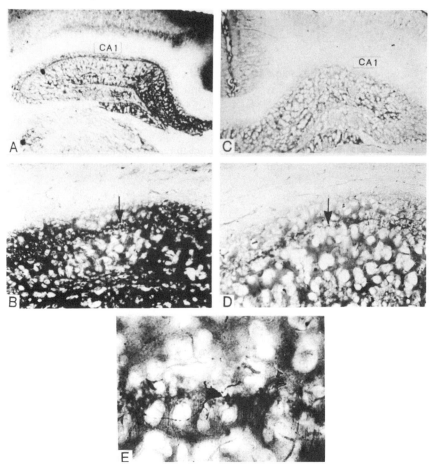

Figure 2. Photomicrographs of brain sections of young (A-B&E) and old (C-D) rats, at the level of the dorsal hippocampus, stained for NADPH-diaphorase (see text for detail). Note the remarkable decrease of staining in the old animals as compared to the intense enzymatic activity in the young animals. A positive pyramidal cell in CA1 region of young rat is seen in high magnification in E. Original magnification: A&C x 10; B&D x 40; E x 100.

DISCUSSION

The results of the present study suggest a close relationship between age-related memory impairments and NOS activity in the hippocampus of Sprague Dawely rats. The data shown hereby indicate that the decline in cognitive performance in aged animals corresponds well with the decrease in NADPH-diaphorase activity in the brain. Although, the involvement of NOS in cognitive processes via LTP was suggested by Bon et al. (1992), there is still a debate as to its specific cellular function in discrete neuronal

Table 1. Regional distribution of NADPH-diaphorase positive cells in the hippocampus of young (3 months) and old (24 months) Sprague Dawely rats.

	Number of stained cells		
Region	**young**	**old**	**% decrease**
CA1 Pyramidal cell layer	28.33 ± 2.33	19.89 ± 2.24*	30
CA3 Pyramidal cell layer	4.99 ± 0.88	3.82 ± 0.30	23
CA4 Pyramidal cell layer	5.70 ± 0.98	3.60 ± 0.89	36
Hippocampal Fissure	23.24 ± 4.14	13.90 ± 2.50	40
Dentate Gyrus			
Upper granular layer	13.65 ± 0.02	6.20 ± 2.45*	55
Lower granular layer	4.50 ± 1.70	2.50 ± 0.43	45

Data are presented as mean ±SEM
* p < 0.05 vs. young group

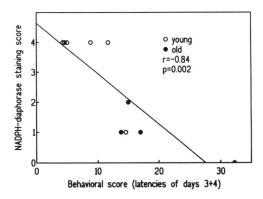

Figure 3. Morpho-behavioral correlation between hippocampal NADPH-diaphorase activity and performance in the MWM on days 3 and 4.

populations. Benedetti et al. (1993) indicated an age-related decline in the levels of amino acids involved in NO synthesis in brains of Wistar rats, thus leading to a decrease in NOS activity. The authors could not determine whether the change in the enzyme level resulted from neuronal loss causing a decrease in the enzyme concentrations, or from modifications of the enzyme properties. The data in the present study clarify this point by showing a significant decline in the number of cells containing NOS within the hippocampus. Moreover, we have shown that the decline was prominent in specific neuronal populations, i.e the CA1 and the dentate gyrus regions which are related to LTP functions. These findings are in accordance with the age-related decline of cognitive function, and support the hypothesis about the possible role of NO in synaptic plasticity and the process of learning and memory.

Acknowledgement

The authors thank Dr S. Shapira for critical reviewing the manuscript.

REFERENCES

Benedetti, M.S., Dostert, P., Marrari, P., and Cini, M., 1993, Effect of ageing on tissue levels of amino acids involved in the nitric oxide pathway in rat brain, J. Neural. Transm. 94:21.

Bon, C., Bohme, G.A., Doble, A., Stutzmann, J.M., and Blachard, J.C., 1992, A role for nitric oxide in long-term potentiation, Eur. J. Neurosci. 4:420.

Bredt, D.S., Glatt, C.E., Hwang, P.M., Fotuhi, M., Dawson, T.M., and Snyder, S.H., 1991, Nitric oxide synthase protein and mRNA are discretely localized in neuronal populations of mammalian CNS together with NADPH diaphorase, Neuron 7:615.

Kadar, T., Silbermann M., Brandies, R., and Levy, A., 1990, Age-related structural changes in the rat hippocampus: correlation with working memory deficiency, Brain Res. 512:113.

Kadar, T., Silbermann, M., Weissman, B.A., and Levy, A., 1990, Age-related changes in the cholinergic components within the central nervous system: working memory impairment and its relation to hippocampal muscarinic receptors, Mech. Ageing. Dev. 55:139.

Levy, A., Dachir, S., Arbel, I., and Kadar, T., 1994, Aging, stress and cognitive function, Ann. N.Y. Acad. Sci. 717:79.

Matsumoto, T., Nakane, M., Pollock, J.S., Kuk, J.E., and Forstermann, U.,1993, A correlation between soluble brain nitric oxide synthase and NADPH-diaphorase activity is only seen after exposure of the tissue to fixative. Neurosci. Lett, 155:61.

SUBJECT INDEX

AUTHORS INDEX